Principles of
Medical Science

Principles of Medical Science

RALPH GOLDMAN, M.D., F.A.C.P.

Professor of Medicine
Assistant Dean for Allied Health Professions
School of Medicine
University of California at Los Angeles

McGRAW-HILL BOOK COMPANY

A BLAKISTON PUBLICATION

New York   St. Louis   San Francisco   Düsseldorf   Johannesburg
Kuala Lumpur   London   Mexico   Montreal   New Delhi
Panama   Rio de Janeiro   Singapore   Sydney   Toronto

Principles of
Medical Science

This book was set in Times Roman by University Graphics, Inc. The editors were Cathy Dilworth and Stuart D. Boynton; the production supervisor was Ted Agrillo. The drawings were done by John Cordes, J & R Technical Services, Inc.
The printer and binder was Kingsport Press, Inc.

Library of Congress Cataloging in Publication Data

Goldman, Ralph.
    Principles of medical science.

    Includes bibliographies.
    1. Nurses and nursing. I. Title.
[DNLM: 1. Medicine—Nursing texts. WY 156 G619p
1973]
RT69.G64   616.07 '024 '613   72-8720
ISBN 0-07-023667-4

To my parents, Henry and May Goldman
and to my wife, Helen

Contents

Preface

There are now more than four million persons employed in the delivery of health services. The physician and the pharmacist were the only health professionals until the first school of nursing was established in 1860. In the past century, laboratory and x-ray technicians, dietitians, sanitary engineers, public health educators, and many other qualified specialists have become necessary for optimum health care. Hospitals, once only for the poor, are now essential for effective diagnosis and treatment. New industries have developed to produce drugs, diagnostic and surgical instruments, and hospital supplies and equipment. A rapidly developing and increasingly complex technology also required biomedical physicists and engineers. This expansion of services has been so great that the health industry, taken as a whole, is one of the three or four largest in the United States. Recent and probable future legislation will undoubtedly increase the public commitment to health and create a demand for even more and better personnel.

Medical scientists have made very little attempt to educate those in the health fields to the general nature of disease. Medical science as a comprehensive discipline has been neglected in favor of the task-oriented development of specific skills. In most curricula individual courses are given, such as nutrition, embryology, genetics, microbiology, and abnormal psychology. Because the emphases are on the subjects taught, the interrelationships are not stressed, and the student cannot evaluate the relative significance in the total pattern. Yet, the number of disease processes is limited, and it seems both appropriate and possible to present a complete and balanced survey of medical science within the confines of a single course.

This book explains the basic principles which may underlie abnormal structure or function and the main mechanisms of injury and disease. In an approximate sequence of possible occurrence, these principles are examined from conception (genetics) through old age (gerontology), including growth and development (birth defects), malnutrition, physical injury, inflammation and repair, immunity and its abnormalities, infections (from virus to helminth), major vascular disorders (including arteriosclerosis), and cancer.

Since the purpose is to assist in the training of those who will be primarily concerned with some aspect of patient care, it seems logical that a clinician should present his view of the clinically needed and useful concepts extracted from the various basic disciplines to be studied. While the presentation cannot be in the same depth as if given by a basic scientist, it is hoped that it is more in accord with clinical needs and perceptions.

It is assumed that students taking this course will have had some introduction to normal anatomy and physiology. Other helpful courses include biochemistry, bacteriology, genetics, embryology, abnormal psychology, parasitology, and nutrition.

Originally, it was planned to include a second section in which specific diseases were examined organ system by organ system. However, a large number of textbooks are already available which describe diseases in varying degrees of depth. What appeared to be needed was not another synopsis of medicine but a synopsis of the underlying principles of medical science. Armed with this information the student can then read disease description at a more profound level of comprehension.

The course will be successful if the student gains this basic knowledge and if, in addition, he can identify the relationship of his role to the total care of the patient and the maintenance of public health. It is hoped that the student will also acquire an appreciation of the fascination and excitement of this complex discipline, which utilizes a vast array of sciences and technologies to identify biologic principles and then applies these principles to the direct benefit of man.

The listing of acknowledgments is doubly pleasant, first, because it makes it possible to thank those who have helped in the preparation of this book and second, because it signifies the completion of the task. Preparation of the manuscript was ably done by Margaret Cole, Gail Hamilton, and Lana Norcross. The original illustrations were prepared by Gwynne Gloege and Sharon Belkin. I would also like to thank Drs. Steven Cederbaum, William H. Hildemann, and B. Lamar Johnson, Jr., for reviewing several chapters to assure that I made no gross errors. The hundreds of students who have taken the course on which this text is based have helped me to understand their needs. Finally, I want to thank my family and friends for their tolerance of social inadequacies during my labors of authorship.

Ralph Goldman

Principles of
Medical Science

Chapter 1

Introduction

To care for a patient without having any knowledge of the nature of the disease process is much like watching a play in a foreign language. One can see what happens, but the significance of the action may not be understood. Science did not start with a fundamental understanding but developed from the observation of phenomena, which were then classified, analyzed, and systematized. This was followed by a penetration to a deeper level and a repetition of the process. New techniques were usually required for each advance. For example, contagion was only a vague concept until the existence of microorganisms could be demonstrated and their role established. It took centuries to advance from the development of glass to the manufacture of lenses and microscopes, and from there to the identification of microbes and to the final establishment of the relationship of bacteria to contagion. In all cases, development has been from the obvious to the obscure. The obvious manifestations of disease are still here for us to examine and to serve as a starting point for further knowledge. What we consider to be fundamental concepts today, while retaining their inherent validity, will undoubtedly yield to more profound concepts as science progresses.

1

An increasing number of people have occupational concerns with disease. These concerns are related to the direct manifestations and underlying causes of disease and to their individual and social effects as well. We shall attempt to characterize the major disease processes and to show how they affect specific organs and organ systems. The approach must of necessity be one of survey rather than depth. It is hoped that this information will serve not only as an operational tool but also as an introduction to a broad and fascinating area of intellectual endeavor.

PROLOGUE TO MEDICAL SCIENCE

There is ample evidence that the life of primitive man was extremely short. Infant and juvenile mortality was high; and the hazards of childbirth, injury, malnutrition, and the elements were extreme. Probably few individuals lived as long as 40 years. When man lived in small and isolated communities, it is unlikely that he suffered from many epidemic diseases. The development of agriculture and of larger and more stable communities reduced the risks of starvation, injury, and the elements; but at the same time it increased the problem of epidemic disease such as smallpox, diphtheria, typhus, and tuberculosis. The conquest of these diseases in the past century has ushered in a new era in which we are increasingly concerned with chronic diseases and the problems of aging. Obviously, in more primitive and rigorous times, individuals with chronic disease and senility could not survive.

Since health was as much a prerequisite for survival as food and protection from the elements, natural hazards, and human enemies, it was one of man's earliest concerns. His knowledge of the obscure was limited, and he naturally assumed that his misfortunes were divine or magical in origin. This combination of the concept of mystic causation and limited knowledge diverted attention away from the patient and toward systems designed to propitiate the gods or to ward off the evil spirits. In this philosophical context the differences between typhoid and typhus, tuberculosis and tumor were relatively unimportant. The history of developing medical knowledge, and with it the characterization and separation of disease entities, has been slow and often intermittent. Even today, previously unrecognized diseases are being described which are relatively common and undoubtedly have existed throughout man's history.

As man's knowledge about himself grew, he became aware of recurrent patterns of disease. Increasing knowledge of anatomy made it possible to recognize anatomical abnormalities, and these began to be correlated with symptoms in the course of disease. As knowledge of physiology developed, abnormalities of function were related to the symptoms and the anatomical changes. Once specific patterns could be distinguished, the search for causes and cures took on new meaning.

DEFINITIONS

The word *disease* means literally "without ease," and disease is thus the opposite of health. However, in medicine the word has a more specific connotation and is used to define a morbid (abnormal) process which has a specific cause, a definite course of development, and typical manifestations. Thus typhoid fever is a disease caused by a specific organism, *Salmonella typhosa,* which is transmitted by food to the intestinal tract, invades the bloodstream, and causes a prolonged fever and intestinal symptoms until it is terminated abruptly by death or, more frequently, by gradual resolution of the symptoms and recovery.

A *syndrome* is a group of abnormalities which occur together in a characteristic pattern. For example, Horner's syndrome is characterized by a small pupil, a droop of the eyelid, and failure of sweating, all affecting only one side of the face. Horner's syndrome may be present in syphilis, some strokes, some cases of cancer of the lung, and a variety of affections that are localized in the neck. The anatomical and physiological defect which ties all these together is a lesion in a portion of the sympathetic nervous system. Thus any disease which produces an appropriate lesion in this structure will have an associated Horner's syndrome. The syndrome serves a useful purpose in calling attention to an abnormal pattern which may lead to the diagnosis of a specific disease. Most frequently, these patterns start out unassociated with any specific disease entity. If, when the total pattern is worked out, it becomes apparent that it is part of a single specific process, the syndrome is reclassified as a disease.

A *symptom* is generally interpreted to mean a specific recognizable abnormality. General use gives it both subjective and objective qualities. However, in medicine the term *symptom* is reserved for only the subjective manifestations which are recognized by the patient himself. Objective evidences of disease are called *signs.* Thus, a pain is a symptom, but if we produce objective evidence of pain as by pressing on the lower right portion of the abdomen in a patient with appendicitis, this is recorded as tenderness, which is a sign. Pain, with its various locations and qualities, is undoubtedly the commonest of symptoms. Other extremely common symptoms include fatigue, weakness, fever, loss of appetite, loss of weight, and shortness of breath. The variety of signs is much greater than the variety of symptoms; because they are objective, they can be analyzed and described in more detail.

It is obvious that clear-cut distinctions cannot always be made among diseases and syndromes or signs and symptoms. Anemia, which is a decrease in the concentration of red cells in the blood, may be a sign—if the patient is sufficiently pallid for it to be apparent—of some disease entity such as a bleeding peptic ulcer. Anemia may be considered a disease, as in the case of pernicious anemia, where it is the major manifestation of a physiological defect in the ability of the intestinal tract to absorb vitamin B_{12}. However, despite these complexities, most illnesses can be classified as specific diseases, although establishment of the diagnosis may at times be difficult and require extended study.

Etiology is the study and description of the causes of disease. We shall see in the next section the variety and usefulness of the concept of etiology. A different concept is rendered by *pathogenesis,* which is the evolution of the abnormal changes in anatomy and physiology during the development of a disease. A knowledge of these changes is useful to facilitate diagnosis, to understand the underlying mechanisms of the clinical manifestations, and to assist in treatment. In many diseases, once the etiological factor sets the process in motion, it is no longer a contributor to the evolution of the disease. Therefore, in these cases, treatment must be directed not to the eradication of the etiological factor, as is most commonly the case in infection, but to the restoration of normal structure and function.

Diagnosis is the process of evaluating the patient and identifying the disease. Modern diagnosis goes further than this and identifies variations in the disease and their implications as well. A number of diagnostic methods will be referred to in the text and in the medical literature. *Clinical diagnosis* refers to the physician's approach to his patient in his attempt to establish the diagnosis. In the usual sense, it implies the use of direct methods with the patient plus a relatively limited number of laboratory procedures. *Differential diagnosis* is a technique whereby the diagnostic possibilities in a given case are listed and the true diagnosis is established by experienced reasoning and appropriate tests. *Pathological diagnosis* may mean the biopsy diagnosis by microscopic examination of a small piece of tissue removed from the body, or it may mean the diagnosis reached as a result of postmortem examination of the body. *Prognosis* means literally "knowledge of the future." Based on the diagnosis, which allows him to know the range of possibilities in a given case, the physician must then make a forecast, or prognosis, of the specific outcome, using his knowledge of the variations in the given patient.

CLASSIFICATION OF DISEASE BY ETIOLOGY

One of the most satisfactory methods of classifying disease is by etiology. This approach makes it possible to examine the disease in relation to the pathological process, which in general tends to be identifiable regardless of the part of the body involved. The etiological classification is used in the *Standard Nomenclature of Diseases and Operations* coding system which is frequently used for classifying diagnoses for medical record purposes. Table 1-1 indicates the major classifications used in this system. We shall use a somewhat modified classification.

Table 1-1 Classification of Disease Used in Standard Nomenclature of Diseases and Operations

Number or letter	Etiological classification
-0	Diseases due to prenatal influence
-1	Diseases due to a lower plant or animal parasite
-2	Diseases due to a higher plant or animal parasite
-3	Diseases due to intoxication
-4	Diseases due to trauma or physical agent
-50	Diseases secondary to circulatory disturbance
-55	Diseases secondary to disturbance of innervation or of psychic control
-6	Diseases due to or consisting of static mechanical abnormality (obstruction, calculus, displacement or gross change in form) due to unknown cause
-7	Diseases due to disorder of metabolism, growth, or nutrition
-8	New growths
-9	Diseases due to unknown or uncertain cause with the structural reaction (degenerative, infiltrative, inflammatory, proliferative, sclerotic, or reparative) manifest; hereditary and familial diseases of this nature
-x	Diseases due to unknown or uncertain cause with the functional reaction alone manifest; hereditary and familial disease of this nature
-y	Diseases of undetermined cause

Number or letter	Topographical classification
0-	Body as a whole (including the psyche and the body generally), not a particular system exclusively
1-	Integumentary system (including subcutaneous areolar tissue, mucous membranes of orifices and the breast)
2-	Musculoskeletal system
3-	Respiratory system
4-	Cardiovascular system
5-	Hemic and lymphatic system
6-	Digestive system
7-	Urogenital system
8-	Endocrine system
9-	Nervous system
x-	Organs of special sense

Genetic Defects   The individual starts with the fertilized ovum, and this cell contains the genetic information which will characterize the structural and functional specificity of the individual.   It is on this specifically defined individual that the environment will react.   The great strides in the recent past in the understanding of the mechanism of genetics have reemphasized the old concept that structure defines function.   Defective genes represent the first mechanism of abnormality which may affect the individual.   However, inherited gene defects are not the only genetic abnormalities, since the number and structure of the chromosomes may also be altered.

Developmental Defects or Congenital Anomalies   These are generally gross anatomical defects resulting from abnormal intrauterine development.   Some of these defects may be genetic in origin, but most are probably due to environmental abnormalities during critical periods of gestation.   Some of these defects are incompatible with life, some are demonstrable externally, but most are externally inapparent and may either reveal themselves by some disability during life or be found only incidentally during a diagnostic procedure or after death.

Trauma   Trauma (injury) may take a variety of forms.   Most commonly it is mechanical trauma manifested by contusion, laceration, and fracture.   Trauma may also be produced by physical agents such as high or low environmental temperature, changes in barometric pressure, ionizing radiation, and electrical injury.   Chemical agents may also produce injury; the most common include alcohol, strong acids and bases, many drugs, heavy metals, and industrial poisons.

Infection   This represents a large group of diseases which have claimed major attention and have responded to successful therapeutic developments since the last quarter of the nineteenth century or roughly during the past hundred years.   Broad classifications within this category include infections produced by viruses, rickettsiae, bacteria, fungi, protozoa, and helminthes (worms).   *Infestation* is caused by a number of parasitic arthropods and is arbitrarily separated from infection because of the greater complexity of the parasites.

Metabolic Diseases   These diseases are due to faulty chemical processes.   It is here that overlapping categories are most apparent.   For example, many metabolic diseases are due to defects in enzymes that control a chemical step, and the defective enzymes may stem from abnormal genes.   However, enzyme defects may also be required later in life due to a variety of disease processes. Metabolic diseases also include most of the endocrine disorders, nutritional diseases, and poisonings. As a result, every system of classification must be somewhat arbitrary.

Hypersensitivity and Allergy   These conditions represent abnormalities of normal immune mechanisms designed to protect the individual against foreign proteins, chiefly those of infecting organisms. Inasmuch as hypersensitivity and allergy will probably be demonstrated to be due to faulty chemistry in the production of antibodies, it is conceivable that they may eventually be considered metabolic diseases as well.

Neoplasia   Neoplasia, or "new growth," is an unsystematic increase in tissue. Most neoplasms are self-limited tumors, do not directly cause death, and are called *benign*. However, between 20 and 30 percent of all individuals will eventually develop a new growth which is not self-limited and may progress to cause death. These new growths are called *malignancies* or, more generally, *cancers*. Carcinomas and sarcomas represent, respectively, the malignancies arising from epithelial structures and those arising from the connective tissue.

Thrombosis   Thrombosis occupies a unique position as a cause of disease. It is a single, specific process in which a blood clot forms in a blood vessel. The obstruction of blood flow to an organ can have a catastrophic effect. By causing heart attacks, strokes, and gangrene, thrombosis is now the greatest single cause of disease and accounts for over half of all deaths in industrial societies.

Functional Disorders   These disorders are associated with defects in function for which there is no apparent anatomical explanation. Common functional disorders are related to failure of smooth muscle to contract or, conversely, failure of contracted smooth muscle to relax. Eventually some of these disorders may be shown to be due to abnormalities of the nervous innervation or of some metabolic function and could then be reclassified more appropriately. There is sometimes the inference that functional disorders are the result of psychic interaction with somatic function. Wherever this is the implication, it will be made clear and the present evidence discussed. A number of mechanical disturbances are of sufficient importance that they can be classed together, although they may be of diverse origins which might also serve as the basis for classification. Thus, obstruction to flow in a blood vessel may be due to a blood clot, in the bile duct to scarring from previous inflammation, in the intestine to failure of proper nervous innervation, in the bladder to a cancer of the prostate blocking the outlet, and in the birth canal to faulty bone structure in the pelvis obstructing the delivery of the child.

Psychic Disorders   These disorders will be classified separately. They are not of uniform origin.   Some are known to be sequelae of specific organic diseases, others may result from the effects of emotional experiences.   The possibility that psychic disorders may be characterized if not caused by metabolic disorders within the brain has been strengthened by the effectiveness of recent drug therapies.

Aging   There is increasing evidence that *aging* is a specific process which affects but is neither caused by nor the cause of specific disease processes.   In a broad sense, the study of aging can examine all functions which are age-related, not only those of senescence but those of growth and development as well.   Like genetics, aging seems to define those inherent structural and functional characteristics of the individual with which the environment interacts.

Finally, there are those diseases and processes whose fundamental origins are still not understood.   Fortunately, these seem to be rapidly decreasing in number.   Many have received the unfortunate descriptive term *idiopathic,* meaning literally "of their own origin."   The inappropriateness of this term is obvious, and it should eventually pass from usage.

CLASSIFICATION BY ANATOMY

Another extremely convenient way to classify disease is by the organ system or part of the body involved.   This method is especially useful for those conditions which are localized.   Traumatic injuries, of course, can be most easily classified in this way.   However, tuberculosis may not be restricted to the lungs, meningitis to the meninges, or gonorrhea to the urethra, and anatomical localization renders etiological classification more precise.   Anatomical classifications divide the body into the organ systems and regional anatomy.   The *Standard Nomenclature of Diseases and Operations* codes the diagnosis by first assigning a number which identifies the anatomical structure involved, followed by the number which identifies the disease etiology (Table 1-1).   In general, this classification is extremely clear-cut, although there is some overlap in the urinary, reproductive, and endocrine systems.

There is relatively little conflict between organ-system and regional anatomical classifications.   Thus, the patient may have a carcinoma of the lung, an amebic abscess of the liver, a fracture of the skull, or arteriosclerotic gangrene of the foot.   It is apparent from these examples that ultimately the most satisfactory diagnoses are those which combine the etiology of the process with its localization. Table 1-1 shows the main topographic divisions as used in the *Standard Nomenclature of Diseases and Operations.* Table 1-2 shows the main categories used in the *International Classification of Diseases,* another system which is widely applied. It will be noted that this system utilizes primarily the topographical approach and reserves the etiological classifications chiefly to disease and injuries involving the body as a whole.

An example will clarify the method. Pulmonary tuberculosis, right upper lobe, moderately advanced, active, would be 363-1232 in *Standard Nomenclature*: Respiratory System, 3; lung, 6; right upper lobe, 3; infective disease, -1; mycobacterium tuberculosis, 23; and moderately advanced, active, 2. If the *International Classification* were used, the code number would be 011.1: tuberculosis, 01; pulmonary, 1; and moderately advanced, active, .1. Although it is more simple to use, the latter is less complete and flexible.

AREAS OF MEDICAL SPECIALIZATION

As medical knowledge becomes more extensive and diagnostic and therapeutic procedures become more technically difficult, it is becoming

Table 1-2   Classification of Diseases and Injuries Used in the International Classification of Diseases*

I	Infective and Parasitic Diseases
II	Neoplasms
III	Allergic, Endocrine System, Metabolic, and Nutritional Diseases
IV	Diseases of Blood and Blood-forming Organs
V	Mental, Psychoneurotic, and Personality Disorders
VI	Diseases of the Nervous System and Sense Organs
VII	Diseases of the Circulatory System
VIII	Diseases of the Respiratory System
IX	Diseases of the Digestive System
X	Diseases of the Genitourinary System
XI	Deliveries and Complications of Pregnancy, Childbirth, and Puerperium
XII	Diseases of the Skin and Cellular Tissue
XIII	Diseases of the Bones and Organs of Movement
XIV	Congenital Malformations
XV	Certain Diseases of Early Infancy
XVI	Symptoms, Senility, and Ill-defined Conditions
XVII	Injuries and Adverse Effects of Chemical and Other External Causes

*Eighth Revision, Department of Health, Education and Welfare, Public Health Service, National Center for Health Statistics.

impossible for a single physician to master the full range of medical knowledge and techniques.   In the era when effective therapeutic techniques were few in number, diagnosis was important only when effective therapy could be applied, and the physician's chief role was to offer a prognosis and to provide reassurance for the patient.   Today, when precise diagnosis often leads to specific treatment with amelioration or cure of the disorder and when potent therapies incorrectly used can create much harm, the level of knowledge must be high, experience extensive, and skill reliable.   As a result, specialization has become imperative.

Despite the recent increasing trends toward specialization, specialization itself is not new.   In fact, the major specialties existed long before the concept and practice of the general practitioner.   Thus, obstetrics was handled by the midwife, trauma by the barber-surgeon, and the more obscure diseases were handled first by the priest and then by the physician. The general practitioner was never truly "general"; he practiced pediatric and internal medicine as well as a limited number of surgical and obstetrical procedures.   The newer specialties have added techniques that he never used.   The general practitioner is now becoming the family physician, a specialist whose role increasingly resembles that of the combined internist and pediatrician.

The term *medicine* is used both in a general sense referring to the study of disease and in the more restrictive sense indicating the study of those diseases which can be treated by medical means.   The specialty of medicine today is divided into two major branches, *pediatrics,* the care of children, and *internal medicine,* the care of adults.*   *Geriatrics,* the care of the aged, is generally considered to be within the realm of internal medicine.   The roles of the pediatrician and the internist are essentially those of the family physician.   It is the family physician's responsibility to guard the health of his patients, to diagnose disease, and to treat those diseases for which his skill is adequate.   He must know what specialized diagnostic and therapeutic skills are available and when his patient would benefit by referral to specialists who can provide these services.

Surgery is concerned with those diseases and conditions for which operative treatment is necessary.   Injury is the obvious and traditional sphere of the surgeon, and such cases often go directly to him.   Textbooks of medicine generally do not cover injuries and their complications. However, with regard to those diseases in which surgical therapy may be important, there may be extensive discussion in textbooks of both medi-

---

* The term *internal medicine* was introduced in the nineteenth century to differentiate medicine from dermatology, or external medicine.

cine and surgery, in each instance from the particular point of view of the presenting specialty. As surgical procedures have become increasingly complex, various surgical subspecialties have become well defined and modern surgeons tend to stay within their areas of technical competence. *Obstetrics,* traditionally a separate specialty, has, with the development of gynecology in the past century, become identified as a subspecialty of surgery.

In this text, we shall be primarily concerned with the processes of disease rather than with treatment. For this reason, we shall not be concerned with whether the disorder is primarily medical or surgical, pediatric or obstetric. However, we shall try to indicate in the course of the discussion how the various specialties relate to each other operationally and how our increased knowledge and skill supplement each other to produce the medical successes we now achieve.

MEDICAL TERMINOLOGY

The vocabulary of medicine is difficult, and physicians are constantly challenged to provide adequate information to patients and their families. Sometimes it is possible to reduce complex concepts to simple language. But precise concepts and precise techniques require precise language. It may be necessary to reduce a complex idea to a simple generalization for the understanding of a layman, but this simple generalization which may be sufficient for the patient is often inadequate for another physician. There is no simple way to define a chromophobe adenoma, renal tubular acidosis, or amyloid disease. "John Jones" is only a name which becomes an identity as we get to know the individual.

Similarly, the study of medicine requires the development of an extensive vocabulary which involves the knowledge not only of the words themselves but also of their underlying connotations. Fortunately, the disease processes which we are to present can be comprehended with a relatively limited vocabulary. Additionally, the existence of numerous words, prefixes, and suffixes which derive from Greek and Latin makes it possible to dissect many of these compound words which serve to identify the concept. A small medical dictionary kept conveniently close at hand should assist in this understanding.

MEDICAL LITERATURE

A textbook of this type, in its attempt to be all-inclusive, must treat each subject with relative superficiality. In order to obtain a deeper and more profound knowledge of a specific subject, it will be necessary for the student to consult the medical literature. It is appropriate to review the various types of medical publications so that the student will have an orientation in his literature exploration. The first level is the medical *textbook* usually prepared for the major specialties of medicine, surgery, pediatrics, and obstetrics and gynecology. These textbooks are generally quite comprehensive and may run to 2,000 pages or more. Concomitant with the increasing medical knowledge and the development of sub-specialization, these texts are usually multiauthored, and the general plan and quality of each chapter is the responsibility of the editors. For further information the student is referred to the texts in the sub-specialties. In medicine these might include volumes on heart disease, gastroenterology, and neurology, while in surgery they might include orthopedics, neurosurgery, or ophthalmology to name but a few. Finally, there is the *monograph,* which is a discussion of a single disease entity or problem. This may be largely a review of the literature; however, more frequently it is based on the author's extensive experience and research on the subject as well.

The advanced student will find it necessary to refer to periodical literature. Because of publication schedules, this represents the most current information. At present, there are probably 6,000 journals which are published regularly on various medical subjects in various parts of the world. Journal articles will not be found in the library card catalog. The most complete listing is that of the *Index Medicus.* This monthly publication lists all current medical articles in 2,500 selected journals by subject and author. This system was adopted in 1960. Similar catalogs in previous years have been the *Current Lists of Medical Literature,* the *Quarterly Cumulative Index Medicus,* and the *Index Catalogue of the Surgeon General's Office.* With these indexes, most of the important articles that have appeared in the past century can be located. A very useful publication is the *Excerpta Medica,* published by the Excerpta Medica Foundation in Amsterdam. This journal abstracts most of the articles from the better journals. Volumes are published in the various specialties, and the abstracts are usually in English. Both the indexes and *Excerpta Medica* are quite expensive and are generally found only on the reference shelves of larger medical libraries.

Journal articles may be divided into a number of different types, and only those of present relevance will be described. The simplest type of article is the *case report.* Here one case, or at the most a few cases, is described in considerable detail in order to call attention to some new or unusual aspect. Rare new entities may first be presented as case reports. While one individual may never gain sufficient experience with a rare entity to characterize it, the analysis of a number of case reports often allows a reviewer to do so. It is always surprising that, despite the intensity of medical observation, new diseases are constantly being described, thereby improving the precision of diagnosis and treatment. For example, Conn described the significance of the aldosterone-secreting tumor of the adrenal gland in 1954. As a result, several hundred people have already been cured of severe hypertension by the removal of these tumors. As another example, a patient may follow an unusual course during the administration of a drug and the case is published to alert the medical profession to the possibility that the drug may have toxic potentialities. If a number of such case reports appear, then the association between the drug and the complication may be established. It then becomes possible to determine whether the seriousness of the disease justifies the risk of the complication.

A second type of article, the *case survey,* is an extension of the case report and examines a large number of cases of the same disease. This may be a review of general or specific clinical characteristics, a clarification of pathogenesis or pathophysiology, an evaluation of a laboratory diagnostic test, or the response to therapy. For example, the advent of kidney biopsy has resulted in the publication of many articles characterizing the pathological changes in the biopsies and correlating them with the clinical manifestations in various diseases.

A *review of the literature* is a response to the increasing number of publications on each subject. The author generally presents no new material but attempts to cover the important past publications and to summarize and synthesize current concepts based on previous investigations. *Monographs* may also be found in the periodical literature, and there are now several journals which specialize in review articles and monographs.

One of the most important types of periodical literature is the *report of research.* This may range from a typical basic study to one evaluating the clinical efficacy of a new treatment. The important characteristic of a research report is that it is structured throughout and that the results are derived from a previously planned program. Retrospective studies are important, but they suffer a lack of precision because no provision was made to collect specific data in a uniform way and to reduce the variables as much as possible.

The medical literature is vast and growing rapidly. No individual can hope to keep up with the developments in more than a small field of specialization. An intensive attempt is being made to devise methods to speed and simplify the dissemination of information, and many promising techniques are being tested. The bibliography at the end of this chapter lists some of the standard textbooks and the more widely read journals available in English. The list represents no attempt at completeness. The references at the end of each chapter in this book will include appropriate textbooks, journals, and, occasionally, a particularly significant journal article.

STANDARD TEXTBOOKS

Anatomy

ANSON, B. J. (ed.): *Morris' Human Anatomy,* 12th ed., New York: McGraw-Hill Book Company, 1966.

GOSS, C. M. (ed.): *Gray's Anatomy of the Human Body,* 29th ed., Philadelphia: Lea & Febiger, 1972.

LOCKHART, R. D., et al.: *Anatomy of the Human Body,* rev. ed., Philadelphia: J. B. Lippincott Company, 1969.

WOODBURNE, R. T.: *Essentials of Human Anatomy,* 4th ed., Fair Lawn, N.J.: Oxford University Press, 1969.

Physiology

BEST, C. H., and N. B. TAYLOR: *Physiological Basis of Medical Practice,* 8th ed., Baltimore: The Williams & Wilkins Company, 1966.

GUYTON, A. C.: *Function of the Human Body,* 3d ed., Philadelphia: W. B. Saunders Company, 1969.

MOUNTCASTLE, V. B. (ed.): *Medical Physiology,* 11th ed., St. Louis: The C. V. Mosby Company, 1961.

VANDER, A. J., J. H. SHERMAN, and D. S. LUCIANO: *Human Physiology,* New York: McGraw-Hill Book Company, 1970.

Pathology

ANDERSON, W. A. D. (ed.): *Pathology,* 6th ed., St. Louis: The C. V. Mosby Company, 1971.

BOYD, W.: *Textbook of Pathology: Structure and Function in Disease,* 8th ed., Philadelphia: Lea & Febiger, 1970.

MOREHEAD, R. P.: *Human Pathology,* New York: McGraw-Hill Book Company, 1965.

ROBBINS, S. L.: *Pathology,* 3d ed., Philadelphia: W. B. Saunders Company, 1967.

Pharmacology

BECKMAN, H.: *Pharmacology: The Nature, Action and Use of Drugs,* 2d ed., Philadelphia: W. B. Saunders Company, 1961.

BEVAN, J. A. (ed.): *The Essentials of Pharmacology: A Textbook for Students,* New York: Hoeber Medical Division, Harper & Row, Publishers, Incorporated, 1969.

DiPALMA, J. R.: *Drill's Pharmacology in Medicine,* 4th ed., New York: McGraw-Hill Book Company, 1971.

GOODMAN, L. S., and A. GILMAN: *The Pharmacological Basis of Therapeutics,* 4th ed., New York: The Macmillan Company, 1970.

GROLLMAN, A.: *Pharmacology and Therapeutics,* 7th ed., Philadelphia: Lea & Febiger, 1970.

MICKS, R. H.: *The Essentials of Materia Medica, Pharmacology and Therapeutics,* 9th ed., London: J. & A. Churchill, Ltd., 1965.

Medicine

BEESON, P. B., and W. McDERMOTT (eds.): *Cecil-Loeb Textbook of Medicine,* 13th ed., Philadelphia: W. B. Saunders Company, 1971, 2 vols.

BLOOM, A. (ed.): *Medicine for Nurses,* 10th ed., Baltimore: The Williams & Wilkins Company, 1967.

BOYD, W.: *An Introduction to the Study of Disease,* 6th ed., Philadelphia: Lea & Febiger, 1971.

WINTROBE, M. W., et. al. (eds.): *Harrison's Principles of Internal Medicine,* 6th ed., New York: McGraw-Hill Book Company, 1970.

Surgery

COLE, W. H., and R. M. ZOLLINGER: *Textbook of Surgery,* 9th ed., New York: Appleton-Century Crofts, Inc., 1969.

DAVIS, L. E. (ed.): *Christopher's Textbook of Surgery,* 9th ed., Philadelphia: W. B. Saunders Company, 1968.

RHOADS, J. E., et. al.: *Surgery: Principles and Practice,* 4th ed., Philadelphia: J. B. Lippincott Company, 1970.

SCHWARTZ, S. I. (ed): *Principles of Surgery,* New York, McGraw-Hill Book Co., 1969.

Obstetrics and Gynecology

EASTMAN, N. J., and L. M. HELLMAN: *Williams' Obstetrics,* 14th ed., New York: Appleton-Century Crofts, Inc., 1971.

GREENHILL, J. P.: *Obstetrics,* from the original text of J. B. DeLee, 13th ed., Philadelphia: W. B. Saunders Company, 1965.

NOVAK, E. R., and G. S. JONES: *Novak's Textbook of Gynecology,* 8th ed., Baltimore: The Williams & Wilkins Company, 1970.

WILLSON, J. R., et. al. (eds.): *Obstetrics and Gynecology,* 4th ed., St. Louis: The C. V. Mosby Company, 1971.

Pediatrics

BARNETT, H. L.: *Pediatrics,* 14th ed., New York: Appleton-Century-Crofts, Inc., 1968.

COOKE, R. E. (ed.): *The Biological Basis of Pediatric Practice,* New York: McGraw-Hill Book Company, 1968.

NELSON, WALDO (ed.): *Textbook of Pediatrics,* 9th ed., Philadelphia: W. B. Saunders Company, 1969.

WATSON, E., and G. H. LOWREY: *Growth and Development of Children,* 5th ed., Chicago: Year Book Medical Publishers, Inc., 1967.

Classification and Nomenclature of Disease

THOMPSON, E. T. (ed.) and A. C. HAYDEN (assoc. ed.): *Standard Nomenclature of Diseases and Operations,* 5th ed., published for the American Medical Association, New York: McGraw-Hill Book Company, 1961.

International Classification of Diseases (Adapted for Indexing of Hospital Records by Diseases and Operation), 8th rev., Washington: U.S. Department of Health, Education and Welfare, 1968.

COMMONLY USED MEDICAL JOURNALS IN ENGLISH

Acta Medica Scandinavica	Acta Med Scand
American Family Physician	Am Fam Physician
American Heart Journal	Am Heart J
American Journal of Cardiology	Am J Cardiol
American Journal of Clinical Nutrition	Am J Clin Nutr
American Journal of Clinical Pathology	Am J Clin Pathol
American Journal of Digestive Diseases	Am J Dig Dis
American Journal of Diseases of Children	Am J Dis Child
American Journal of Human Genetics	Am J Hum Genet
American Journal of the Medical Sciences	Am J Med Sci
American Journal of Medicine	Am J Med
American Journal of Obstetrics and Gynecology	Am J Obstet Gynecol
American Journal of Ophthalmology	Am J Ophthalmol
American Journal of Pathology	Am J Pathol
American Journal of Physical Medicine	Am J Phys Med
American Journal of Physiology	Am J Physiol
American Journal of Psychiatry	Am J Psychiatry
American Journal of Public Health and the Nation's Health	Am J Public Health
American Journal of Roentgenology, Radium Therapy and Nuclear Medicine	Am J Roentgenol Rad Ther Nucl Med

American Journal of Surgery	Am J Surg
American Journal of Tropical Medicine and Hygiene	Am J Trop Med Hyg
American Review of Respiratory Diseases	Am Rev Resp Dis
Anaesthesia	Anaesthesia
Anesthesiology	Anesthesiology
Annals of Internal Medicine	Ann Intern Med
Annals of Otology, Rhinology and Laryngology	Ann Otol Rhinol Laryngol
Annals of Surgery	Ann Surg
Annals of Thoracic Surgery	Ann Thorac Surg
Archives of Dermatology	Arch Dermatol
Archives of Environmental Health	Arch Environ Health
Archives of General Psychiatry	Arch Gen Psychiatry
Archives of Internal Medicine	Arch Intern Med
Archives of Neurology	Arch Neurol
Archives of Ophthalmology	Arch Ophthalmol
Archives of Otolaryngology	Arch Otolaryngol
Archives of Pathology	Arch Pathol
Archives of Physical Medicine and Rehabilitation	Arch Phys Med Rehabil
Archives of Surgery	Arch Surg
Arthritis and Rheumatism	Arthritis Rheum
Blood; Journal of Hematology	Blood
Brain; Journal of Neurology	Brain
British Heart Journal	Br Heart J
British Journal of Radiology	Br J Radiol
British Journal of Surgery	Br J Surg
British Medical Journal	Br Med J
Canadian Medical Association Journal	Canad Med Assoc J
Cancer	Cancer
Chest	Chest
Circulation; Journal of the American Heart Association	Circulation
Clinical Pharmacology and Therapeutics	Clin Pharmacol Ther
DM: Disease-a-Month	DM
Diabetes	Diabetes
Endocrinology	Endocrinology
Gastroenterology	Gastroenterology
Gut	Gut
Journal of Allergy and Clinical Immunology	J Allergy Clin Immunol
Journal of the American Dietetic Association	J Am Diet Assoc

Journal of the American Geriatrics Society	J Am Geriatr Soc
Journal of the American Medical Association	JAMA
Journal of Applied Physiology	J Appl Physiol
Journal of Bone and Joint Surgery; American Volume	J Bone Joint Surg [Am]
Journal of Bone and Joint Surgery; British Volume	J Bone Joint Surg [Br]
Journal of Clinical Endocrinology and Metabolism	J Clin Endocrinol Metab
Journal of Clinical Investigation	J Clin Invest
Journal of Clinical Pathology	J Clin Pathol
Journal of Experimental Medicine	J Exp Med
Journal of Gerontology	J Gerontol
Journal of Immunology	J Immunol
Journal of Infectious Diseases	J Infect Dis
Journal of Investigative Dermatology	J Invest Dermol
Journal of Laboratory and Clinical Medicine	J Lab Clin Med
Journal of Laryngology and Otology	J Laryngol
Journal of Medical Education	J Med Educ
Journal of Nervous and Mental Diseases	J Nerv Ment Dis
Journal of Neurosurgery	J Neurosurg
Journal of Obstetrics and Gynaecology of the British Commonwealth	J Obstet Gynaec Br Comm
Journal of Oral Surgery	J Oral Surg
Journal of Pediatrics	J Pediatr
Journal of Thoracic and Cardiovascular Surgery	J Thorac Cardiovasc Surg
Journal of Trauma	J Trauma
Journal of Urology	J Urol
Lancet	Lancet
Medical Clinics of North America	Med Clin North Am
Medical Letter on Drugs and Therapeutics	Med Lett Drugs Ther
Medicine	Medicine (Baltimore)
New England Journal of Medicine	N Engl J Med
Obstetrics and Gynecology	Obstet Gynecol
Pediatrics	Pediatrics
Physical Therapy; Journal of the American Physical Therapy Association	Phys Ther
Physiological Reviews	Physiol Rev
Plastic and Reconstructive Surgery	Plast Reconstr Surg

Postgraduate Medicine	Postgrad Med
Progress in Cardiovascular Diseases	Prog Cardiovasc Dis
Public Health Reports	Public Health Rep
Radiology	Radiology
Rheumatology and Physical Medicine	Rheumatol Phys Med
Surgery	Surgery
Surgery, Gynecology and Obstetrics	Surg Gynecol Obstet
Surgical Clinics of North America	Surg Clin North Am

Some Essential Structural and Functional Properties of the Human Organism

The fundamental biological unit is the *cell,* a microscopic structure with a central nucleus surrounded by cytoplasm and bounded by a cell membrane. Every individual starts as a single cell; some species persist as single-celled organisms and others multiply their cells to achieve the diversity of size and structure seen in nature. The cell of a single-celled organism is relatively unspecialized and can perform all the functions necessary for survival. As organisms become larger, with more cells, the structure becomes more complex, and groups of cells take over specific functions. In so doing these cells give up the capacity for universal action. Specialized groups of cells are known as *tissues.* Some aggregates of tissues, such as the brain, heart, and liver, are structurally and functionally so unique and well identified that they are called *organs.*

Although the functional living unit of the individual is the cell, it is a mistake to believe that the tissues are made up entirely of cells. The cell itself has no rigidity, and a collection of cells would have no form. The characteristic structure exhibited by various forms of life is due primarily to materials produced by specialized cells which are then laid down outside and between the cells. The most obvious of these in man is bone, and in plants, cellulose. Therefore it is important to examine not only the cell and the intracellular structure and function but also the extracellular components.

THE CELL

The original meaning of the word *cell,* "a little room," is still applied to the rooms of a prison or monastery. The word was first used in the present meaning by Robert Hooke, who, in the seventeenth century, made a microscope and examined thin slices of cork. However, he gave the name not to the cell itself but to the open space bounded by the hard, extracellular material which was left after the cell died. It was not until the early part of the nineteenth century that Schleiden and Schwann first presented the theory that all life was based on the cell as a fundamental structural unit. The publication in 1858 of Rudolph Virchow's textbook *Cellular Pathology* was a revolutionary step. It brought the end of the classical humoral concepts of disease* and provided a framework on which modern structural and functional concepts could be developed. Subsequently, improvements in the microscope, the development of staining techniques to improve the examination of tissues, and the recent development of the electron microscope and techniques for its use have all resulted in a multifold expansion of our knowledge and understanding of structure and function in the normal and diseased states.

Cellular Chemistry

Before proceeding with the discussion of the structure of the cell, we must examine some of the essential chemical components of cells and tissues. We are all generally aware that the normal diet contains proteins, fats, and carbohydrates; vitamins and minerals; and water as the major components. Since most foodstuffs are derived from plant or animal substances which are organized as cells, their composition is essentially similar to that of human tissues. We are also aware that industrial polymers and synthetics are long-chain compounds made up of smaller units. Because they are extremely large, they are termed macromolecules. The tissues similarly are made up primarily of long-chain macromolecules. The *polysaccharides* are chains of sugars. *Glycogen,*

---

* According to Western concepts there were four humors—blood, mucus, yellow bile, and black bile—and all disease was due to an alteration in the relationships between them. The Chinese went one better and believed in five humors.

an important animal polysaccharide, is a long-chain storage form of glucose. The *mucopolysaccharides* are structural sugars combined with protein.

The *proteins* make up the most important structural components of the body. Proteins are extremely long macromolecules formed by the linkage of relatively small molecules known as *amino acids*. The amino acids are organic acids, but in addition they possess a nitrogen-containing amino group, which has the properties of a base. Since a base and an acid can combine, the base of one amino acid can join the acid of the next to form a chain. These chains are called *polypeptides*. There are only 20 different amino acids, but they can be combined and recombined into an infinite number of sequences. A protein may contain several thousand amino acids. In the next chapter we shall see how these sequences are formed and some of the problems that arise when the sequences are formed incorrectly. Two types of proteins are recognized. The *structural proteins* give the body its form and include such compounds as the myosins of muscle, the keratins of skin, nails, and hair, and the protein matrix of bone. The *enzymes* are protein catalysts; like all catalysts, they are capable of greatly accelerating chemical reactions. Each chemical reaction in the body is regulated by a specific enzyme; the adequacy or inadequacy of a specific reaction in the overall body metabolism is thus extremely dependent upon the proper action of the appropriate enzyme.

The *nucleic acids* are long-chain compounds made up of a pentose sugar, phosphoric acid, and purine and pyrimidine bases. Two general forms of nucleic acid are recognized: *deoxyribonucleic acid* (DNA) and *ribonucleic acid* (RNA). DNA is found entirely in the cell nucleus and makes up the chromosomes; the RNA is found in both the nucleus and the cytoplasm. The actions of DNA and RNA will be discussed in the next chapter.

An important component of the cell is the group of *lipids*. The lipids are fatty substances and include fatty acids, neutral fats, phospholipids, cholesterol, and similar compounds. Unlike sugars and amino acids, they do not form chains, although lipid molecules may be incorporated into some macromolecules of protein and carbohydrate.

The body contains 60 to 70 percent water, of which not quite two-thirds is within the cells and the remainder is outside of the cells. In addition to the macromolecules, this aqueous solution contains a variety of inorganic materials as well as a large number of smaller organic compounds which serve various physiologic functions. The fluid state of the cellular contents and of the material outside the cell facilitates the metabolic processes within the cell and makes possible the transportation

of nutrients, wastes, and metabolic products. The body fluid composition
will be examined in more detail later in this chapter.

CELLULAR ANATOMY AND PHYSIOLOGY

With this very sketchy description of the chemical aspects of tissue structure, it is now possible to examine the cellular anatomy in more detail. The characteristics of two typical cells are illustrated in Figs. 2-1,
2-2, and 2-3. The material making up the cell is given the general name
protoplasm. Each cell is divided into two distinct components, the
nucleus and the cytoplasm. As seen by ordinary light microscopy, the
nucleus is a relatively compact, dark mass which is surrounded by a
larger volume of less dense cytoplasm. Depending upon the type of cell,
the nucleus varies somewhat as to its shape, location, and density. However, it is the cytoplasm which exhibits the greatest degree of variability
and which generally characterizes the specific type of cell.

The Nucleus

The nucleus is the administrative center for the cell. It contains the
genes which, like instructions on the tape of a computer, are lined up on
the chromosomes and carry the information necessary to manufacture
the necessary proteins. Structure and function are determined by the
composition and organization of the structural proteins and the enzymes. An intact nucleus is necessary for cell survival. (In one important instance a cell survives without a nucleus: During the course
of development, the nucleus of the red blood cell disintegrates. Yet
the cell continues to function for an average of 120 days as an oxygen
carrier. The red blood cell can, of course, neither repair itself nor
reproduce.)

The nucleus is composed of four main structures: the nuclear membrane, the chromatin, the nucleolus, and the nuclear sap. The *nuclear
membrane* has been demonstrated by electron microscopy to be a definite
structure. (At the light microscopic level, it is often difficult to be certain when a membrane is present or when, as with droplets of oil mixed
in water, the apparent membrane is only an interface between two substances that do not mix.) Pores are visible in the membrane, but there
is no visual evidence of a free interchange either across the membrane or
through the pores. During mitosis, or cell division, the membrane disappears and reforms only after the division of chromosomal material. The
chromosomes are identifiable only during mitosis. During the resting

phase, the density of the nucleus is due to the presence of many small granules of *chromatin*.   The recent demonstration that each chromosome is an extremely long strand of DNA makes it highly improbable that the strand breaks up during the resting period; reassembly in the proper sequence would seem to be an extremely difficult process, with many chances for error.   It is now believed that during mitosis each DNA

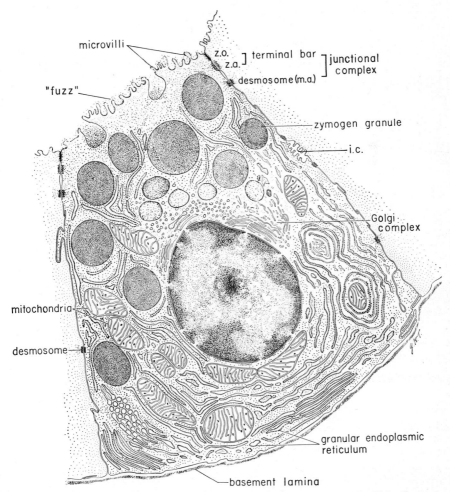

Figure 2-1   The internal structure of a typical cell.   This diagram illustrates a cuboidal or columnar epithelial cells specialized as a glandular secretory cell.   [*From E. D. Hay in R. O. Greep (ed.), Histology, McGraw-Hill, New York, 1966, p. 85. By permission of the publishers.*]

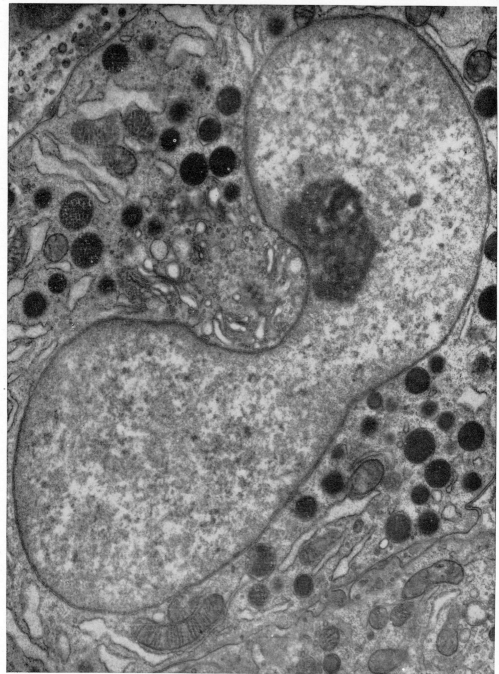

Figure 2-2 Electron micrograph of a myelocyte, or immature white blood cell. [*From L. Weiss in R. O. Greep (ed.), Histology McGraw-Hill, New York, 1966, p. 4. By permission of the publishers.*]

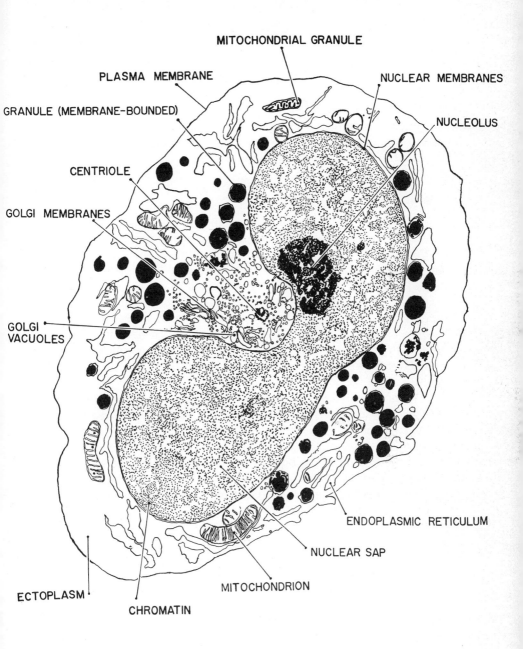

MITOCHONDRIAL GRANULE

PLASMA MEMBRANE

NUCLEAR MEMBRANES

GRANULE (MEMBRANE-BOUNDED)

NUCLEOLUS

CENTRIOLE

GOLGI MEMBRANES

GOLGI VACUOLES

ENDOPLASMIC RETICULUM

NUCLEAR SAP

ECTOPLASM

MITOCHONDRION

CHROMATIN

Figure 2-3   Myelocyte. Key to the intracellular structures seen in Fig. 2-2. [*From L. Weiss in R. O. Greep (ed.), Histology, McGraw-Hill, New York, 1966, p. 5.   By permission of the publishers.*]

strand becomes more tightly coiled and is stainable as a compact structure, the chromosome. During the resting phase between mitoses, the
coil unwinds, but areas of tight coiling are visible as granular chromatin
material. The *nucleolus,* literally the little nucleus, appears within the
larger nucleus. It is probable that it is the site of synthesis of *RNA ribosomes.* The remainder of the nuclear material is termed the *nuclear sap.*
The nucleus manufactures the ribosomes and the messenger RNA. These
two structures enable the cytoplasm to produce proteins and perform all
the other necessary activities of the cell.

The Cytoplasm

The cytoplasm is the site of most of the metabolic activity of the cell.
The cytoplasm surrounds the nucleus and is surrounded in turn by the
cell membrane. As with the nuclear membrane, the definite existence
of a cell membrane apart from an inert extracellular shell was not confirmed until the development of the electron microscope. With this
instrument it has been demonstrated that the cell membrane consists of
three layers. The cell membrane is often extremely specialized, depending
on the function of the cell. In the case of absorbing cells, as in the intestine, there may be thousands of fingerlike processes which increase the
cellular absorptive surface, just as the more visible villi of the intestinal
tract increase the intestinal surface.

     Within the cytoplasm a number of structures can be demonstrated.
The *endoplasmic reticulum* is a series of fine membranes. Anchored
to the endoplasmic reticulum are the granules known as *ribosomes.* The
ribosome consists of RNA apparently synthesized in the nucleolus. Its
exact role is not known, but it has been clearly shown that it is at the
ribosome that the messenger and transfer RNA act to produce new
proteins. The *Golgi apparatus* has been recognized for many years, but
now it has been demonstrated to be a series of membranes rather than a
cluster of fibers. The Golgi apparatus appears to be the site of carbohydrate macromolecule production. When mixed molecules of carbohydrates and proteins, such as mucus, are synthesized, it is found that
the protein is produced at the endoplasmic reticulum. It then migrates
to the Golgi apparatus, where the carbohydrate is added, and at the
Golgi apparatus it is enclosed in a secretory vesicle, which is eventually
extruded by the cell. The whole process has an assembly line precision,
with the raw materials entering the cell on the capillary side and the
finished product delivered on the secretory side of the cell.

     The *mitochondria,* of which there are many hundreds in most cells,
are infrequently seen by light microscopy, but they are well demonstrated

by the electron microscope.   They are small vesicles (droplets) containing many shelflike cristae (ridges).   The mitochondria appear to be responsible for oxidative respiration in a sequence known as the *Krebs cycle.*   The fuel is pyruvic acid, which is derived from carbohydrates, fats, and some amino acids.   The direct combustion of pyruvic acid with oxygen would produce large amounts of heat, which would be dissipated rapidly.   In order to limit heat production and to save the energy, the combustion is performed in a careful stepwise process.   Energy is stored by the production of *adenosine triphosphate* (ATP).   Energy is released by ATP with the formation of *adenosine diphosphate* (ADP) and phosphoric acid.   This energy release is at the site of need and not necessarily in the mitochondria.

Cytoplasmic inclusions are defined as vesicles which are not part of the metabolic machinery of the cells.   Three types can be identified: stored foods, secretion granules, and pigment.   Protein is available from cell turnover and is ordinarily not stored.   Carbohydrates are stored as glycogen, almost entirely by cells of the liver and muscle.   Fat is normally stored by special cells in tissues between major organs and in special fat depots, as beneath the skin of the abdomen and in the mesentery, the membrane which supports the intestines within the abdominal cavity.   In disease states the fat may be stored in organ cells, particularly those of the liver.   Fat vesicles may become so large that there is only a thin rim of cytoplasm and a markedly displaced nucleus, the storage cell looking much like a signet ring.

Secretion granules are vesicles which contain proteolytic (protein dissolving) enzymes.   Some cells, such as those of the pancreas and intestinal glands, produce enzymes which are used in the digestion of foodstuffs.   However, these vesicles are found in many other cells and are called *lysosomes* because they are capable of lysing (dissolving) the cell itself; in fact, the lysosomes are probably responsible for cell dissolution after cell injury or death.   Because of their capacity for cell destruction, they have been referred to as "suicide bags."   Their usual function is not known, but it seems possible that they can digest particulate matter which accidently enters the cells or which in an old cell must be destroyed and replaced.   Their most obvious function is in the phagocytes, to be discussed in the chapter on inflamation, which ingest and destroy bacteria and other foreign proteins.

Pigment granules may have a variety of sources.   *Lipochrome,* one type of pigment, accumulates in cells as they age, particularly in nerve, heart, and liver cells.   Pigments arising from the body include hemosiderin and hemotoidin, from blood breakdown, and melanin, which produces the skin color of a tan or racial pigmentation.   Other pigments, arising from

outside the body and stored to render them inactive, include such substances as coal dust, silver, lead, and carotene.

Cellular Functions

Although more complex classifications of cellular function have been
made, it seems reasonable to divide all cell functions into three major
groups: (1) the basic maintenance functions of a cell, (2) reproduction,
and (3) specialized functions. In the first category can be included
absorption and assimilation, respiration and energy transfer, anabolism
and catabolism (constructive and destructive processes), and excretion.

Normal reproduction and growth in response to stress or injury may
take on specialized forms. *Hypertrophy* is the enlargement of a cell or
organ beyond the usual normal size. This is the frequent response of
cells which do not reproduce, particularly muscle cells. *Hyperplasia*
is a response to stress by cells capable of reproducing and results in an
increase in the number of cells. Often there is both hypertrophy and
hyperplasia. When kidney substance is lost, new nephrons, the functional units of the kidney, cannot be regenerated. Therefore the residual
nephrons show hypertrophy, which is due both to enlargement of the
original cells and to hyperplasia, which is a total increase of the number
of cells in each remaining nephron unit. *Atrophy* is a decrease in size
due to injury, disease, or disuse. *Necrosis* is death of cells or tissues;
somatic death is death of the organism.

The functions of specialized cells are determined by the cell structure
and the consequent capacity for response to physiological stimulation.
Thus the muscle cell contracts, the nerve cell conducts, and the glandular
cell secretes. Since all cells in an individual have the same genetic
material in the nucleus, they have the same initial potentialities. The
mechanisms for differentiation are not known yet, but once differentiation
occurs, the cell can carry out only those residual functions which the
chemical and physical structure will allow. The basic metabolic functions persist, and reproduction may or may not be possible. Thus specialization represents a limitation and intensification of cellular capacity
rather than the development of a new or unique function.

TISSUES

The word *tissue* derives from the French word *tissu,* meaning "weave"
or "texture." It was first applied by Bichat, a French pathologist, in
the early nineteenth century. Bichat based his definition and initial
classifications on the gross characteristics of tissues and scorned the

use of the microscope.   Surprisingly, microscopic examination has supported and extended the concept.   In essence, a tissue is an aggregation of similarly specialized cells united in the performance of a particular function.   It is evident that the distinction between a tissue and an organ is somewhat arbitrary, although the former term is probably more comprehensive.   It is general practice to divide all tissues into four major groups: (1) epithelium, (2) connective tissue, (3) muscle, and (4) nerve.

Epithelial Tissue

Epithelium   Epithelial tissue forms the surface covering or lining of all body surfaces and cavities (Fig. 2-4).   Epithelium becomes modified in response to the type of surface to which it is applied.   Simple epithelium is only one cell thick.   Squamous epithelium is an extremely thin layer of

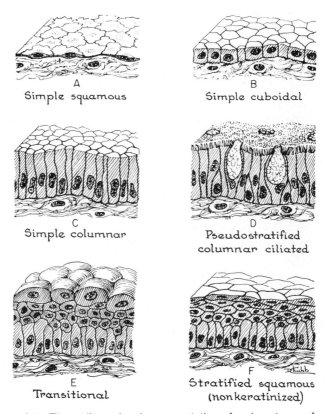

A
Simple squamous

B
Simple cuboidal

C
Simple columnar

D
Pseudostratified columnar ciliated

E
Transitional

F
Stratified squamous (nonkeratinized)

Figure 2-4   Three-dimensional representation of various types of epithelial tissues. *(From A. W. Ham, Histology, 6th ed., Lippincott, Philadelphia, 1969, p. 170.   By permission of the publishers.)*

simple epithelium which, like a layer of tile, acts chiefly to protect the surface. Cuboidal and columnar simple epithelium consists of cells which have depth and have obvious functional capacity beyond that of a protective covering. Often, especially in the case of columnar epithelium, the epithelial cells also have secretory capacity.

Stratified epithelium consists of epithelium which is several cells deep. The epidermis of the skin is the most important example of this type of epithelium (Fig. 2-5). There is a basal, germinal layer of cells which is

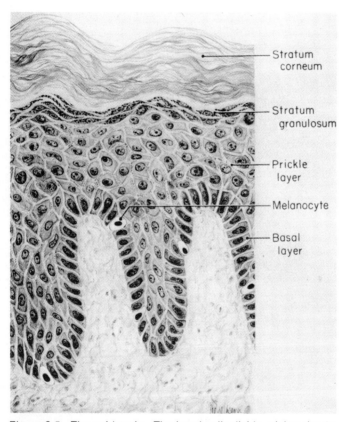

Figure 2-5 The epidermis. The basal cells divide, giving rise to daughter cells which are gradually pushed to the surface. In the process, the cells become less active and are converted to keratin, which provides surface protection. The melanocytes produce melanin, which provides pigmentation. *(From D. M. Pillsbury, W. B. Shelly, and A. M. Kligman, Dermatology, Saunders, Philadelphia, 1956, p. 8. By permission of the publishers.)*

relatively cuboidal in shape.   As the cells are piled on each other toward the surface, they become increasingly thin and more squamous.   These cells also produce *keratin,* a protein material which is hard, relatively waterproof, and serves as a protection from the environment.   The outer cells are dead and composed almost entirely of keratin.   These cells gradually wear off and are replaced by cells from the next lower level.   Hair, nails, and feathers are all modifications of keratin produced by appropriately specialized cells.   The urinary bladder and some other organs contain a specialized type of stratified epithelium.   The great distensibility of the bladder requires that the cells be adapted for this purpose.   Therefore, bladder epithelium is covered by transitional epithelial cells.   When the bladder is contracted, these cells are relatively cuboidal.   However, during the distension of the bladder, they are capable of being stretched almost to the thinness of squamous cells.

Two types of epithelium require special comment.   *Endothelium* is an extremely thin, squamous epithelium which lines the blood vessels and, indeed, represents almost the entire structure of the capillaries. These cells are so thin that, although they form the capillary tube and completely encircle the vessel, the cytoplasm is represented by only a single line on light microscopy.   This thin layer separates the blood from the tissue cells yet allows easy diffusion of solutes in both directions. The major body cavities—the pericardial cavity, pleural cavity, and peritoneal cavity—are also lined by a layer of thin, squamous epithelium which in this position is termed *mesothelium.*

It should be noted that epithelium is not invaded by blood vessels. The vascular supply of epithelium is derived from vessels which lie adjacent to the epithelium, and exchange is achieved by processes of diffusion.   The epithelial portion of the skin, the *epidermis,* is avascular and does not bleed when injured.   However, the epidermis does not rest on the *dermis* (the connective-tissue portion of the skin) as a smooth layer but as an irregularly thick layer which fits into the dermis like parts of a jigsaw puzzle (Figs. 2-6 and 2-7).   The bottom layers of the stratified squamous epithelium thus surround and are surrounded by blood vessel loops.   When epithelium is injured, it must be replaced by epithelial cells which grow in from the surrounding undamaged epithelium.   In the case of skin, extensive destruction is often associated with retention of some of the deep-lying epithelium, the so-called *rete pegs,* and especially the hair follicles and glands which penetrate quite deeply into the subcutaneous tissue.   Thus, skin can be repaired not only by ingrowth from the outside but also by hyperplasia of deep-lying cells from the rete pegs and hair follicles (see Fig. 2-6).

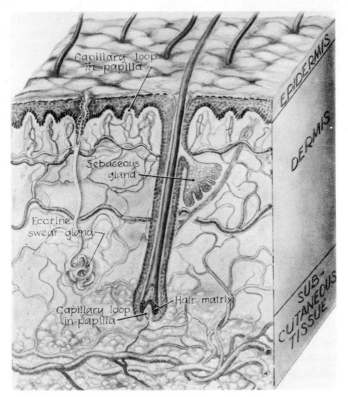

Figure 2-6 Three-dimensional representation of the skin. The epidermis is stratified squamous epithelium. The dermis and subcutaneous tissues are connective tissues which give support, particularly for the hair follicles and glands, and are much less cellular. The blood vessels terminate in the dermis as capillary loops, which do not penetrate the epidermis. *(From D. M. Pillsbury, W. B. Shelly, and A. M. Kligman, Dermatology, Saunders, Philadelphia, 1956, p. 3. By permission of the publishers.)*

Glands In addition to forming a covering tissue, the epithelial tissue also composes the functional secretory tissue of all glands (see Figs. 2-8 and 2-9). Pockets of epithelial cells burrow into the deeper tissue, forming sacs in the larger secretory organs. If the original duct remains open, so that the secretory products are delivered through this duct, the gland is termed an *exocrine* gland. However, if the duct is lost, the secretory products must then diffuse into the adjacent blood vessels. Such a gland is known as an *endocrine* gland. The most important glands of the epidermis are the sweat glands, the sebaceous glands, and the mammary glands. The most important glands of the gastrointestinal tract

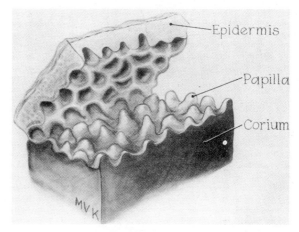

Figure 2-7 The relationship of the epidermis to the dermis. The cross-section of the epidermis seen in Fig. 2-5 suggests that projections of epidermis (rete pegs) penetrate into the dermis. The reverse is actually the case, and each dermal papilla brings capillaries in close approximation to the epidermis. *(From D. M. Pillsbury, W. B. Shelly, and A. M. Kligman, Dermatology, Saunders, Philadelphia, 1956, p. 9. By permission of the publishers.)*

include the salivary glands, the liver, and the pancreas. The endocrine glands which were originally derived from the intestinal epithelium include the pituitary, the thyroid, and the parathyroid glands.

Connective Tissue

It is surprising that the connective tissue as such does not receive the attention which it deserves. In addition to performing its literal function, the connective tissue gives the body its form, both by providing structural rigidity and by filling the spaces between specific tissues and organs. One of the chief characteristics of this tissue is its ability to produce extracellular substances which provide the rigidity of the body. The extracellular substance of connective tissue in which the cells are imbedded is known as the *matrix* of that tissue. The connective tissue is classically divided into four components: (1) connective tissue proper, (2) blood and lymph, (3) cartilage, and (4) bone.

Connective Tissue Proper The connective tissue proper is the most characteristic and least specialized of the connective tissue group. The typical cell of the connective tissue is the *fibroblast,* a cell with a long, slender nucleus which when young has an active ameboid cytoplasm and when old becomes quiescent, with a scanty, spindle-shaped cytoplasm (Fig.

EPITHELIAL TISSUE

Glandular Division

How Glands form from epithelial surfaces.

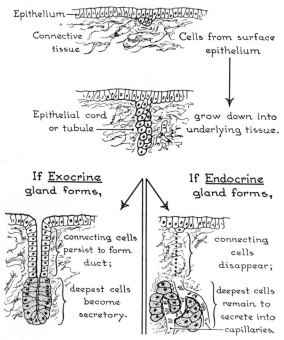

Epithelium

Connective tissue — Cells from surface epithelium

Epithelial cord or tubule — grow down into underlying tissue.

If **Exocrine** gland forms,

If **Endocrine** gland forms,

connecting cells persist to form duct;

deepest cells become secretory.

connecting cells disappear;

deepest cells remain to secrete into capillaries.

Figure 2-8   The development of the glands. *(From A. W. Ham, Histology, 6th ed., Lippincott, Philadelphia, 1969, p. 192. By permission of the publishers.)*

2-10).   The fibroblast produces the two characteristic types of extracellular fiber of the connective tissue.   The first of these is *collagen,* which may, in total quantity, be the most important protein of the body.   Collagen fibers are macromolecules of protein measuring some 2,800 angstroms in length (Fig. 2-11 A).   Collagen is usually laid down in bundles of fibers which average 10 micrometers in width, or approximately equal to the diameter of a small cell.   Under the electron microscope these fibers have an interesting and quite characteristic banding every 640 angstroms, which makes collagen easily identifiable.   Examples of almost pure collagen are the tendons, ligaments, and scar tissue.

Sheets of connective tissue, largely collagen, are called *fascia,* and

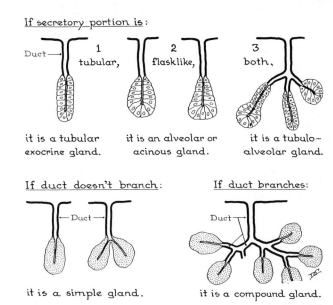

If secretory portion is:

1 tubular,
it is a tubular exocrine gland.

2 flasklike,
it is an alveolar or acinous gland.

3 both,
it is a tubulo-alveolar gland.

If duct doesn't branch:
it is a simple gland.

If duct branches:
it is a compound gland.

Figure 2-9   Types of secretory (exocrine) glands. *(From A. W. Ham, Histology, 6th ed., Lippincott, Philadelphia, 1969, p. 193. By permission of the publishers.)*

these serve to separate compartments of the body and bundles of muscles. Leather is almost entirely collagen; the epidermal tissue is removed and the already tough collagen of the dermis is made even stronger by the chemical process of tanning. It is interesting that the characteristics of leather are due to the long-chain polymers which make up the macromolecules, and thus both the structural and functional characteristics are similar to those of some modern synthetics. There are many tissues where a loose-binding connective tissue is needed but where strength and rigidity are not so important. In the loose connective tissue, smaller strands of collagen are laid down in an irregular manner. These are called *reticulum* fibers, from the Greek word *rete,* meaning "net."

The second type of fibers produced by the fibroblast, the elastic fibers, are composed of *elastin* and are found in the tissues where resilliency is necessary (Fig. 2-11B). Thus there is considerable elastin in the walls of arteries, which are subject to the repeated force of the heartbeat. As we shall see later, important changes in the vascular system can result from injury to or aging of the elastic fibers. The same is true of the skin, which wrinkles with age as youthful elasticity is lost.

One of the questions regarding connective tissue is the degree of specialization of the connective-tissue cell. Some believe that the fibro-

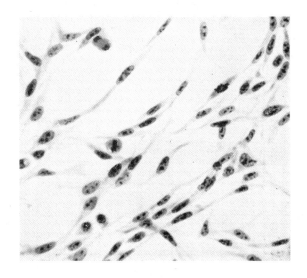

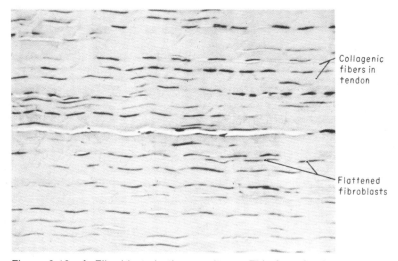

Collagenic
fibers in
tendon

Flattened
fibroblasts

Figure 2-10 *A:* Fibroblasts in tissue culture. This form is also assumed by fibroblasts in loose connective tissue. [From K. R. Porter in R. O. Greep (ed.), *Histology, McGraw-Hill, New York, 1966, p. 114. By permission of the publishers.*] *B:* Fibroblasts in tendon. The fibroblasts have laid down large quantities of collagen to form dense connective tissue and have become compressed by the mass of collagen and the stresses placed upon it. *(From A. W. Ham, Histology, 6th ed., Lippincott, Philadelphia, 1969, p. 375. By permission of the publishers.)*

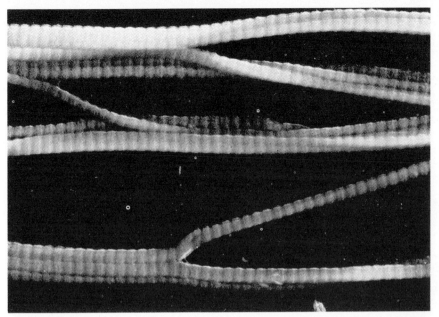

A

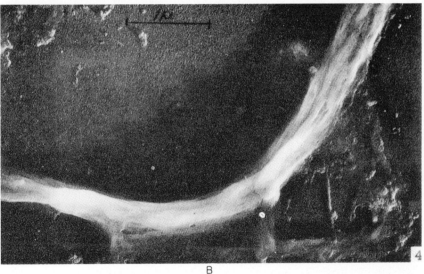

B

Figure 2-11 Collagen and elastin. *A:* Electron micrograph of collagen fibrils. Note the highly organized structure with cross-banding at intervals of 640 angstroms. x45,000. [*From K. R. Porter in R. O. Greep (ed.), Histology, McGraw-Hill, New York, 1966, p. 103. By permission of the publishers.)* *B:* Elastic fibers. These fibers are amorphous as compared to collagen and give no structural indication of their elastic capacity. x37,000. *(From J. Gross, J. Exp. Med., 89:699, 1949. By permission of the publishers.)*

blast is a primitive cell, capable of differentiating into all the other more specialized connective-tissue cells to be described in subsequent paragraphs. Another important cell in the connective tissue, whose origin has not been completely clarified, is the *histiocyte,* or *macrophage,* about which much more will be said in the discussion of inflammation. *Fat tissue* is a modified connective tissue in which the cells become swollen with large storage drops of neutral fat (Fig. 2-12).

Blood and Lymph   The blood and lymph systems can be divided into the circulating components and the hematopoietic tissues, or the tissues in which the blood cells are formed. The circulating blood makes up about 7 percent of the total body weight or 5 liters in the average adult male of 70 kilograms (154 pounds). If the blood is allowed to settle and clotting is prevented, the cells will be found to comprise about 45 percent, and the fluid, or plasma, makes up the remaining 55 percent of the blood volume. The blood plasma will be examined later in this chapter, with the discussion of the body fluids.

The cellular components of the blood consist of 4.5 to 5.0 million red blood cells (RBC) and 5,000 to 10,000 white blood cells (WBC) per cubic millimeter. Mature blood cells are shown in the color plate (see page 210). Microscopic examination of the red cells shows them to be of characteristic shape and to contain no nuclei. The principal components of the red cells are the cell membrane; the hemoglobin, which acts as an efficient transport mechanism of oxygen between lungs and the tissues; and the enzymes, which speed the attachment and detachment of oxygen from the hemoglobin and carbon dioxide from the blood water. It has been demonstrated that the shape of the red cell gives a maximum surface-to-volume ratio, which is in accord with the gas-transport functions of the cell. Although they are without nuclei, the average life-span of the red cells is 120 days.

The white blood cells are usually examined by spreading a drop of blood on a microscope slide, staining the cells, and then examining them under the microscope. A count of the various types of white cells is termed a *differential* white-cell count. The most common cell is the *polymorphonuclear neutrophil.* This cell has an unusual nucleus. Instead of being in one mass, the adult cell generally has the nuclear material divided into three masses joined by a thin protoplasmic strand (see color plate). The cytoplasm of this cell is filled with fine neutrophilic granules, so called because they stain with a neutral dye. Normally, the polymorphonuclear neutrophil (neutrophil or PMN) makes up 50 to 70 percent of all the white cells. The *polymorphonuclear eosinophil* (eosinophil or PME) resembles the PMN in general structure. However, the nucleus is generally in only

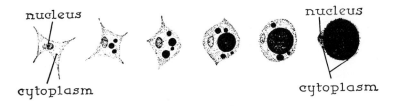

A

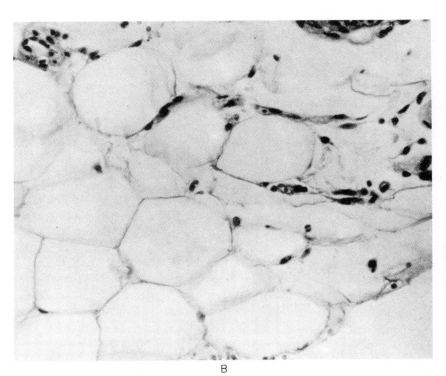

B

Figure 2-12 Fat cells. *A:* The accumulation of fat by a mesodermal cell, showing the displacement of the nucleus and cytoplasm by the large central globule of fat. *(From A. W. Ham, Histology, 6th ed., Lippincott, Philadelphia, 1969, p. 233.) B: Section*
of typical fatty tissue containing clusters of fat cells. *(From D. M.
Pillsbury, W. B. Shelly, and A. M. Kligman, Dermatology, Saunders,
Philadelphia, 1956, p. 73. By permission of the publishers.)*

two segments, and the cytoplasm contains large, characteristic granules which stain brilliantly with eosin. These cells make up 1 to 4 percent of the white blood cells. The third type of polymorphonuclear cell, the *basophil* (or PMB), also resembles the others; however, its cytoplasm contains a moderate number of basophilic granules. This cell makes up 1 percent or less of the white-blood-cell count. The *monocyte* is a somewhat larger cell which characteristically has a kidney-shaped, relatively lightly staining nucleus. It makes up 5 to 7 percent of the white-blood-cell count. Finally, the remaining 30 percent or so of the white blood cells are the *lymphocytes.* The small lymphocyte is hardly larger than the red blood cell and contains a spherical, densely staining nucleus and a scanty cytoplasm which stains a lighter blue with the usual dyes. The much less frequent large lymphocyte contains more cytoplasm and a less dense nucleus. (See color plate facing page 210.)

The blood cells are also divided into two major groups on the basis of their site of origin: the myeloid cells and the lymphoid cells. The myeloid cells are those which are produced in the bone marrow. They include all the polymorphonuclear cells, the monocytes, and the red blood cells. The lymphocytes are produced in the spleen and lymph nodes. In many blood diseases it is useful to examine the bone marrow, since changes in the nature of cell production may clarify the terminal phenomenon demonstrated by the circulating blood. The bone marrow contains stem cells for the red blood cells, polymorphonuclear cells, and monocytes. The more primitive the blood cell, the more difficult the individual cells are to differentiate. The red blood cell contains a nucleus until a relatively short time before its discharge into the circulation. The dense nucleus gradually disintegrates, first leaving a fine nuclear reticulum (network) in a cell called the *reticulocyte,* and finally even the reticulum disappears in the adult cell. A sudden loss of red blood cells, as by hemorrhage, may result in the release of immature cells into the circulation. Most commonly these are the reticulocytes, although in situations of greater stress nucleated cells may also appear. The early polymorphonuclear cells, or myelocytes, appear to arise from the same stem cell, and it is relatively late in their development that the characteristic granules appear. The nucleus originally is single, then progressively assumes a kidney shape, a horseshoe shape, and finally the segmented form. Immature polymorphonuclear white cells are released into the circulation during infection and in myeloid leukemia. However, different types of cells are released in each of these conditions, and they can generally be distinguished by examination of the stained slide.

A cell not previously mentioned which is present only in the bone marrow is the *megakaryocyte.* This is an extremely large cell whose major

function is the production of platelets.   The *platelet* is a small cell fragment which circulates in the bloodstream.   It has the capacity for occluding small leaks in the vascular endothelium and is especially important in
the proper clotting of blood, where its chief role seems to be that of causing
the fibrin of the blood clot to contract and thereby strengthen the anti-
hemorrhagic mechanism.

Cartilage   Cartilage is the third major component of the connective
tissue and an important supporting structure of the body (Fig. 2-13).
Indeed, in the infant the skeleton is almost entirely composed of cartilage,
which contains within it small areas of bone formation.   This arrangement
makes it possible for the infant and child to grow at a rapid rate without
requiring the extensive and slower remodeling of calcified bone.   These
cells of cartilage are widely separated by an intercellular substance.   One
of the main components of this intercellular substance is *collagen;* how-

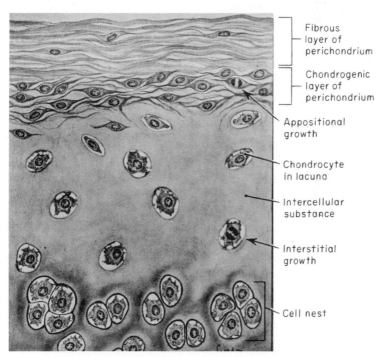

Figure 2-13   Cartilage. The cells are separated by the glycoprotein intercellular material. Nests of cells represent division of the
isolated cells. Since cartilage has no blood supply, metabolic
activity is limited and there is little tissue repair. *(From A. W. Ham,
Histology, 6th ed., Lippincott, Philadelphia, 1969, p. 378. By permission of the publishers.)*

ever, there are also other substances present which are glycoproteins, that is, proteins linked to long-chain carbohydrates. In the adult most of the cartilaginous skeleton is replaced by bone, and the chief cartilaginous remnants are on the surface of the joints, where the elasticity and smoothness of the cartilage make smooth joint movement possible. Other important sites of adult cartilage are in the ears, the nose, and the costal cartilages which join the ribs to the sternum.

Bone Bone makes up the adult skeleton, and its rigidity is due to the presence of calcium salts. Because of these salts, bone often resists the usual processes of postmortem decay and creates the impression that it is

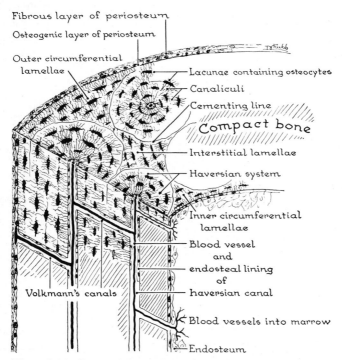

Figure 2-14   Bone. A three-dimensional diagramatic representation of the shaft of a long bone. Bone cells, or osteocytes, lie in lacunae, or clefts, in the calcified bone. Concentric rings of cells surround the blood vessels in the haversian canals. The layers of calcification between the cells are called lamellae. Each blood vessel with its osteocytes and lamellae makes up a haversian system. Surrounding the bone is a fibrous layer of periosteum containing osteoblasts, which make new bone. Also present are osteoclasts, which destroy old bone. Thus the bone undergoes continuous replacement and repair. *(From A. W. Ham, Histology, 6th ed., Lippincott, Philadelphia, 1969, p. 431. By permission of the publishers.)*

made up of nonviable tissue. However, during life bone is very much alive and undergoes constant metabolism. Bone contains from 14 to 44 percent water and from 30 to 35 percent protein in addition to the calcium salts. The bone cells are called *osteocytes.* The matrix is similar to that of cartilage and contains collagen and a glycoprotein. Living bone is well supplied with blood vessels. Surrounding the bone there is a dense fibrous tissue known as the *periosteum. Osteoblasts,* or bone-building cells, are derived from the periosteum and appear to be able not only to produce the matrix but also to initiate calcification. Other cells which also appear to be derived from the resting cells of the periosteum develop into *osteoclasts,* or bone-destroying cells. Both these cells are important in the remodeling and development of bone during growth and play a role in bone repair. The complex structure of the bone is diagramed in Fig. 2-14.

Long bones have an efficient and admirable mechanism for calcifica-

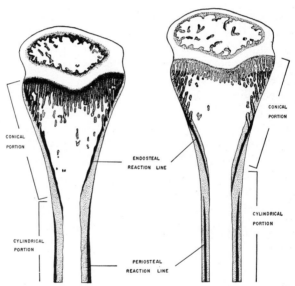

Figure 2-15 Bone growth. Diagrams of radioautographs of the head of the tibia of a young, growing rat. *A:* Rat killed a few hours after receiving radioactive phorphorus. The blackened area shows that the radioactive phosphorus has been incorporated into the bone of the epiphyses, into the metaphysis just below the epiphyseal cartilage, and beneath the periosteum of the shaft. *B:* Rat killed several days after injection of radioactive phosphorus showing further growth. The metaphysis has lengthened, replacing earlier bone at the epiphyseal cartilage, and new bone has been deposited under the periosteum, burying the portion with radioactive phosphorus deeper within the shaft. *(From M. L. Moss, Am. J. Anat., 86:289, 1950. By permission of the publishers.)*

tion and growth. Centers of ossification develop in the diaphysis, which is the shaft of the bone, and in the epiphyses, which are the ends of the bone. The diaphysis and epiphyses are separated by a cartilage known as the epiphyseal plate (Fig. 2-15). This mechanism gives strength to the bone and at the same time allows growth without interfering with joint movement. When full growth is obtained, the epiphyseal cartilage becomes completely ossified and the epiphyses are said to close. The appearance of ossification centers and the closure of the epiphyseal plates occur at different ages at different sites, and the age of an immature skeleton can usually be accurately estimated by knowledge of the ages at which these events occur.

The probable interrelationships of the various connective-tissue cells are shown in Fig. 2-16.

Muscle

Muscle is tissue in which the function of contractility has become specialized. Three types of muscle are recognized: voluntary, cardiac, and smooth muscle. *Voluntary muscle* makes up the largest bulk of the muscle tissue in the body. It is also called skeletal muscle, since these muscles are attached to the skeleton. Voluntary muscle is made up of large, ribbonlike cells which appear to possess a number of nuclei lying on the periphery, or outer surface, of the cell (Fig. 2-17A). The principal protein of the cell is actomyosin. This long-chain molecule has the capability of rearrangement so that it acts like a coiled spring. It is the molecular rearrangement which causes the muscle to contract and allows it to relax. The cytoplasm of the muscle cell contains easily visible lines which at intervals cross the cytoplasm. For this reason this muscle is frequently called striated muscle. Groups of muscle cells are gathered together by strong sheets of dense connective tissue which are attached to tendons and, in turn, to bone. The contractile power of the muscle is thus transmitted through the connective tissue to the bone to produce movement. *Cardiac muscle* very much resembles voluntary muscles in the shape of the cells and the presence of cross-striations (Fig. 2-17B). However, there are recognizable differences and, of course, cardiac muscle contractions are involuntary.

Smooth muscle cells, on the other hand, are relatively small and spindle-shaped and contain elongated nuclei (Fig. 2-17C and D). In general size and shape, they very much resemble fibroblasts. They perform a variety of functions where minor muscular power is necessary, such as pulling on the base of the hair follicle to make the hair stand on end. Their most consistent function is to cause contraction of various tubes and vesicles. Thus they are present surrounding the bronchi, the gastrointestinal

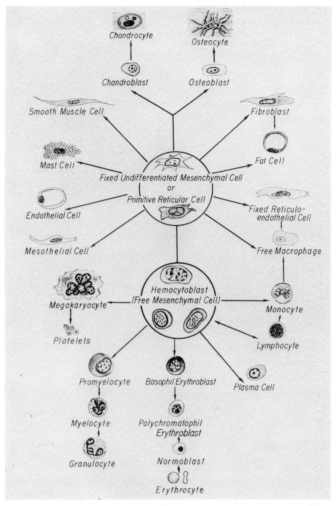

Figure 2-16   The genealology of connective tissue cells.   *(From C. R. Leeson and T. S. Leeson, Histology, Saunders, Philadelphia, 1970, p. 153.   By permission of the publishers.)*

tract, the ureter, the uterus, the blood vessels, the gall bladder, the urinary bladder, and a number of other organs.   Their most important stimuli for contraction or relaxation arise from the autonomic nervous system and the presence of mediating chemicals such as acetylcholine and epinephrine. In general, muscle cells are postmitotic; that is, they survive for the lifetime of the individual and are not replaced.   A specific exception is the apparent development of smooth muscle cells in the production of new blood vessels following injury.

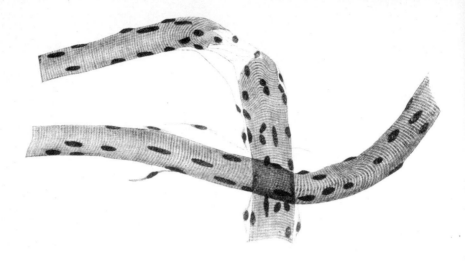

A

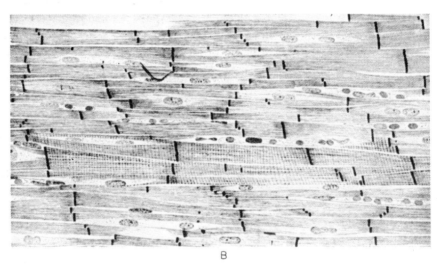

B

Figure 2-17   Muscle tissues.   *A:* Two separated fibers of voluntary muscle.   *(From A. A. Maximow and W. Bloom, A Textbook of Histology, 3d ed., Saunders, Philadelphia, 1938, p. 151.)*   *B:* Section of human cardiac muscle.   *(From W. Bloom and D. Fawcett, A Textbook of Histology, 6th ed., Saunders, Philadelphia, 1968, p. 289.   By permission of the publishers.)*   *C:* Isolated smooth muscle

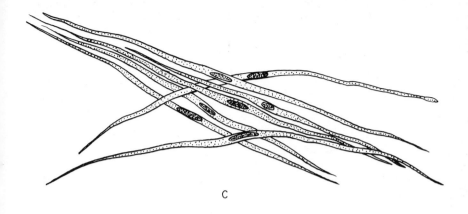

C

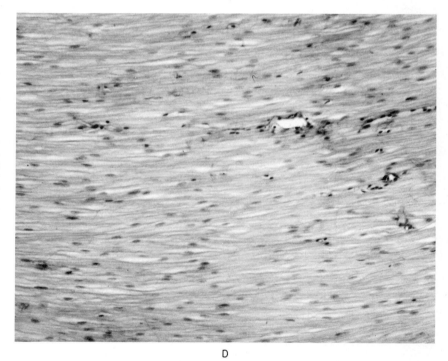

D

cells from the intestinal tract. *(After W. Bloom and D. Fawcett, A Textbook of Histology, 6th ed., Saunders, Philadelphia, 1968, p. 264. By permission of the publishers.)* D: Longitudinal section of smooth muscle cells of human intestine. [*From R. J. Barrnett, in R. O. Greep (ed.), Histology, McGraw-Hill, New York, 1966, p. 195. By permission of the publishers.*]

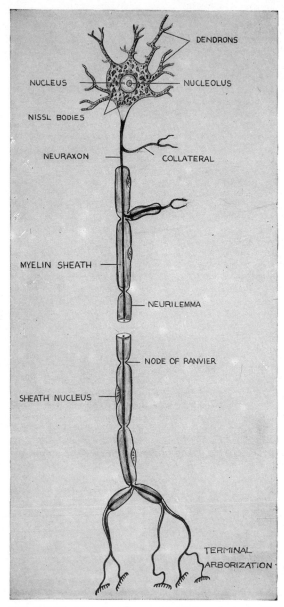

Figure 2-18   Diagramatic representation of a typical (motor) nerve
cell and its myelin sheath. *(From M. Singer and M. M. Salpeter,
in R. O. Greep (ed.), Histology, McGraw-Hill, New York, 1966,
p. 207.   By permission of the publishers.)*

Nervous Tissue

The nervous tissue is made up of two principal types of cells: the neurons and the supporting cells. The *neurons,* or nerve cells, have specialized the capacity of irritability and conduction. Structurally, the cytoplasm has been drawn out into one or more extremely long strands which, in the nerves supplying the leg, can be over a meter in length (Fig. 2-18). Strands which carry nerve impulses to the nuclear region of the cell are called *dendrites* or *dendrons,* while strands conducting the impulse from the nuclear region to another neuron or to an effector cell are termed *axons.* Effector cells are those, such as muscle or glandular cells, which carry out the action stimulated by the nerve impulse. Many neurons do not have dendrites but are directly stimulated by fibers from the preceding neuron in the chain; other neurons may have multiple dendrites. The axon must always be present in a functional cell but is limited to one per cell. The supporting cells of the nervous system, although of different origin, perform the same function as the connective tissue in other parts of the body. The characteristic cell is the *glial* cell. Like muscle, nerve cells are postmitotic and are not replaced after injury or death.

THE FLUID AND ELECTROLYTE COMPOSITION OF THE BODY

The Body Fluids

In the subsequent paragraphs we shall examine a different aspect of the body structure. A lean young man is made up of approximately 10 parts water, 2 parts protein, 1 part mineral or inorganic substances (including sodium, potassium, calcium, magnesium, chloride, phosphorus, and sulfur, as the principal components), 1 part fat, and a small fraction of a part of carbohydrate. With the exception of fat, these ratios remain remarkably constant. Thus, the normal young man is some 70 percent water, 14 percent protein, 7 percent minerals, and 7 percent fat. With increasing obesity, the ratios of all components with the exception of fat remain constant to each other, although they become progressively smaller fractions of the whole. Since all women and most men have more fat than the lean young man, the average body water is probably closer to 60 percent of the body weight. The total body water is divided into two major components, the intracellular water and the extracellular water. The *intracellular water* is the water inside the cells and makes up 33 percent of the body weight or about 55 percent of the total body water, whereas the *extracellular water* comprises 27 percent of the body weight and 45 percent of the total body water. The extracellular water, in turn, is divided into a number of components including the plasma water, tissue water, cerebrospinal fluid, aqueous humor of the eye, and water trapped in the intestinal tract. For purposes of the present discussion, it is convenient to consider only the plasma water, tissue water, and intracellular water.

Electrolytes

The various constituents of the body are dissolved in the fluid compartments. These include the macromolecules previously discussed, electrolytes, and a large variety of smaller organic molecules. *Electrolytes* are charged particles or ions in solution. Under almost all circumstances the number of positively and negatively charged electrolytes must be equal. We shall be primarily interested in the number of charges, rather than in the size and weight of each particle. An *equivalent* is the number of charges, positive or negative, equal to the number of charges of 1 gram of hydrogen ion in solution. Since an equivalent is a much larger concentration than is usually found in nature, a quantity one-thousandth as large, or 1 *milliequivalent,* is used as the reference concentration.

Examination of plasma, tissue, and cell water reveals the concentrations of electrolytes shown in Table 2-1 and Fig. 2-19. With the exception

Table 2-1   Composition of Body Fluids and Comparison to Seawater

| Milliequivalents per liter | Seawater | Extracellular fluid | | Intracellular fluid* |
		Blood plasma	Interstitial fluid	
Na^+	470	140	142	
K^+	10	5	5	150
Ca^{++}	20	5	2.5	
Mg^{++}	107	3	1.5	45
Total cation	607	153	151	195
HCO_3^-	2	25	28	8
Cl^-	548	103	115	2
$HPO_4^=$	1	2	2	100
$SO_4^=$	56	1	1	20
Organic acid$^-$		6	5	
Protein$^-$		16		65
Total anion	607	153	151	195

* Muscle

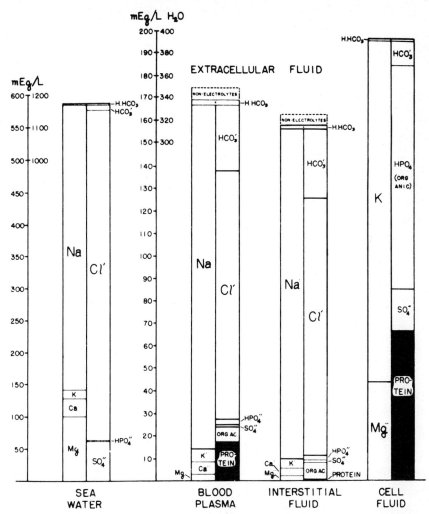

Figure 2-19   Diagram of the body fluid compartments showing the relative concentrations of the various components. The positively charged cations are shown in the left side and the negatively charged ions are shown on the right side of each pair. The solute concentrations are compared to those of seawater. Note that the scale for seawater is more than three times as concentrated as that for the body compartments. *(From J. L. Gamble, Chemical Anatomy, Physiology and Pathology of Extracellular Fluid, 6th ed., Harvard University Press, Cambridge, Mass., 1954. By permission of the publishers.)*

of the protein concentration, plasma and interstitial (tissue) fluid components and concentrations are essentially the same. The principal positively charged ion is sodium and the negatively charged ion is chloride, the components of table salt. On the other hand, the chief positively charged ions within the cell are potassium and magnesium, while phosphate and protein make up the chief negatively charged ions. Thus it is apparent that while many substances can move freely from the tissue fluids into the cells or in the opposite direction, others are extremely limited in such movement. The cell wall has the capacity to regulate this movement, and the principal factors involved appear to be: (1) the size of the molecule (large molecules, such as protein, cannot penetrate the cell wall); (2) the charge (positive and negative charges must be balanced); and (3) the specific solute attempting to cross the cell membrane (potassium ion seems to be able to enter the cell freely, while sodium cannot).

By way of a brief digression, it can be pointed out that the extracellular fluid has a composition very similar to that of ocean water, although much less concentrated. It has been postulated that these extracellular concentrations are much the same as those that would have been found in ocean water at the time the first animals left the ocean for a terrestrial or freshwater existence. There is considerable logic to the argument that terrestrial animals are not, in fact, out of the water. The body can be likened to an aquarium in which the skin is the container and the extracellular fluid the aqueous environment.

The regulation of the electrolytes in the various body fluids is quite precise. For example, if the concentration of serum potassium is outside the range of 3.5 to 5.5 milliequivalents per liter, serious physiological abnormalities and even death can result. The exact mechanisms which determine the quantity of each electrolyte which can enter the cell are not known. However, it is quite certain that considerable cellular energy must be required. It has been demonstrated that several of the hormones of the adrenal cortex, as well as pitressin from the posterior portion of the pituitary gland, are necessary to maintain normal fluid and electrolyte balance. The recent development of instruments which can determine electrolytes quickly and inexpensively has resulted in the demonstration that there are fluid and electrolyte disorders associated with many disease conditions and that the correction of these abnormalities is often essential for adequate treatment.

Osmotic Pressure

An important factor governing the distribution of fluid in the various body compartments is *osmotic pressure*. If a membrane separates two solutions of the same composition and is permeable to water and the solutes, the level of solution in the container on both sides of the membrane will be equal. If, however, a substance which cannot pass through the membrane is placed in one compartment, the following phenomena will occur. The amount of water and solutes going across the membrane from the side containing the nondiffusible molecule will be decreased as the large molecules obstruct passage of the diffusible molecules. However, because of a ball-valve effect, the water and solutes from the other compartment will have no difficulty in entering from the other direction. As a result, the fluid-level on the side of the nondiffusible molecule will rise and that on the solute-free side will fall. This will produce a hydrostatic pressure on the concentrated side due to the increased weight of the solution. Eventually the hydrostatic pressure will become equal to the osmotic pressure and a new equilibrium will result. The osmotic pressure is therefore equal to the weight of the excess solution which it can sustain. This mechanism is illustrated in Fig. 2-20.

It can be seen that in relation to the interstitial fluid (tissue fluid), the

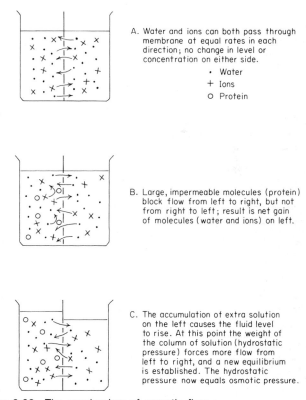

A. Water and ions can both pass through membrane at equal rates in each direction; no change in level or concentration on either side.

· Water
+ Ions
O Protein

B. Large, impermeable molecules (protein) block flow from left to right, but not from right to left; result is net gain of molecules (water and ions) on left.

C. The accumulation of extra solution on the left causes the fluid level to rise. At this point the weight of the column of solution (hydrostatic pressure) forces more flow from left to right, and a new equilibrium is established. The hydrostatic pressure now equals osmotic pressure.

Figure 2-20   The mechanism of osmotic flow.

protein in the blood plasma will exert an osmotic effect and therefore will tend to draw water from the tissue space into the circulation. On the other hand, the hemodynamic pressure produced by the heartbeat tends to push water in the other direction, from the blood vessels into the tissues. The mechanism functions in the following manner: On the arterial end of the capillary loop, the hemodynamic pressure exceeds the osmotic pressure and fluid enters the tissue space. On the venous end of the capillary and in the small venules, the hemodynamic pressure appears to be exhausted. At this point the osmotic pressure exceeds the hemodynamic pressure and fluid reenters the capillaries. A number of factors can alter this relationship. Some of the most obvious are (1) a change in the hemodynamic

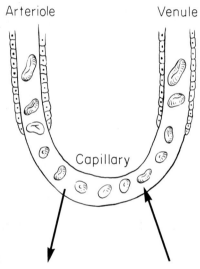

Hemodynamic pressure 32 mmHg	Osmotic pressure Tissue pressure	20
Osmotic pressure Tissue pressure – 20	Hemodynamic pressure – 8	
Filtration pressure 12	Reabsorptive pressure 12	

Plasma fluid forced out of capillary by excess of hemo-dynamic pressure from heart over osmotic and tissue pressures.	Interstitial fluid re-enters capillary, since osmotic and tissure pressures now exceed hemodynamic pressure.

Figure 2-21 Factors controlling shifts between the plasma and interstitial fluids. On the arterial side, the cardiodynamic pressures are sufficient to force fluid out of the blood vessels and into the tissues. On the venous side, the cardiodynamic force has been expended and, in the presence of sufficient blood protein, which is unable to cross the capillary wall, there is an osmotic pressure which draws the tissue fluid back into the blood vessels.

relationships, such as, for example, would occur with venous obstruction and which would increase the vascular hydrostatic pressure; (2) a decrease in the serum protein, which would result in a reduction in the osmotic pressure; and (3) a disruption of the capillary endothelium. In all these conditions excess fluid would collect in the tissue space and would not be returned to the circulation. Similar factors regulate the exchange of water between the tissue space and the cell (see Fig. 2-21).

An inadequacy of water leads to *dehydration* (Fig. 2-22B). If the loss is general, the intracellular and extracellular losses may be proportional. However, usually the first loss is by the extracellular fluid, which then becomes more concentrated. Since the sodium chloride cannot enter the cell, an osmotic force is set up, and water leaves the cell to reestablish

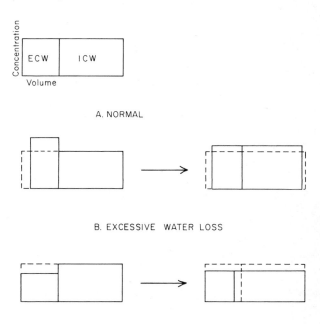

Figure 2-22 Shifts in body compartment volume and concentration. Excessive water loss affects the extracellular compartment first. This results in increased concentration but decreased volume in the extracellular space. Water then flows from the less concentrated cells. The result is a decrease in volume of both the extra- and intracellular spaces and an increase in the final concentration of both. If there is excessive sodium loss from the extracellular space, the extracellular fluid then becomes dilute and moves into the more concentrated cells. There is a reduction in concentration of both spaces but an enlargement of the intracellular space, leading to cellular overhydration.

equilibrium. This same loss of cellular fluid would result if the extracellular fluid became more concentrated from any cause, particularly the excessive intake of salt, even though the total body water were not reduced.

Excessive collection of fluid in the interstitial space is known as *edema*. This is a common abnormality and may be due to local causes such as injury and the inflammatory response or to more remote causes such as heart failure, liver disease, and kidney disease. *Intracellular overhydration* is usually due to a fall in concentration of the extracellular fluid (Fig. 2-22C). This may follow the excessive intake of water, but more frequently it is due to excessive sodium chloride losses. Under these circumstances the cellular osmotic pressure exceeds the extracellular pressure, and fluid moves into the cell. The cell swells as a result, and cellular functions may become disorganized (Fig. 2-23).

Acid-Base Regulation

Normally, the extracellular fluid is very slightly alkaline and the intracellular fluid is slightly acidic. In biology, the acidity of a solution, or its concentration of hydrogen ions (H^+), is generally reported in pH units. The numerical value of the pH is equal to the log of the reciprocal of the hydrogen ion concentration. The lower the pH, the greater the hydrogen ion concentration and the greater the acidity. Water is neutral; that is, the concentration of hydrogen ions is equal to the concentration of hydroxyl ions (OH^-). Thus water which has a hydrogen ion concentration of 1×10^{-7} has a pH of 7.0. The pH of the plasma (as representative of extracellular water) is pH 7.4, with a narrow range from 7.35 to 7.45. Since

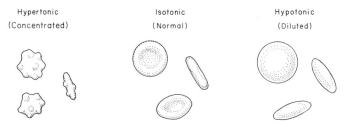

Hypertonic	Isotonic	Hypotonic
(Concentrated)	(Normal)	(Diluted)

Figure 2-23   The effect of hypertonic and hypotonic solutions on the red blood cell. If the red blood cell is placed in a solution more concentrated than normal plasma or in an abnormally concentrated plasma and the dissolved material cannot enter the cell, the water will diffuse out of the cell and the cell will shrink, or become crenated. If the cell is placed in dilute plasma or in a solution more dilute than normal plasma, water will diffuse into the cell, which will then swell. If the swelling is sufficient, the cell will hemolyze, or rupture. These changes correspond to those described in Fig. 2-22.

the pH is greater than 7.0, the H^+ is less than the OH^- and the solution is slightly alkaline. The pH of the intracellular water is much more difficult to determine, and techniques suitable for clinical use have not been devised. The intracellular pH is on the order of 6.8, slightly acidic. The extremely narrow range of hydrogen ion concentration is maintained by a series of buffers or chemicals which hold the hydrogen in unionized form until it can be excreted. The two most important buffers are proteins, especially hemoglobin, and bicarbonate. Carbon dioxide, a major metabolic end product, combines readily with plasma water to produce carbonic acid. However, the extracellular fluid contains a large concentration of sodium bicarbonate. As a result, the presence of a large amount of bicarbonate ion (HCO_3^-), by its mass action effect, causes most of the carbonic acid to remain in the form H_2CO_3 and prevents its dissociation into the more acidic form H^+ and HCO_3^-. When the carbonic acid reaches the lungs, the carbon dioxide is blown off in the expired air, leaving a neutral water residue. Other products of metabolism may include acids and bases which must be excreted in the urine. Strong acids may be excreted by buffering with phosphate salts and by the production of ammonia, whereas basic residues are excreted as carbonate and bicarbonate salts.

BIBLIOGRAPHY

BLOOM, W. and D. W. FAWETT: *A Textbook of Histology,* 9th ed., Philadelphia: W. B. Saunders Company, 1968.

GAMBLE, J. L.: *Chemical Anatomy, Physiology and Pathology of Extracellular Fluid; A Lecture Syllabus,* 6th ed., Cambridge, Mass.: Harvard University Press, 1954.

GREEP. R.: *Histology,* 2d ed., New York: McGraw-Hill Book Company, 1966.

HAM, A. W.: *Histology,* 6th ed., Philadelphia: J. B. Lippincott Company, 1969.

MONTAGNA, W.: "The Skin," *Scientific American,* February, 1965.

WELT, L. G.: *Clinical Disorders of Hydration and Acid-Base Equilibrium,* 3d ed., Boston: Little, Brown and Company, 1971.

Heredity and Genetics

The fertilization of the egg and its subsequent development into a more or less predictable adult is one of the most remarkable achievements of nature. The human ovum is 0.14 millimeter in diameter and weighs 0.00015 milligram, or approximately one twenty-millionth of an ounce. The male spermatozoon is 0.004 millimeter in diameter excluding the tail, and the weight is proportionately less. We know that the genetic contribution of the male is equivalent to that of the female. Curt Stern has estimated that all the spermatozoa necessary to produce 4 billion people can be contained in a volume equivalent to that of an aspirin tablet. Therefore all the genetic material necessary for the 4 billion people who will be alive in the year 2000 can be contained in two such tablets. This genetic information must define not only the physical characteristics of the adult but also the functions of all the cells, tissues, and organs, and it must further characterize those differences which make each individual unlike other members of the species. It must replicate the parents yet at the same time allow enough variation so that the individual is not an exact duplicate. The significance of this phenomenon must be understood. The environment can affect the individual only in relation to his fundamental structure and his predetermined ability to respond to these stimuli. Our understanding of the nature of the genetic mechanisms has developed only since 1900, when the work of Gregor Mendel, done 34 years before, was rediscovered. The interaction between heredity and environment will be seen repeatedly in our subsequent discussion.

The Chromosomes

Cells reproduce by dividing. At the beginning of this process the nuclear membrane disappears and the irregular material which characterizes the nucleus of the cell rearranges itself so that a number of discrete structures may be identified. These rod-shaped structures are known as *chromosomes* (Fig. 3-1). Their number is characteristic for each species,

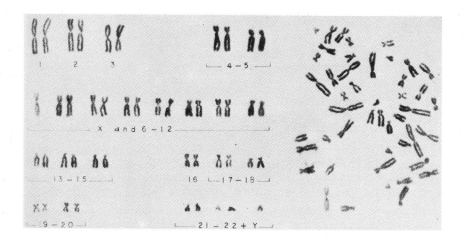

Figure 3-1 Normal male chromosomes. On the right is a photograph of a single cell taken during the metaphase of cell division. The individual chromosomes are then cut out and arranged in descending order of size and configuration, as at left. Individual pairs often cannot be specifically identified. This can be seen in the group which includes the X chromosomes and the pairs numbered 6 to 12. The male has 15 chromosomes in this group; the female has 16. The Y chromosome resembles the twenty-first and twenty-second pairs. In the male there are 5 chromosomes in the group; in the female, 4. *(From V. A. McKusick in Harrison's Principles of Internal Medicine, McGraw-Hill, New York, 1970, p. 10. By permission of the publishers.)*

and in man the number has now been definitely determined to be 46. As the process proceeds, it can be determined that although the chromosomes are of different shapes, they can be arranged into 23 similarly shaped pairs. Each chromosome then divides longitudinally, and half of each chromosome migrates into each of the two daughter nuclei. When the two nuclei are reconstituted, the cytoplasm divides and each of the two cells begins a separate existence. This process is known as *mitosis* (Fig. 3-2). Each of the two daughter cells has exactly the same genetic material, which in turn is the same as that of the parent cell.

In sexual reproduction there is a fusion of two cells, the ovum and the spermatozoon. If these were two ordinary cells, the genetic composition would be twice that of the normal cell and therefore there would be 92 chromosomes. In order to avoid this multiplication of chromosomes with each generation, a mechanism has evolved in which the ova and spermatozoa undergo a process known as *meiosis* (Fig. 3-2), during which the number of chromosomes is reduced to half of the original number. Briefly, in meiosis the paired chromosomes do not divide. Instead, one each of the pair goes to a different daughter nucleus. Thus, each of the sex cells (gametes) has 23 chromosomes, one from each pair. On fertilization, the spermatozoon and the ovum each contribute 23 chromosomes and the pairs are reconstituted. However, it is apparent that (1) the fertilized ovum (zygote) has received one chromosome of each chromosome pair from a different parent, and (2) of the original pair contained by the parent, the chromosome donated is random.

X and Y Chromosomes   Of the 23 pairs of chromosomes in the human, 22 pairs can be quite comparably matched and are called *autosomes.* The twenty-third pair are the *sex chromosomes.* In the female these chromosomes are identical and are called X chromosomes. The male, however, has one X chromosome and another much smaller chromosome known as the Y chromosome. Since only the male has the Y chromosome, it is the male that determines the sex of the offspring. In meiosis, 50 percent of the spermatozoa receive the X chromosome and 50 percent the Y chromosome. The female has only X chromosomes, and all the ova carry the X chromosome. Therefore, a spermatozoon carrying an X chromosome produces a female and one carrying a Y chromosome produces a male. Although the number of X-carrying spermatozoa must equal the number of Y-bearing spermatozoa, the number of male conceptions is 1.2 to 1.5 times the number of female conceptions. This is balanced by a greater male mortality in intrauterine life, and the birth ratio is approximately 1.06 males to 1.0 females. The male mortality continues high throughout life, and by the age of 50, females outnumber males.

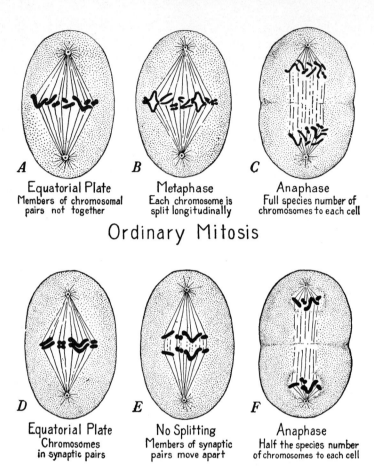

A	B	C
Equatorial Plate	**Metaphase**	**Anaphase**
Members of chromosomal pairs not together	Each chromosome is split longitudinally	Full species number of chromosomes to each cell

Ordinary Mitosis

D	E	F
Equatorial Plate	**No Splitting**	**Anaphase**
Chromosomes in synaptic pairs	Members of synaptic pairs move apart	Half the species number of chromosomes to each cell

Reduction Division

Figure 3-2   Comparison of mitosis and meiosis (reduction division).   In mitosis, each chromosome divides longitudinally and
each new chromosome migrates to a different daughter cell.   In
the meiotic division, the chromosomes do not divide, but one member of each chromosome pair migrates to a different daughter
cell, which then has half the species number of chromosomes.
*(From B. M. Patten, The Early Embryology of the Chick, 3d ed.,
McGraw-Hill, New York, 1929, p. 26.   By permission of the publishers.)*

Chromosome Structure   As the result of a brilliant series of experiments and deductions, much is now known about the structure of the
chromosome and its mode of action.   The basic material making up the
chromosome is deoxyribonucleic acid (DNA).   Each molecule of DNA

is made up of a large number of units called *nucleotides.* Each nucleotide is in turn made up of a nitrogenous base, a molecule of sugar, and a molecule of phosphoric acid. The nitrogenous bases are adenine and guanine, which are purines, and cytosine and thymine, which are pyrimidines. Therefore four different nucleotides are possible. The nucleotides are then linked together by sugar to phosphate bonds to produce a long spiral molecule which may have as many as a million nucleotides in the chain. Since the molecule is made up of sugar-to-phosphate linkages,

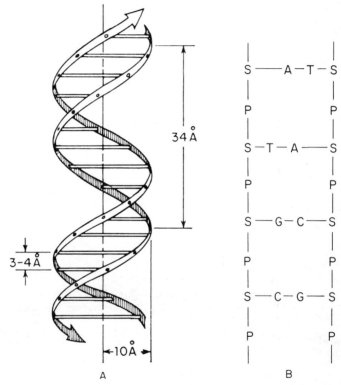

Figure 3-3 Diagramatic representation of the DNA molecule as proposed by Watson and Crick. The uprights of the spiral ladder are composed of alternate molecules of phosphoric acid (P) and a simple pentose sugar (S). The rungs of the ladder are composed of two nitrogenous bases. Each of the bases is linked on one end to the sugar molecule and on the other to its paired base; the size of the bases and the distance between the upright spirals dictates that the pairs must always be adenine and thymine or guanine and cytosine. Thus, reading from left to right, four types of rungs are possible: adenine-thymine, thymine-adenine, guanine-cytosine, and cytosine-guanine. *(From J. D. Watson and F. Crick, Nature 171:737, 1953. By permission of the publishers.)*

the purine and pyrimidine portions of each nucleotide stick out from the chain like the base of a T. These point inward to the center of the spiral (Fig 3-3). Each of the nitrogenous bases then links with a nitrogenous base projecting from a second DNA strand, which winds around the first. The distance separating the two strands and the length of the purine and pyrimidine bases dictates that each cross-linkage between the strands be made up of one purine and one pyrimidine. The thymine of one chain is always cross-linked with an adenine from the other, and the guanine is always linked with cytosine. Reproduction of each chromo-

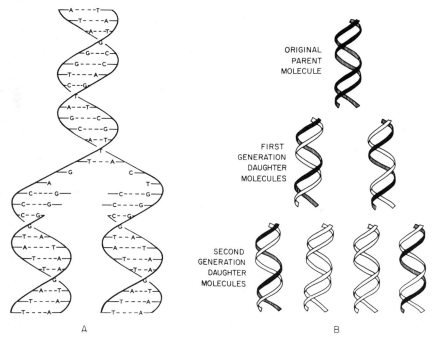

Figure 3-4   Replication of DNA. *A:* During ordinary cell division and mitosis, there must be a replication of the chromosomal material. The double spiral unwinds, separating at the base-base bonds. As the helix uncoils, a new complementary strand is formed which, because of the spatial requirements, duplicates the original. *(From H. E. Sutton, Genes, Enzymes, and Inherited Diseases, Holt, Rinehart and Winston, New York, 1961, p. 36. By permission of the publishers.)*   *B:* The integrity of the original strand has been confirmed by radioisotope labeling of the original components (dark strands). If the original strands broke up, each of the second-generation daughter molecules would be radioactive and each of the cells would contain radioactive material. *(From M. Meselson and F. W. Stahl, Proceedings National Academy of Sciences, 44:671, 1958. By permission of the publishers.)*

some strand *(replication)* is performed by the unwinding and separation of each strand of the pair, which then duplicates its opposing strand (Fig. 3-4).

The chromosome transmits its information to the remainder of the cell by the following mechanism. According to the template hypothesis, the chromosome causes the production of similar molecules known as *ribonucleic acid* (RNA). This process is termed *transcription* (Fig. 3-5). RNA differs from DNA only by the substitution of uracil for thymine. These chromosome products, known as messenger RNA, then migrate outside the nucleus into the cytoplasm of the cell. At this point the importance of the sequence of nucleic acids becomes apparent. Proteins are made up of long chains of amino acids known as *polypeptides*. There are 20 different amino acids, and the combinations which can be made up from these 20 different components is almost infinite. It has been found that each amino acid is represented on the chromosome by a sequence of three nucleotides known as a *codon*. Since there are four different nucleotides, there are 64 possible sequences of three, more than enough for the available amino acids. In fact, most amino acids are represented by more than one codon. Two codons appear to serve as punctuation, separating gene sequences, and the purpose of one codon has not been identified. The messenger RNA thus transmits to the manufacturing portion of the cell the sequence of amino acids necessary for a particular polypeptide in much the same manner as a computer tape activates the computer mechanisms. The production of polypeptides from this genetic code (Table 3-1) is called *translation* (Fig. 3-6).

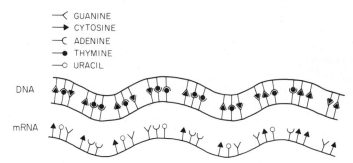

Figure 3-5 Transcription. A strand of RNA is formed in the nucleus complementary to one of the strands of the DNA helix. The RNA strand differs from DNA most importantly in that *uracil* replaces *thymine* as one of the four nitrogenous bases. Once this strand has formed, it is termed messenger RNA (mRNA) and migrates to the cytoplasm, where it attaches to a ribosome.

Table 3-1   The Genetic Code for RNA*

Amino acid	Abbreviation	Codons					
Alanine	ala	GCU	GCC	GCA	GCG		
Arginine	arg	CGU	CGC	CGA	CGG	AGA	AGG
Asparagine	asn	AAU	AAC				
Aspartic acid	asp	GAU	GAC				
Cysteine	cys	UGU	UGC				
Glutamic acid	glu	GAA	GAG				
Glutamine	gln	CAA	CAG				
Glycine	gly	GGU	GGC	GGA	GGG		
Histidine	his	CAU	CAC				
Isoleucine	ile	AUU	AUC				
Leucine	leu	UUA	UUG	CUU	CUC	CUA	CUG
Lysine	lys	AAA	AAG				
Methionine	met	AUA	AUG				
Phenylalanine	phe	UUU	UUC				
Proline	pro	CCU	CCC	CCA	CCG		
Serine	ser	UCU	UCC	UCA	UCG	AGU	AGC
Threonine	thr	ACU	ACC	ACA	ACG		
Tryptophan	try	UGG					
Tyrosine	tyr	UAU	UAC				
Valine	val	GUU	GUC	GUA	GUG		
Punctuation (?)		UAA	UAG				
Unknown		UGA					

*Adapted from Nirenberg et al., 1965.

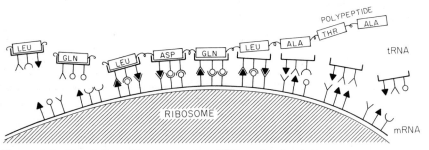

Figure 3-6   Translation.   The messenger RNA molecule determines the sequence of amino acids which go into the production of protein molecules.   Molecules of transfer RNA (tRNA) pick up specific amino acids and bring them to the mRNA-ribosome complex.   Each tRNA molecule contains a code complementary to an mRNA codon.   As these complementary units combine, the appropriate amino acids are brought into proximity for linkage in producing the programmed protein.

The Genes

It is recognized that each chromosome contains more than one piece of information. The individual items of information on the chromosome are known as *genes*. The exact number of genes on each chromosome is unknown. A reasonable minimal estimate is that there are about 1,250, making a total of about 30,000 for the human. However, there is enough nucleoprotein available for a total of about a million genes. Each gene is probably responsible for the production of a single polypeptide.

The polypeptides of the body are of two general types, enzymes and structural proteins. An enzyme is an organic compound which has the property of catalyzing a chemical reaction. These enzymes determine the function and much of the structure of the organism by regulating the rate and direction of the various chemical reactions within the body. The structural proteins include such proteins as collagen, keratin, myosin, and hemoglobin. The genes which control the production of the polypeptides are known as *structural genes*. However, it is apparent that at least one other form of control is necessary. Since every cell gets the same genetic information but different classes of cells have different structure and different functions, it is proposed that there are some genes known as *regulator genes* which in some way control the expression of the genetic information. For example, all cells must carry the capacity for the production of genetically specific hemoglobin, yet hemoglobin is produced only in the red blood cells. This capacity must then be suppressed in all other cells. At the same time the red blood cell cannot carry out the specialized functions that are possible in other cells.

RULES OF INHERITANCE

We have previously noted that the chromosomes occur in pairs. Each of these pairs of chromosomes contains a similar sequence of genes. The position of a gene on the chromosome strand is known as its *locus*. The two genes at the same locus on paired chromosomes affect the same function, although perhaps not in exactly the same way. Each gene of such pair is known as an *allele*. If each of the genes of a pair of alleles is the same, they are said to be *homozygous*. If they are different, they are called *heterozygous*.

One of Mendel's contributions to genetics was the recognition that if there is a possibility of two characteristics in the heterozygous state, then one may be dominant and the other recessive. That is, the one which is dominant will be expressed. Only a homozygous recessive will show the recessive trait. If a homozygous dominant mates with a homozygous recessive, all their offspring will manifest the particular dominant characteristic. The *phenotype,* or appearance, will be that of the dominant. However, the *genotype,* or gene characteristic, will be heterozygous because both the dominant and the recessive gene will be present in each of the offspring. A heterozygous individual will produce gametes at the meiotic division in which 50 percent will carry the dominant gene and 50 percent the recessive gene. By the laws of chance, if two heterozygotes are mated, 25 percent of their offspring will be homozygous dominant, 25 percent homozygous recessive, and 50 percent will be heterozygous but will express the dominant phenotype. The fact that despite the phenotype the genes retain their individuality gave rise to the first law of Mendel, which is known as the law of segregation.

The family relationships of humans contain a large number of variables, and it is important to be able to present the genetic information in as clear and precise a manner as possible. In order to achieve this, a series of conventional symbols has been developed. These are shown in Fig. 3-7. The propositus, index case, or proband is the individual

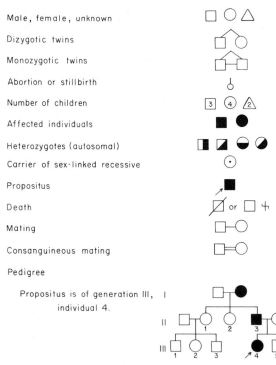

Figure 3-7 Common genetic symbols and conventions for pedigree charts.

under initial study who led to the exploration of the interrelationship. A diagram of this type is known as a pedigree.

Dominant Inheritance

We have noted that if a dominant gene is present, the dominant characteristic will be expressed. However, the genotype for the dominant characteristic may be either homozygous or heterozygous. If an offspring does not show a dominant trait which was present in a parent, it can be assumed that the parent was heterozygous for the trait and that the offspring is now homozygous for the recessive characteristic. Therefore this dominant trait has been lost to the individual, and no future generation will show the dominant characteristic unless it is reintroduced. Thus the dominant characteristic will be apparent from generation to generation in a vertical pattern. If either or both parents are homozygous for the dominant characteristic, all their children will manifest this characteristic. If both are heterozygous, three-fourths of the children will manifest the trait (one-fourth homozygous and one-half heterozygous) and one-fourth will not manifest the trait. If one parent is heterozygous and the other homozygous recessive, half the children will manifest the dominant trait and half the recessive trait (Fig 3-8).

Recessive Inheritance

Recessive inheritance follows a different pattern. Most abnormalities due to recessive inheritance are relatively rare in the population. When a recessive characteristic becomes apparent, it is usually due to the

Figure 3-8 Inheritance patterns and ratios. Solid symbols represent homozygous and split symbols represent heterozygous individuals. The black genes are dominant, the white genes are recessive. If a gene is dominant, that characteristic will be manifest whether the individual is homozygous or heterozygous. If a gene is recessive, only the homozygous individuals will manifest that characteristic. Mating number 5 is the usual mating which produces offspring with the recessive characteristic; the apparently unaffected parents are heterozygous, one-fourth of the offspring will have the characteristic, one-half will be heterozygous without the trait, and one-fourth will be homozygous dominant. Consanguinity is frequent in the parents of individuals with recessive characteristics.

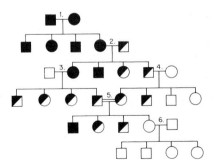

mating of two individuals who are heterozygous for the particular trait. One-fourth of their children will show this particular characteristic. Because most recessive diseases are relatively rare, such a disease, after its appearance in one generation, is not likely to appear again for many generations. In communities where intermarriage is relatively common, the possibility of marriage between heterozygotes for the recessive characteristic is consequently greater and the trait may reappear. Since the recessive manifestation is likely to be concentrated in a single generation, it is often spoken of as a familial trait. As only one in four individuals will be affected, manifestations of the trait in multiple members of a family are most likely to be seen in large families. Small families with relatively few children may not manifest the characteristic, and these heterozygotic matings may be missed. Correction factors have been developed for the loss of visibility of heterozygotic matings for different family sizes, and these can be applied to correct for the number of heterozygotes in the community. It is obvious that in most instances only one individual in a family will be affected, and therefore random cases of an unusual disease may not be recognized as genetic in origin until a large number of cases have been collected (Fig. 3-9).

Sex-linked Inheritance

Most of the previous discussion has been related to the characteristic features of inheritance based on the mechanism of paired autosomal chromosomes and genes. The X chromosome seems to act independently. It is, of course, unpaired in the male. According to the Lyon hypothesis, one of the X chromosomes is inactive in the female. The choice of which one is random in each cell. The female cells can be recognized by the fact that in the resting nucleus there is a small dark spot, a clump of chromatin known as the *Barr body*. There is strong evidence that this represents the inactive X chromosome. The Barr body has practical

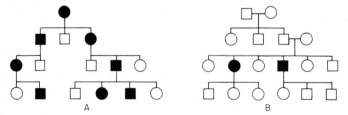

Figure 3-9 Simplified genealogies. Affected individuals are shown in black. *A:* Dominant inheritance, showing continuation from generation to generation. *B:* Recessive inheritance, showing tendency for limitation to one generation.

significance which will be discussed subsequently. Because the X chromosome acts independently, a recessive trait can become manifest by the presence of a single gene in the male. In the female, however, it can become only partially manifest if at all. Since all X chromosomes in the male come from the maternal organism, 50 percent of the male offspring will receive the gene from a heterozygous mother and manifest the characteristic. At the same time, 50 percent of the daughters will receive the gene and act as recessive, heterozygous carriers. The male cannot transmit X-linked genes to his sons, but all his daughters will be affected. At present, about a hundred X-linked traits have been recognized (Fig. 3-10).

The Y chromosome is necessary for the manifestations of male primary and secondary sexual features. Other than this isolated but important effect, very few factors are known or suspected to be transmitted by the Y chromosome.

Multiple-gene Inheritance

If all characteristics were inherited by single-gene pairs, then each characteristic would be expected to show only two qualities, the dominant or the recessive. At most, there would be three qualities, dominant, recessive, and intermediate. There are many qualities, however, which show a continuous gradation, and the distribution within this gradation often has a normal distribution curve. There is now much evidence to show that many factors are produced by the random assortment of a number of genes. This can be likened to the shuffling of a deck of cards. An occasional hand will be extremely high or extremely low. Most hands will

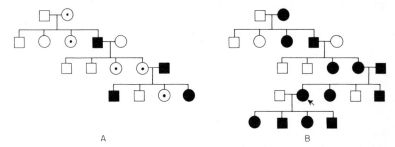

A   B

Figure 3-10 *A:* Sex-linked recessive pedigree. Since the male has only one X chromosome, inheritance of only one affected gene will produce the defect; however, in the female, both X chromosomes must contain the affected genes. *B:* Sex-linked dominant pedigree. In this example, the propositus is probably homozygous, since all her sons and daughters inherit the trait.

cluster around the average values, with gradations based on the laws of probability falling between the two extremes. The result will be a normal distribution curve. Height might be considered a typical example. Obviously, genetic factors determine only the potential for height, and environmental factors such as malnutrition and disease may modify the eventual outcome.

A number of methods have been devised to isolate the genetic and environmental factors. One of these techniques is to use identical twins, for their genetic material is identical, and to compare them with nonidentical twins, siblings, parents, and the random population. This technique has proved especially valuable in the study of twins who were reared apart, particularly when their environments were also divergent.

Statistical treatment of population data has also been effective in evaluating the relative importance of genetic and environmental components. For example, it has been demonstrated that there is a normal distribution curve for blood pressures. If ordinary high blood pressure were due to genetic factors, then an individual with a maximum high blood pressure would be expected to have the least favorable combination of genes possible. However, he also has a number of genes that are not expressing themselves. If he were to marry another individual with similar high blood pressure, on the basis of a chance assortment of their combined genes some of the hidden genes would express themselves in the offspring. While the blood pressure of the children might be high, the statistical odds are that their pressure would not be as high as that of their parents. In addition, since extremely high blood pressure is rare, it is statistically improbable that an individual with an extremely high blood pressure would marry another individual with an equally high blood pressure. Therefore in the combined mating, an even larger number of genes in the pool would lead away from this extreme value. The same factors would operate at the extremely low end of the blood pressure curve. As a result, there would be a tendency for the offspring of members of the extreme ends of the curve to have blood pressures which range toward the mean. On the other hand, inidividuals with average blood pressures would have a completely random assortment of genes and there would always be the possibility that, on mating with another random assortment, a combination would evolve which would either increase or decrease the pressure in their offspring. Because of the multiple genes involved and the random nature of human mating, it would be impossible to select in such a way as to perpetuate any particular combination. Extremely large populations have been studied in regard to blood pressure, and the mathematical predictions have held true. These data should not be interpreted to indicate that environment is not a factor but only that environment must act on an inherent, genetically determined range of possibilities.

GENETIC DISEASES

It should be realized at the outset of this discussion that most human genes produce enzymes which control chemical reactions common to most mammals, if not to lower orders as well. Therefore these genes and their enzymes must be similar, if not identical. A lesser number of genes serve to characterize the species. A still smaller number differentiate the individual from other members of the species. A very small number of genes will be abnormal. The changes in genes which alter the gene product are known as *mutations.* A change of one nucleotide in the DNA chain may alter the sequence of amino acids so that the effect of the enzyme produced is entirely different from normal. Naturally occurring mutations are infrequent, although they have been estimated to occur about once in every hundred thousand cell reproductions. A number of factors are known to cause mutations, including radiation energy and a variety of chemicals. Most mutations tend to be hostile to the organism; the beneficial mutations probably result in the evolutionary process. Many mutations which produce abnormal genes are recurrent. That is, the same mutation may independently affect a number of individuals in a species. Similarly, the abnormal gene may mutate back to the normal form. Once a gene has mutated, all cells derived from the cell containing the mutated gene will be affected by this genetic alteration.

In vertebrates the germ cells, those cells which eventually produce new individuals, are isolated relatively early in the *gonads,* that is, in the ovaries and testes. Therefore only mutations in these cells can be transmitted to the progeny. These mutations are known as *germinal mutations.* Mutations within nonreproductive cells are known as *somatic mutations.* It is for this reason that acquired characteristics cannot be transmitted, because acquired changes are manifest in somatic cells. There is evidence that somatic mutations also occur in the frequency indicated, and that mutant cells accumulate with the aging of the individual. In fact, one theory of aging is that the accumulation of mutant somatic cells is the cause of the manifestations of the aging process.

Dominant Disorders

A dominant mutation generally becomes immediately evident, and if it is seriously detrimental, it will be rapidly eliminated. Many of these individuals may die in infancy or fail to reproduce, and the genetic character of their disease may be unrecognized. An excellent example is that of achondroplastic dwarfism. This is the type of dwarfism in which the head and torso are of normal size (although the head may be enlarged), but the arms and legs are markedly shortened. In 1941, Morch did an extensive study of achondroplasia in Denmark in which almost every such dwarf in the country was identified. It was found that there was approximately one achondroplastic dwarf in every 10,000 births. Eighty percent were found to die during their first year of life. However, the remainder had approximately a normal life expectancy. The 20 percent survivors were found to marry less frequently and to have fewer children than normal individuals. Since the trait is due to a heterozygous dominant genotype, half of the children of a dwarf and a normal individual would be expected to be achondroplastic. Assuming a stable population, an achondroplastic parent would have an average of two children, one of whom would also be achondroplastic. Thus of 1,000 achondroplastic births in which there was no ancestral history, 80 percent would die and 20 percent at the most would produce one achondroplastic child each, and there would be 200 second-generation achondroplastics. The third generation would contain less than 40, and in very few generations the strain would die out.

A number of genetic principles are demonstrated by this example, but only a few will be pointed out. First, it is obvious that for this particular disorder to persist, there must be a relatively high mutation rate, since affected families have a low reproduction rate. Second, without extensive and careful case surveys, it would be impossible to recognize the disease as being genetic in origin. Third, the number of individuals affected by most common dominant diseases remains relatively constant. The rate of mutation can thus be estimated directly by the summation of all affected individuals or indirectly by knowing the effective fertility of affected individuals as compared to normals.

Dominance of minor traits may be followed for many generations. Fraser Roberts reports an interesting case which may have been traced as far as 15 generations. His patient had absence of the joints of the middle, ring, and little fingers of the left hand, with webbing and incomplete separation of the middle and ring fingers. The family had known of this minor disability for a number of generations. A distant ancestor was the first Earl of Shrewsbury, born in 1390 and killed in battle in 1453. He was one of the figures in Shakespeare's Henry VI, although he lived 20 years longer than the play indicates. His tomb was being repaired in 1874, and the skeleton was examined and found to have the same bony defects which had been seen in the current members of the family.

A very interesting form of dominant defect is a central nervous system disorder called Huntington's chorea. This disease appears late in life and is characterized by bizarre and uncontrollable twitching of the arms and face. Mental deterioration may follow. Almost all the cases in the United States appear to be traced back to three individuals who came from the same rural area in England during the seventeenth century. There is good evidence to suggest that the first witches of Salem were afflicted with this disease. It is easy to visualize the reasonableness, in a less sophisticated era, of attributing the manifestations of the disease to possession by the devil. One of the unfortunate factors is that, because the manifestations come late, the individual cannot tell whether or not he is affected and cannot make wise decisions regarding procreation. The personal conflicts which can arise in such a family have been dramatized by Eugene O'Neill in the play *Strange Interlude.*

Recessive Disorders

An important and fascinating recessive disease is sickle-cell anemia. This is a disease which originated in populations inhabiting subsaharan Africa and is associated with a peculiar deformity in the shape of the red blood cells (Fig. 3-11). This disease is so severe that few affected individuals live to maturity. In 1949, Pauling and Itano demonstrated that patients with sickle-cell disease have an abnormal hemoglobin (subsequently several dozen other types of abnormal hemoglobins were found, most of which produced characteristic diseases). Hemoglobin, a pigment contained in the red blood cell, facilitates the transportation of oxygen from the lungs to the tissues. It is made up of a heme pigment center and four globin chains attached somewhat like tentacles. Normally there are two alpha and two beta chains. Further study revealed that in sickle-cell disease, the beta chain is replaced by a different globin. Globins are polypeptide chains, and this abnormality represents one of the nonenzyme polypeptide abnormalities that gene defects can produce. The difference between the two chains is in the substitution of valine for glutamic acid in the sixth position from the free end of the globin molecule. It is represented as follows:

Hb A (normal)   valine-histidine-leucine-threonine-proline-*glutamic acid-*
glutamic acid-lysine-

Hb S (sickle)   valine-histidine-leucine-threonine-proline-*valine-*glutamic
acid-lysine-

Examination of the genetic code shows that the RNA triplet for glutamic acid is GAA, while that of valine is GUA. Thus the single substitution of uracil for adenine in one of the triplets of the genetic code was sufficient to produce this change. Of further theoretic importance is the fact that in addition to sickle-cell disease, sickle-cell trait has long been recognized. Individuals with the trait show some evidence of sickling of red blood cells, although not as much as those with the disease. They show few other clinical manifestations. Examination of the hemoglobin of patients with

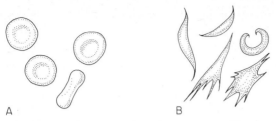

Figure 3-11   Characteristic sickle red cells.   The normal red cell
is a regular disc *(A);* the sickled cells assume the bizarre forms *(B).*
The distorted forms become more evident when the blood is stored
in an atmosphere without oxygen.

the trait shows that they have both normal and S-type hemoglobins.   By
genetic analysis it had been recognized that patients with the trait are
heterozygous and those with the disease are homozygous.   The present
information reinforces this interpretation and goes further in explaining the
genetic mechanics.

Sickle-cell disease has presented an interesting area for speculation.
It has been demonstrated that patients with sickle-cell globin may have an
increased resistance to the malarial parasite.   The geographic area in
which sickle-cell disease originated is one in which malaria is universal and
severe.   There is evidence that the protection offered by the trait to the
individuals with malaria more than counterbalanced the disabling effects
of the relatively infrequent appearance of the fully developed homozygous
disease.

Repeated mention has been made of the fact that genes control
enzyme formation.   Many of the principles of normal and abnormal gene
and enzyme action can be exemplified by examination of the metabolism of
phenylalanine, one of the amino acids.   The normal route of phenylalanine
metabolism is indicated by the solid arrows (Fig. 3-12).   Normally phenylalanine is converted to tyrosine by the action of the enzyme phenylalanine
hydroxylase.   In the disorder of phenylketonuria (PKU), or phenylpyruvic
oligophrenia, this enzyme is defective.   As a result, phenylalanine takes
alternative metabolic pathways and is converted to phenylpyruvic acid and
other phenylketone acids.   These individuals have lighter pigmentation
than normal and severe mental retardation; most patients have an IQ of
less than 20.   The is not a rare disorder, and patients make up about 1
percent of the inmates of institutions for the mentally retarded.   With
modern nutrition, antibiotics, and other treatment, they may have a normal
life-span.   The tremendous social cost of these individuals is obvious.

There have been a number of important developments in the past few

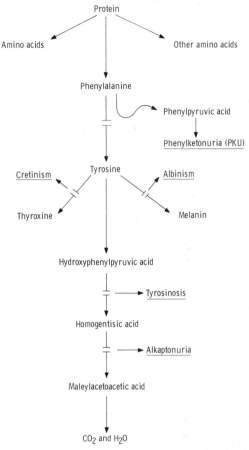

Figure 3-12 Pathway of phenylalanine metabolism. Phenylalanine, an amino acid, is derived from protein. It normally serves
as a precursor of the skin pigment, melanin, and of thyroid hormone. Excess phenylalanine is eventually degraded to carbon
dioxide and water. A variety of enzyme defects are possible in
the metabolic pathway. Broken arrows indicate sites of possible
enzyme defect, and the resultant diseases are underlined.

years which may modify the outlook for persons with this disorder. First,
it has been found that if these infants are fed phenylalanine-deficient diets,
they may achieve normal or near-normal intelligence. Second, extremely
simple tests for phenylketones in the blood and urine have been devised,
and several states have passed laws making testing mandatory for all
infants. This is important, since early dietary treatment is necessary in
order to achieve the best results. Third, it has been found that the heterozygous parents of patients with phenylketonuria show a higher blood level

of phenylalanine after phenylalanine feeding than do normal individuals. Thus it is theoretically possible to screen for potential parental combinations. At present, the difficulty of the test and the infrequency of the disease makes this course somewhat impractical.

Returning to the metabolism of phenylalanine, we see that tyrosine may be converted to melanin, a dark brown pigment which gives the skin its normal color and which accounts for racial pigmentation. Phenylketonuric children are pale because the only tyrosine available to them for melanin formation is that present in the diet. In *albinism* there is an enzymatic block in the step from tyrosine to melanin. Albinism is known in many mammals as well as man. The skin and hair of albinos is pure white, and the retinal fundi are pink and usually visible. The common white rabbits are albinos, and the pink reflection of their eyes is well known. The absence of pigment in the skin and eyes renders albinos especially susceptible to light injury.

Tyrosine is also converted to thyroxine, which is the active thyroid hormone. If the enzymes for this conversion are deficient, *hypothyroidism* will result. Inadequate thyroid hormone results in a slowing of all metabolic processes, and when it occurs in children, growth retardation and mental deficiency result. Childhood hypothyroidism is known as *cretinism* and can be satisfactorily treated with thyroid hormone by mouth. Not all cretinism is due to this genetic defect, which is actually quite rare.

Alkaptonuria is a defect due to the failure of normal metabolism of homogentisic acid. The necessary enzyme is homogentisic acid oxidase; as a result of a defect in this enzyme large amounts of homogentisic acid are present in the blood and tissue, and there is an overflow into the urine. Homogentisic acid has the characteristic that it turns black on oxidation. Thus, the urine turns black on standing, and in children it may produce a staining of the diapers. Retention of homogentistic acid within the body results in its deposition, chiefly in the cartilages. The cartilages then turn black and tend to become brittle. This discoloration may become apparent in the cartilages of the ears, or it may become indirectly apparent by the production of an arthritis in middle-aged individuals known as *ochronosis*. Neither albinism or ochronosis are particularly benefited by present therapy. However, as compared to phenylketonuria, the disabilities induced are relatively minor.

Figure 3-13, adapted from McKusick, indicates a number of patterns by which enzymatic abnormalities may become manifest. The first pattern represents the normal situation. The second is the situation seen in alkaptonuria; there is an accumulation of the metabolite at the point of the metabolic defect, as if a dam were placed in the stream. This metabolite produces its own deleterious effects and, in this case, spills into the urine,

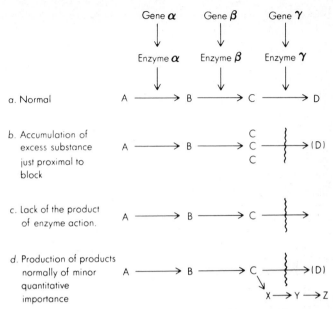

Figure 3-13 Types of metabolic abnormalities resulting from enzyme defects. *A:* Normal. *B:* Accumulation of excess substance at the block, as in tyrosinosis and alkaptonuria. *C:* Lack of the product, as in albinism and cretinism (juvenile hypothyroidism). *D:* Abnormal metabolites such as in phenylketonuria. [*From V. A. McKusick (ed.), Human Genetics, 2d ed., 1969. Prentice-Hall, Englewood Cliffs, N.J., p. 69. By permission of the publishers.*]

where the characteristic features cause recognition. In the third sequence the normally produced substance is not in the main metabolic stream. However, the absence of the normal metabolic precursor results in a defect, as in albinism or hypothyroidism. The fourth pattern is that presented by phenylketonuria. The failure of the normal pathway results in the increased production of alternative metabolites, which are toxic in the resultant concentrations.

The previous two sets of examples—(1) sickle-cell disease, representing a defect in a gene directing structural protein production, and (2) the sequence of genes controlling the enzymes regulating the metabolism of phenylalanine—show how, as our knowledge progresses, the clear concept of the nature of recessive transmission has changed. This is particularly true in the case of enzyme production. The heterozygous individual has some normal enzyme, and the defect is clinically undetected. Only when there is stress may it be possible to uncover the manifestation of heterozygosity. Thus when a normal individual is fed an excess of phenylalanine, it is all quickly metabolized to tyrosine. A heterozygous individual will also achieve this conversion, but usually at a measurably slower rate. The homozygous individual, lacking the enzyme, will fail to convert phenylalanine to tyrosine, and phenylpyruvic acid will appear.

Genes which produce protein structures can do so even if heterozygous, and if these products are visible, will be called "dominant", even though the product may be defective. If the gene product is an enzyme, the presence of only one normal gene will result in enough enzyme function to mask the presence of a defective gene. Thus, a defect in both genes is necessary to demonstrate an obvious functional defect, and the condition is termed recessive. Even though a recessive disorder is said to be homozygous, the two defective genes may not be the same; it is only necessary that neither can produce the required protein. It is obvious that the classical concepts of dominance and recessivity must be modified and that the differences are literally more apparent than real.

Since homozygosity is necessary for the expression of a recessive trait, the presence of such a gene in a normal individual would ordinarily go undetected. It is estimated that almost every individual carries at least one to three seriously harmful recessive genes. If a serious recessive disorder had a frequency of only one in a million births, a low frequency for many recessive disorders, the gene would have to be present in one of every five hundred individuals. The logic is as follows: A heterozygous individual has two alleles, therefore only one of his two genes would carry the trait and the gene frequency would be one in a thousand sex cells. If there is one chance in a thousand that the gene is present in the sperm and one in a thousand that it is present in the ovum, the probability of homozygosity in the fertilized ovum would be $1/1,000 \times 1/1,000$, or one in a million. More than five hundred recessive disorders have been identified, so each individual could carry an average of at least one defective gene. Thus, although recessive genetic disease is rare, the frequency of defective heterozygotes must be quite common.

Sex-linked Disorders

It must be remembered that sex-linked genes can be transmitted by the mother to half her sons and half her daughters and by the father only to his daughters, all of whom are affected, but to none of his sons. Only a few X-linked dominant diseases are known. If dominant, the gene produces the disorder in both males and females. Most X-linked diseases are recessive. Since homozygosity is rare, women rarely manifest these diseases. However, only one gene is necessary to cause the disease in males, as the X-chromosome is unopposed. Therefore, males receive the disease from their unaffected mothers and transmit the gene to their daughters.

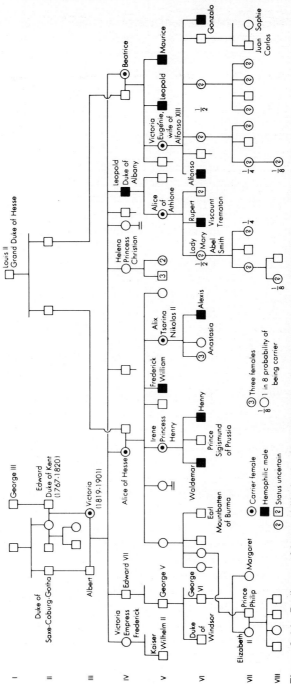

Figure 3-14 Pedigree of hemophilia in the descendants of Queen Victoria. [*From V. A. McKusick (ed.), Human Genetics, 2d ed., 1969. Prentice-Hall, Englewood Cliffs, N.J., p. 40. By permission of the publishers.*]

The most famous pedigree of sex-linked disease is that of Queen Victoria and her descendants. Apparently, a new mutation in one of Queen Victoria's parents created a gene for hemophilia on one of her X chromosomes. The relevant pedigree is present in Fig. 3-14. Classical hemophilia is caused by the absence of a specific protein necessary for blood clotting. This protein is known as antihemophilic globulin, or factor VIII. In an emergency it can be partially replaced with fresh blood. Pure antihemophilic globulin is now available as a single blood component. Unfortunately, the first is not entirely effective and the latter can only be produced in extremely small amounts and is quite expensive.

About a hundred characteristics have been recognized as transmitted through the X chromosome. Most of these represent rare recessive abnormalities. In addition to the classical hemophilia, there is another bleeding disease, a clinically indistinguishable type of hemophilia known as hemophilia B, which is due to factor IX deficiency. There is also a type of muscular dystrophy; several types of skin disease, including one which produces thickening and scaling of the skin (the reptile man of the circus side shows); color blindness; and a type of kidney disease known as nephrogenic diabetes insipidus in which large volumes of urine, between 10 and 20 quarts, are produced daily. A number of sex-linked recessive traits have lethal characteristics, and many of the more serious diseases may result in the death of the patient before he reaches the reproductive age. This, of course, is evident particularly in the cases of hemophilia and muscular dystrophy.

Multiple-gene Disorders

Almost all the diseases so far described have been the result of variations in single genes. We have previously observed that a number of individual characteristics may be the result of polygenic factors which result in a gradation between two extremes usually following a normal distribution pattern. Because of the difficulty in evaluating the interacting influences of genetic constitution and environmental exposure, it is difficult at present to identify the relationship of these factors to disease. The example of the blood pressure has already been discussed. A number of other factors are known to affect blood pressure, such as emotional characteristics and variations in diet such as the amount of salt ingested.

Another characteristic of the individual is the concentration of his serum cholesterol. In each person the serum cholesterol concentration shows considerable variation from time to time, but the range of variation is fairly consistent. Stress, diet, and level of thyroid activity all affect the cholesterol concentration.   The recent enthusiasm for unsaturated fats in the diet stems from the observation that they result in the lowering of the serum cholesterol.   Nevertheless, there is good evidence that genetic factors also affect the concentration of the serum cholesterol even when environmental factors are appropriately evaluated.   Both high blood pressure and high serum cholesterol values are associated with an increased frequency of arteriosclerosis and coronary artery disease.   This association is still stronger when both factors vary in the same direction.   Thus, while coronary artery disease is not a genetic disease, it is probable that certain genetic factors in association with environmental factors are responsible for the disorder.   If we can be sure that a given individual has a high inherent risk of the disease, we can be justified in intensifying attempts to lower the blood pressure by applying current methods of treatment, and to lower the serum cholesterol with the proper use of drugs and diet.

Chromosome Abnormalities

So far the genetic disorders which we have discussed have been the result of the expression of abnormal genes or combinations of genes.   Recent techniques which have made it possible to examine the chromosomes have revealed that a number of disorders are associated with an abnormal number or structure of the whole chromosome.   One of the first disorders to be clarified was *Klinefelter's syndrome*.   Persons with this disorder appear to be males; however, their testes are small and on microscopic examination show no evidence of spermatogenesis (the formation of sperm).   Their extremities are generally long and occasionally there may be moderate enlargement of the breasts (gynecomastia).   Often they cannot be told from normal males (Fig. 3-15).   Obviously reproduction is impossible.   This disorder appears in about one out of five hundred male births.   The first clue to the nature of the disorder was the observation of Barr bodies in the nuclei.   These are thought to be the second X chromosome in the female nuclei and should not appear in the male, who normally has but one X chromosome (Fig. 3-16).   Subsequently, chromosome counts of patients with Klinefelter's syndrome revealed 47 rather than the normal 46.   The extra chromosome is an X chromosome, so that the sex chromosome pattern is XXY instead of the normal XY.   It is probable that the presence of the extra chromosome is due to a phenomenon called nondisjunction.   This is the failure of two chromosomes to separate during nuclear cleavage, with the result that both go into one daughter nucleus while they are unrepresented in the other.   Nondisjunction may occur

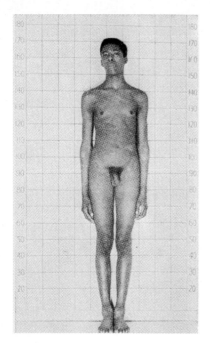

Figure 3-15 *A:* Patient with Klinefelter's syndrome. Note the tall, slender build with long extremities, mild gynecomastia, and female hair distribution. *B:* Chromosomes of the syndrome. There are 47 chromosomes with both the Y chromosome and two X chromosomes (16 chromosomes in the 6 to 12 group). *(From V. A. McKusick in Harrison's Principles of Internal Medicine, McGraw-Hill, New York, 1970, p. 12. By permission of the publishers.)*

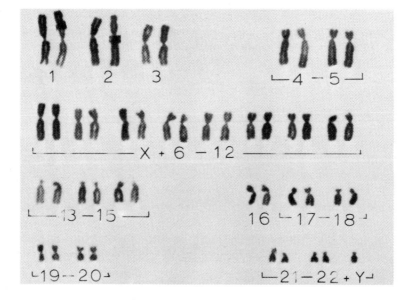

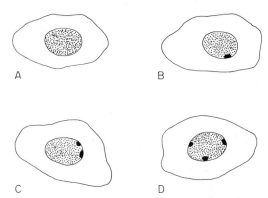

Figure 3-16   Barr bodies in cell nuclei.   *A:* No Barr body evident. One active X chromosome.   *B, C,* and *D:* One, two, and three Barr bodies representing cells with two, three, and four X chromosomes.   These are said to be chromatin-positive.   Normal male cells (XY) and patients with Turner's syndrome (XO) lack the Barr body.   Normal females (XX) and patients with Klinefelter's syndrome (XXY) have one Barr body.   Two and three Barr bodies are seen in the combinations XXX, XXXY, and XXXX, XXXXY.

in either one of the miotic divisions or in one of the mitotic divisions during the early development of the embryo.

Several important facts emerge from the development of knowledge regarding this syndrome.   First, the presence of the Y chromosome, despite its small size and otherwise unknown functions, appears to determine the male phenotype regardless of the number of X chromosomes.   This means that the male characteristics are under positive control and are not merely due to the absence of female characteristics.   Second, the presence of the Barr body is strong evidence that it represents the inactive extra X chromosome.   Syndromes in which three and four X chromosomes have been found have been associated with two and three Barr bodies respectively.

Klinefelter's syndrome has a female counterpart in *Turner's syndrome.* These patients appear once in every five thousand or so female births and are characterized by short stature, failure of development of secondary sexual characteristics, a peculiar "shield shape" chest, web neck, and the frequent association of cardiovascular abnormalities (Fig. 3-17).   They are not fertile.   Examination of resting nuclei fails to reveal the presence of a Barr body.   Whereas patients with Klinefelter's syndrome are phenotypically males with a female sex chromatin, patients with Turner's syndrome are phenotypically females with a male sex chromatin (i.e., no Barr body).   However, more careful examination shows that these patients have only 45 chromosomes and that the Y chromosome is absent.   There-

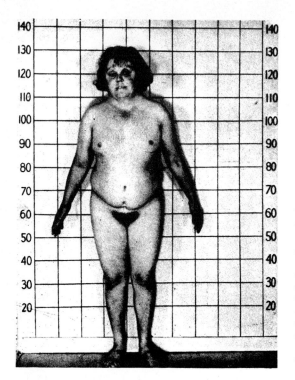

Figure 3-17 *A:* Patient with Turner's syndrome. The patient has a short stature, broad, short neck, and characteristic shieldlike chest. *B:* Chromosomes of this syndrome. There are only 45 chromosomes; there is only one X and no Y. *(From V. A. McKusick in Harrison's Principles of Internal Medicine, McGraw-Hill, New York, 1970, p. 13. By permission of the publishers.)*

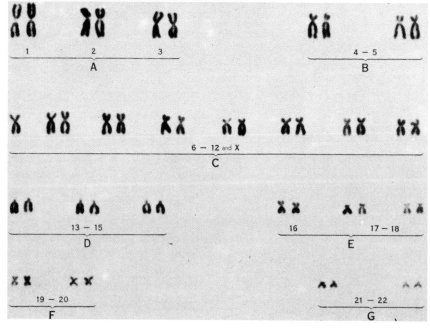

fore, it is the absence of the Y chromosome, not the presence of the paired XX chromosomes which determines the female sexual phenotype. The sex chromosome pattern is designated XO.

Mosaicism is a term used to indicate that, within the same individual, different nuclei have different numbers of chromosomes. When such a situation is present in Klinefelter's or Turner's syndromes, it is an indication that the nondisjunction took place after fertilization and the beginning development of the embryo. Apparently the Y chromosome may be absent, resulting in Turner's syndrome; however, it is probable that the absence of one of the autosomes is not compatible with life. On the other hand, there are syndromes associated with a greater number than 46 chromosomes.

Several chromosomal abnormalities have now been recognized in the autosomes. The first to be described in man was in *Down's syndrome,* previously known as mongoloid idiocy. This syndrome is characterized by severe mental retardation; a defect in the eyelids which makes the eyes appear oriental; short hands, feet, and stature; frequent congenital malformations, especially of the heart; and a characteristic "simian" line in the palms. Examination of the individual chromosomes showed that the total number was 47 and that the extra chromosome was probably of the twenty-first pair (Fig. 3-18).

One form of chronic leukemia is associated with the loss of part of chromosome 22. This abnormality is noted in the white cells of the blood and not in any of the other body cells. Therefore it probably represents damage to one blood cell, which then reproduces the abnormal line. If this defect were inherited, then it should be manifest in all the cells. It cannot be determined whether the chromosome abnormality is the cause or the effect of leukemia. This will have to await further study.

MANAGEMENT OF GENETIC DISORDERS

Much of the difficulty in accepting genetic concepts in humans is the natural reluctance to accept predestination. It must be repeated that heredity and environment are not exclusive but interact upon each other. Genetic diseases can be treated only if we recognize them, characterize their defects, and proceed to work out solutions to the specific problems. The number of these solutions which have already been developed is far greater than is generally realized, and accelerated interest promises even greater results. A number of examples will be given. Successful blood transfusions depend upon the understanding of genetic principles. Clarification of the genetic mechanisms related to the Rh factor has made it possible to predict the development of erythroblastosis fetalis and to devise

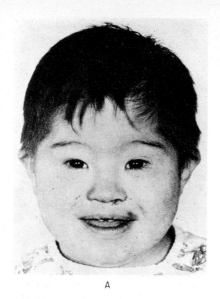

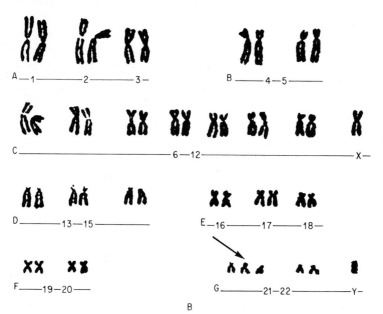

A — 1 ——— 2 ——— 3 —   B —— 4—5 ——

C ———————— 6—12 ———————— X —

D ——— 13—15 ———   E —16——17——18—

F ——19—20——   G ——— 21—22 ——— Y—

B

Figure 3-18 *A:* Patient with Down's syndrome. These patients have severe mental retardation, short stature and extremities, eyes which appear mongoloid, and a "simian" fold in the palm (a single line which extends all the way across the palm instead of the usual human double line). *B:* Chromosomes of this syndrome. There is an extra chromosome in the 21–22 group which is usually assigned to 21. [*From L. Lockhart in H. T. Lynch (ed.), Dynamic Genetic Counseling for Clinicians, Charles C Thomas, Springfield, Ill., 1969, p. 52. By permission of the publishers.*]

methods to prevent it and to treat it when it occurs. Hemochromatosis is a hereditary disease which results in excessive accumulation of iron within the body, and Wilson's disease is one which results in excessive retention of copper. Hemochromatosis is effectively treated by frequent withdrawal of blood, requiring the individual to use up iron stores for blood replacement. Wilson's disease is treated by the use of penicillamine, which increases the excretion of copper.

Dietary management may be effective, either by elimination diets or by dietary supplementation depending upon the disease. We have seen that phenylketonuria can be treated by the drastic reduction of phenylalanine in the diet. Galactosemia is a recessive disease due to deficiency of the enzyme galactose-1-phosphate uridyl transferase, which results in extremely high levels of galactose in the blood. These infants develop severe liver disease. The common source of galactose is milk, and elimination of galactose by the removal of dairy products from the diet effectively controls the disorder. McKusick points out that many species of mammals produce amino acids which man must obtain from other sources, and the same is true for vitamins; this dietary necessity represents a "genetic defect" which is ordinarily remedied by an appropriate diet.

Some patients have an X-linked genetic deficiency of the erythrocyte glucose-6-phosphate dehydrogenase. These individuals cannot tolerate certain drugs and are sensitive to the fava bean. Yet they are perfectly normal if they observe appropriate precautions. Antihemophilic globulin can be used in hemophilia, insulin in diabetes, and thyroid hormone in genetic defects of thyroid hormone synthesis. Surgical therapies are possible in some disorders. Splenectomy of patients with hereditary spherocytosis corrects the hemolytic anemia. Removal of the colon in cases of hereditary polyposis reduces the chance for the development of cancer, and kidney transplantation is a promising possibility for the treatment of certain hereditary types of kidney disease.

Finally, genetic counseling, although certainly not precise, offers increasing possibilities. Occasionally potentially dangerous genetic combinations can be recognized before procreation. Most important, however, is genetic counseling after the recognition of a diseased member of the family. In many instances fairly precise estimates as to the risk of repetition of the defect can be given, and the potential parents can then make decisions based on this information. Amniocentesis is a very recently developed technique which makes it possible to identify a number of serious defects early in embryonic development. It may be of greatest value in diagnosing cases when the risk is known to be high. If this technique is successful, recent changes in social policy may make it possible to consider abortion of some of these defective fetuses.

BIBLIOGRAPHY

CARTER, CEDRIC O.: *Human Heredity,* Baltimore:Penguin Books, Inc., 1962.

CRICK, F. H. C.: "The Structure of the Hereditary Material," *Scientific American,* October, 1954.

——: "Nucleic Acids," *Scientific American,* September, 1957.

——: "The Genetic Code," *Scientific American,* October, 1962.

——: "The Genetic Code III," *Scientific American,* October, 1966.

GOODMAN, R. M. (ed.): *Genetic Disorders of Man,* Boston: Little, Brown and Company, 1970.

LERNER, I. M.: *Heredity, Evolution and Society,* San Francisco: W. H. Freeman and Company, 1968.

McKUSICK, VICTOR A.: *Human Genetics,* 2d ed., Englewood Cliffs, N.J.: Prentice-Hall, Inc., 1969.

MONTAGU, ASHLEY: *Human Heredity,* 2d rev. ed., New York: Signet Books, New American Library Inc., October, 1963 (2d printing revised).

NIRENBERG, M. W.: "The Genetic Code: II," *Scientific American,* March, 1963.

ROBERTS, J. A. F.: *An Introduction to Medical Genetics,* 5th ed., London: Oxford University Press, 1970.

STERN, CURT: *Principles of Human Genetics,* 2d ed., San Francisco: W. H. Freeman and Company, 1960.

THOMPSON, J. S. and M. W. THOMPSON: *Genetics and Medicine,* Philadelphia: W. B. Saunders Company, 1966.

WHITTINGHILL, MAURICE: *Human Genetics and Its Foundations,* New York: Reinhold Book Corporation, 1965.

Congenital Anomalies

All abnormalities which are present at the time of birth are congenital defects. These include not only genetic abnormalities such as those discussed in Chap. 3 but also environmental abnormalities caused by postconceptual influences from fertilization to birth. The term *congenital* does not distinguish between hereditary and environmental influences; it merely signifies that the abnormality under discussion was present at the time of birth. Congenital syphilis, for example, is due not to any hereditary component but to transmission of a maternal infection to the fetus. This distinction between *congenital* and *hereditary* is often misunderstood. The present discussion shall be limited to *congenital anomalies*, namely structural abnormalities present at the time of birth.

Many of these anomalies are immediately obvious. Examples include microcephaly (small-headedness, the "pinhead" of the sideshow), cleft lip and cleft palate, clubfoot, spina bifida (a condition in which the arches of the vertebrae do not fuse and parts of the spinal nervous system may protrude into sacs just under the skin), and a number of rarer but very obvious defects such as failure of the chest wall to completely enclose the heart or of the abdominal wall to completely enclose the bladder.

Other defects may not be found until a specific clinical abnormality develops or unless special examinations are performed. Thus many heart anomalies are first detected by the presence of abnormal heart sounds or signs of heart failure, and kidney and urinary tract abnormalities may be found only when special x-ray studies are done. Most congenital anomalies are best discussed with disorders of the appropriate organ systems; however a few will be discussed here in some detail in order to describe the general mechanisms involved.

EMBRYOLOGY

The nature of congenital anomalies can only be appreciated by an understanding of the normal development of the fetus and especially of the development of the organ involved. The ovum is ejected from the ovary

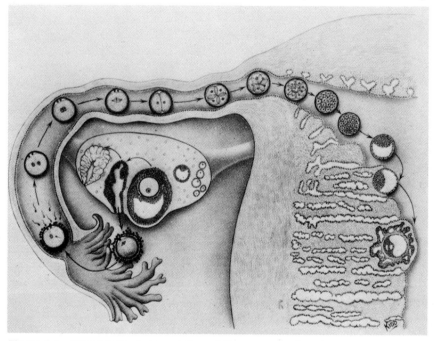

Figure 4-1 Diagramatic representation of the process of ovulation, fertilization, and implantation. After ovulation, the ovum enters the fallopian tube, where it is fertilized. Cell multiplication begins immediately and the trophoblast is identifiable by the time of implantation. *(From R. G. Harrison, Textbook of Human Embryology, 2d ed., Blackwell, Oxford, 1963, p. 58. By permission of the publishers.)*

during ovulation and enters the fallopian tube, where, if it is fertilized, the genetically reconstituted single cell begins to divide (Fig. 4-1). A ball of cells forms which gradually evolves into an outer shell of cells and an inner cluster. During this period the early embryo migrates down the fallopian tube into the cavity of the uterus, and during the second week it becomes implanted in the mucosal lining of the uterus. The thin-walled

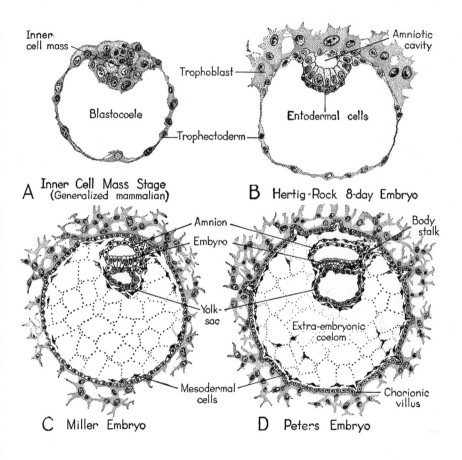

Figure 4-2   Early development of the human embryo. *A:* Blastodermic vesicle prior to implantation. *B:* Hertig-Rock 8-day embryo. Early implantation with beginning differentiation of embryonic cells. *C:* Miller 12-day embryo. Ectoderm (amnion) and endoderm (yolk sac) showing early differentiation. *D:* Peters embryo. Approximately 14 days. Mesodermal cells surrounding the ectoderm and the endoderm have become apparent. *(From B. M. Patten, Foundations of Embryology, 2d ed., McGraw-Hill, New York, 1964, p. 318. By permission of the publishers.)*

sphere is known as the *trophoblast,* and during the further development of the embryo, the portion facing the uterus becomes thickened and complex to form the placenta, whereas the remainder becomes a thin-walled covering for the embryo. The placenta and its thin-walled extension, as well as some structures to be added later, are known as the *chorion* (Fig. 4-2).

The ball of cells within the trophoblast now differentiates. The cells in contact with the chorion form a sphere. These cells become the ectoderm, and the cavity within is known as the amniotic cavity (Fig. 4-2B). Another sphere of cells forms which is in contact with the ectoderm but not with the chorion. These cells become the endoderm and the cavity becomes the yolk sac (Fig. 4-2C). The embryo itself develops at the tangential point of contact between these two spheres of cells. A third major group of cells, the mesoderm, develops outside the ectodermal and endodermal vesicles. The amniotic cavity becomes greatly enlarged and, much like turning a glove inside out, eventually surrounds almost the entire remainder of the embryo and becomes the bag of waters. This fluid-filled environment equalizes the intrauterine pressures and allows for free expansion and movement of the developing fetus (Fig. 4-3).

At this very early stage the potentiality of the various cells is already well established. The ectoderm eventually gives rise to the skin and its appendages—including the hair, teeth, skin glands, nails, lens of the eye, and auditory vesicle—as well as the entire nervous system. The endoderm gives rise to the esophagus, stomach and intestinal tract, trachea, bronchi and lungs, pancreas, and liver. The mesoderm gives rise to all the other body structures including the supportive tissues of the organs derived from the ectoderm and endoderm. It might be noted that during the fifth week, primordial germ cells can already be identified in the gonads, and it is from these cells that the ova and sperm are derived for subsequent reproduction. Figure 4-4 gives a detailed summary of the origins of most organs and tissues.

The embryo now undergoes rapid differentiation, and by the end of the third month, although only 2½ inches (68 millimeters) in crown-rump length, is readily identifiable as a human and almost all the basic structures have been established (Figs. 4-5 to 4-8). The conceptus is generally termed the *ovum* until implantation, the *embryo* until the end of the eighth week, and the *fetus* until birth. Subsequent development involves increase in size and refinement in structure in preparation for extrauterine life. Limitations in space do not allow a detailed discussion of the development of the individual structures. However, most congenital anomalies can be explained by a knowledge of this development. Wherever possible an attempt will be made to present this evolution as related to specific anomalies.

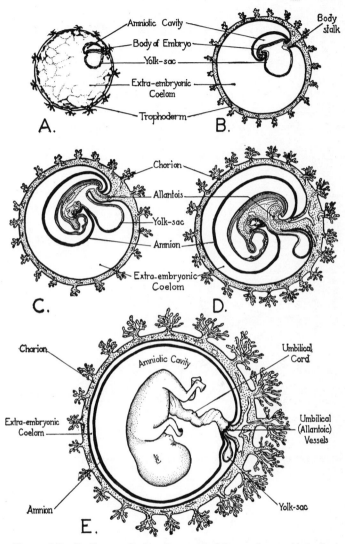

Figure 4-3   Further early development of the embryo.   Note that
the expanding ectodermal amniotic cavity folds over the embryo
and results in the enclosure of the mesodermal and endodermal
components within the fetal structure.   The residual yolk sac becomes an internal component of the umbilical cord, as do the
mesodermal umbilical vessels which carry nutrition and waste
products to and from the placenta.   The amniotic fluid equalizes
the pressure on the fetus and allows it some degree of movement.
The amnion is popularly known as the bag of waters.   *(From B. M.
Patten, Foundations of Embryology, 2d ed., McGraw-Hill, New
York, 1964, p. 331.   By permission of the publishers.)*

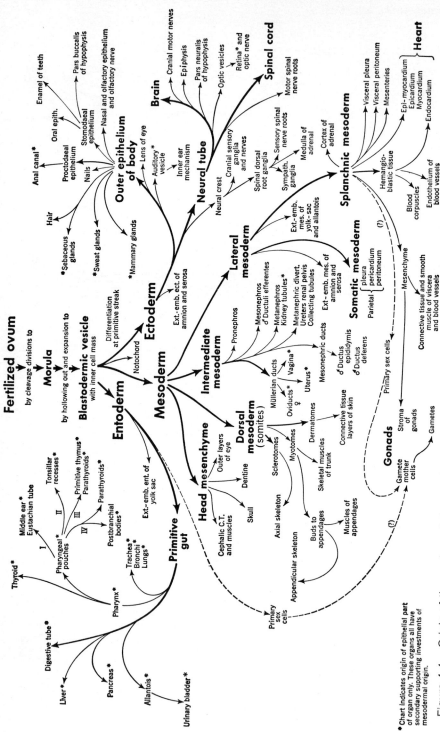

Figure 4-4   Origin of tissues by cellular specialization. (From B. M. Patten, Human Embryology, 3d ed., McGraw-Hill, New York, 1968, p. 59. By permission of the publishers.)

*Chart indicates origin of epithelial part of organ only. These organs all have secondary supporting investments of mesodermal origin.

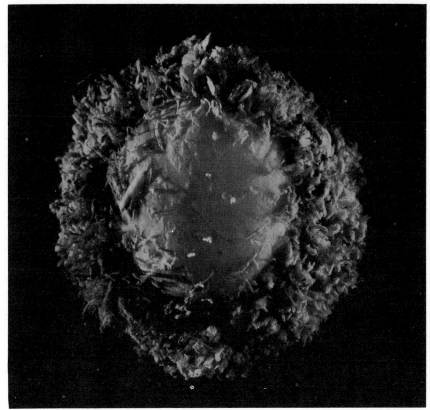

Figure 4-5 Twenty-eight-day chorion. *(From L. L. Langley, E. Cheraskin, and R. Sleeper, Dynamic Anatomy and Physiology, 2d ed., McGraw-Hill, New York, 1963, p. 646. By permission of the publishers.)*

COMMON MAJOR ANOMALIES

As previously defined, the concept of congenital anomalies will be restricted to anatomical defects present at the time of birth and demonstrable grossly without requiring microscopic identification. Many anomalies are externally visible and readily apparent at birth. Internal anomalies may not be recognized without special examination unless they produce appropriate symptoms and disability. A significant number of anomalies produce no malfunction and are recognized only on autopsy or incidentally to other examinations. Many minor, easily demonstrated anomalies may not be recorded and therefore fail to be listed in statistical studies. Since they cause no difficulty, this is probably of no signifi-

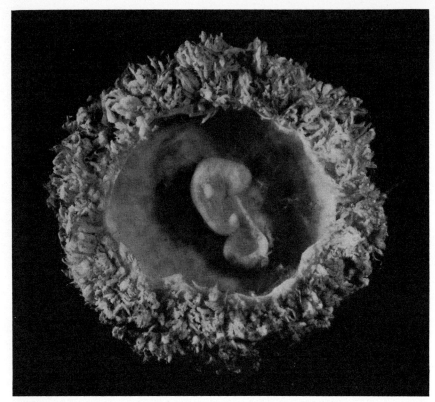

Figure 4-6 Twenty-eight-day embryo. The embryo is entirely enclosed in ectoderm and the limb buds are apparent. The yolk sac is much reduced in size. *(From L. L. Langley, E. Cheraskin, and R. Sleeper, Dynamic Anatomy and Physiology, 2d ed., McGraw-Hill, New York, 1963, p. 647. By permission of the publishers.)*

cance. Examples are extra nipples, present in a high percentage of the population, and the so-called torus palatinus, a raised ridge on the hard palate due to an overgrowth of the palatine processes at the time of formation of the hard palate. Somewhat more important anomalies such as polydactyly (an excessive number of digits) and syndactyly (fusion of digits) are quite common but produce little disability and are often amenable to surgical repair. Specific attention will be paid to only a small group of common and relatively severe defects.

Anencephaly

The structures of the nervous system are derived from the ectoderm. At about the sixteenth day a neural, or medullary, groove forms along

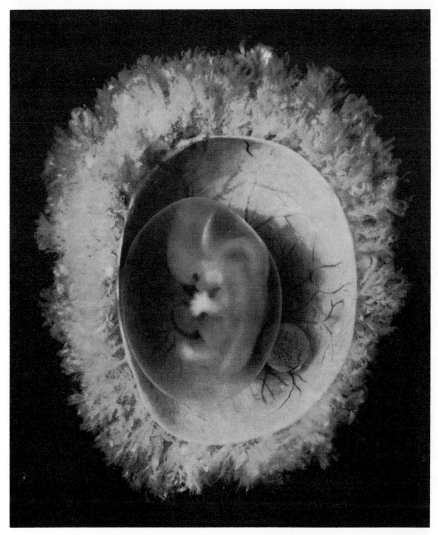

Figure 4-7 Forty-day embryo with intact amnion and yolk sac at lower right. *(From L. L. Langley, E. Cheraskin, and R. Sleeper, Dynamic Anatomy and Physiology, 2d ed., McGraw-Hill, New York, 1963, p. 649. By permission of the publishers.)*

the back of the embryo (Fig. 4-9). This groove becomes deeper and gradually tubular in shape as the ectodermal lips of the groove grow medially over the groove and cover it. By the twenty-sixth day the ectoderm has reestablished its continuity, and just beneath it lies a now completed tube which eventually develops into the nervous system. The tube is then surrounded by mesoderm, which gives rise to the neural

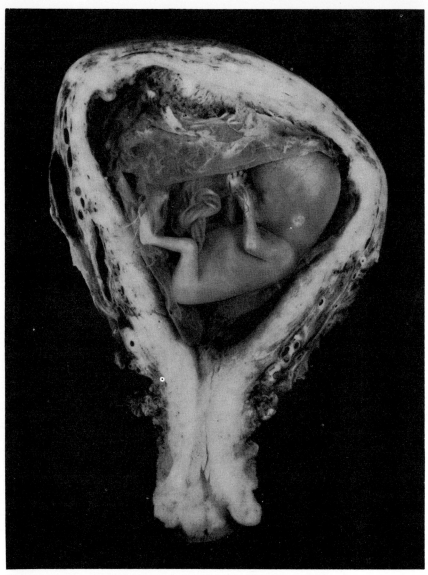

Figure 4-8   Seventy-day embryo in uterus.   All structures are now
well differentiated and growth will be the major change until the
time of birth.   *(From L. L. Langley, E. Cheraskin, and R. Sleeper,
Dynamic Anatomy and Physiology, 2d ed., McGraw-Hill, New York,
1963, p. 650.   By permission of the publishers.)*

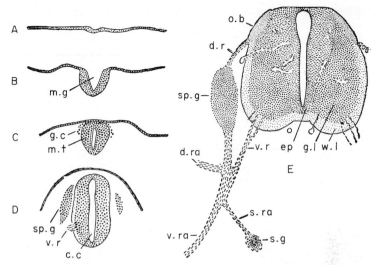

Figure 4-9 The development of the neural (medullary) tube as seen in cross-sections of dorsal ectoderm. A: Beginning thickening of epithelium and groove formation. B: Further development of the medullary groove (m.g.). C: Closure of the groove with formation of the medullary tube (m.t.), reestablishment of continuity of the ectoderm, and appearance of ganglion cells (g.c.), which will eventually form peripheral nerves. D and E: Further development, showing the dorsal root (d.r.) and spinal ganglion (sp.g.), which will form the peripheral sensory system; the ventral root (v.r.), which will form the peripheral motor system; and the sympathetic ramus (s.ra.) and sympathetic ganglion (s.g.), which will form part of the autonomic nervous system. [*From M. Singer and M. N. Salpeter in R. O. Greep (ed.), Histology, McGraw-Hill, New York, 1966, p. 265. By permission of the publishers.*]

arches of the vertebrae and the skull. These protect the neural tissue. Failure of proper development of the head end of the neural tube and of its bony covering gives rise to an *anencephalic* (brainless) *monster* (Fig. 4-10). The remainder of the fetus may be well formed, but due to failure of development of the brain or its subsequent deterioration because of the absence of a skull, this portion of the central nervous system is greatly reduced and distorted. This abnormality occurs approximately once in a thousand births and is incompatible with life for more than a few hours.

Spina Bifida

A related abnormality is spina bifida (Fig. 4-11). This abnormality occurs in approximately three of a thousand births and is due to failure of development of the neural arches. The commonest sites for this defect are the cervical and lumbar regions. In one form, spina bifida

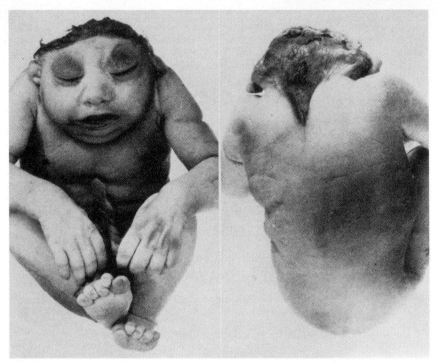

Figure 4-10 Anencephaly. Anterior and posterior views demonstrating failure of proper development of the neural tube. *(From
A. L. Smith, Microbiology and Pathology, 9th ed., Mosby, St. Louis,
1968, p. 445. By permission of the publishers.)*

occulta, the arch may be almost complete and no abnormality may be
detected. In meningocele, a subcutaneous cyst of varying size may be
present which contains no nervous tissue but only the cerebrospinal
fluid which normally bathes the brain and spinal cord. This form of
abnormality lends itself to surgical repair and minimal residual disability.
The severest and unfortunately the most common defect is the meningo-
myelocele, in which the cyst contains nerves and portions of the spinal
cord. Severe and irreversible neurological lesions are common in children
with this defect and many have other anomalies as well. Almost half of
them develop hydrocephalus within the first year. Therapy has not been
particularly successful.

Hydrocephalus

Hydrocephalus is an extremely characteristic disorder in which the
cranial vault becomes greatly expanded, very much resembling illustrations of the supergeniuses of science fiction (Fig. 4-12). Tragically,

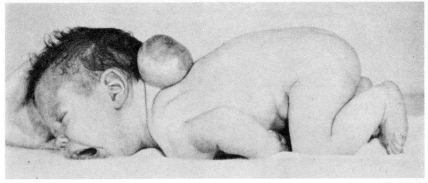

A

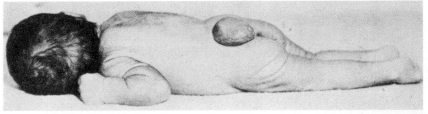

B

Figure 4-11   Spina bifida.   *A:* Meningocele in the cervical region.
B: Meningocele in the lumbosacral region.   *(From J. C. Meakins,
The Practice of Medicine, Mosby, St. Louis, 1940, p. 989.   By
permisssion of the publishers.)*

these individuals invariably have a reduced mentality.   The brain and
spinal cord are enclosed in a tough and relatively inelastic three-layered
sheath known as the meninges.   The cerebrospinal fluid is produced in
cavities within the brain and flows through three small openings in the
brain stem into the space between the nervous tissue and the meninges.
Normally the rate of fluid production in the brain is equaled by the rate
of reabsorption by blood vessels in the meninges.   Generalized increases
in cerebrospinal fluid can result from excessive production or inadequate
reabsorption.   The usual immediate cause of hydrocephalus is a block
in the flow of fluid from the cavities within the brain to the submeningeal
space.   As the fluid is retained, the brain enlarges.   The bones of the
skull in the infant are not attached to each other, and they spread as a
result of the pressure, producing the characteristic head shape.

Hydrocephalus can arise from a number of causes, but almost half
are due to congenital malformations.   Most of these are associated with
spina bifida cystica; the combination is also known as the Arnold-Chiari
anomaly.   Recently it has been recognized that the protozoan *Toxoplasma*
is an important cause of hydrocephalus.   Although this parasite usually

105

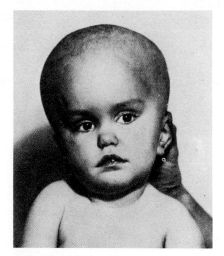

A

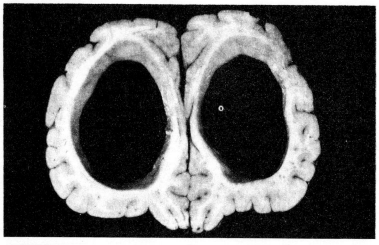

B

Figure 4-12 Hydrocephaly. *A:* External appearance. *(From J. C. Meakins, The Practice of Medicine, 3d ed., Mosby, St. Louis, 1940, p. 1072. By permission of the publishers.)* *B:* Cross-section of brain showing internal tissue destruction. The ventricles, normally relatively small slits, have been expanded by the presence of fluid which has caused pressure destruction of most of the brain tissue. *(From R. P. Morehead, Human Pathology, McGraw-Hill, New York, 1965, p. 1467. By permission of the publishers.)*

Figure 4-13 (Opposite) Development of the face. *(From B. M. Patten, Human Embryology, 3d ed., McGraw-Hill, New York, 1968, p. 346. By permission of the publishers.)*

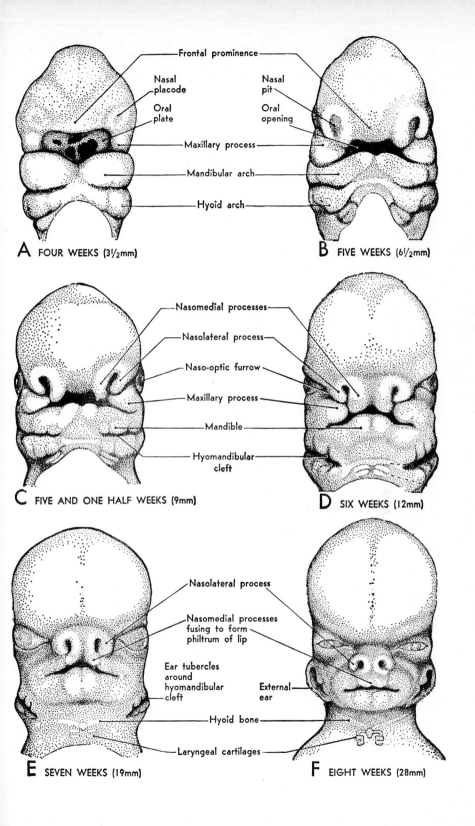

A FOUR WEEKS (3½mm)

Frontal prominence
Nasal placode
Oral plate
Maxillary process
Mandibular arch
Hyoid arch

B FIVE WEEKS (6½mm)

Nasal pit
Oral opening

C FIVE AND ONE HALF WEEKS (9mm)

Nasomedial processes
Nasolateral process
Naso-optic furrow
Maxillary process
Mandible
Hyomandibular cleft

D SIX WEEKS (12mm)

E SEVEN WEEKS (19mm)

Nasolateral process
Nasomedial processes fusing to form philtrum of lip
Ear tubercles around hyomandibular cleft
Hyoid bone
Laryngeal cartilages

External ear

F EIGHT WEEKS (28mm)

produces no signs or symptoms in the adult, the fetus can be infected across the placenta and significant abnormalities can result. The commonest combination is that of hydrocephalus, chorioretinitis, convulsions, and intracerebral calcification. Microcephalus, spasticity, microphthalmus, large ears, and mental defects have also been reported. Because of the recency of this observation, the frequency of the disorder, methods of diagnosis, and techniques of treatment have not been well established.

Cleft Lip and Cleft Palate

Cleft lip, or harelip, and *cleft palate* are well known. Cleft lip occurs about once in a thousand births. Two-thirds of the cases are in males and about half have an associated cleft palate. Cleft palate unassociated with harelip occurs in one of 2,500 births. The mechanism of the defect in formation of the harelip can be easily appreciated by examination of Fig. 4-13. Initially the nasopharynx is a single large cavity. A nasal process grows down from above and meets two maxillary processes growing in from the sides. Harelip results from a failure of proper fusion. Shortly after the beginning of development of the nasal and maxillary processes, two lateral palatine processes develop and move inward to create separate nasal and oral cavities, eventually restricting their communication to the nasopharynx. Cleft palate results from failure of fusion of these two palatine processes. Patients with harelip and cleft palate have the obvious difficulties with appearance, respiration, eating, and speech. In addition, the improper pressure relationships produce further difficulty as a result of improper dentition and improper development of the upper jaw. Most of these difficulties can now be overcome by improved surgery, speech therapy, and orthodontia (Fig. 4-14).

Clubfoot

Clubfoot is generally referred to in the medical literature as talipes, a word derived from *tallus,* "ankle"; and *pes,* "foot." Varieties include varus, where the foot is turned inward; valgus, where it is turned outward; equinus, where it is fixed with the toes pointed down; and calcaneus, where the foot is bent upward so that the weight is borne on the heel. Combinations also occur, and about 75 percent of clubfeet are of the talipes equinovarus type, in which the foot is pointed with the toes down and the foot turned inward (Fig. 4-15). A certain amount of deformity may be present at birth and is probably due to intrauterine position. This usually corrects itself shortly without special therapy. The more severe types are usually recognized quite early and treatment should be started promptly. Treatment is usually accomplished by gradually cor-

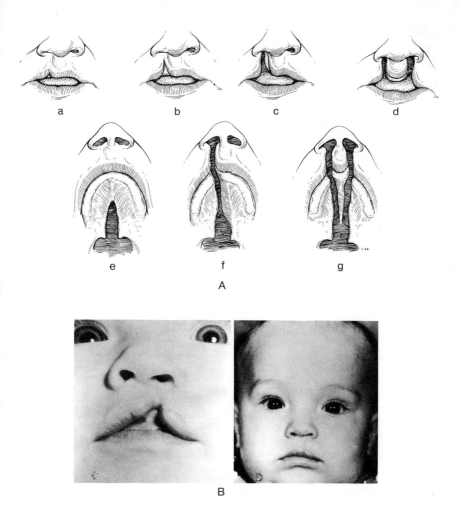

Figure 4-14 *A:* Classification of cleft lip and palate. a. Minimal incomplete cleft of the lip (primary palate).   Note nostril asymmetry. b. Moderately severe incomplete cleft of the lip (primary palate). Note nostril asymmetry. c. Complete unilateral cleft lip and palate (primary and secondary palate). d. Complete bilateral cleft lip and palate (primary and secondary palate). e. Incomplete cleft of the palate (secondary palate). f. Unilateral complete cleft of lip and palate (primary and secondary palate). g. Bilateral complete cleft of lip and palate (primary and secondary palate). *B.* Repair of cleft lip. Notice the relationship of the defects to development in Fig. 4-13D. *[From R. A. Chase in S. I. Schwartz (ed.), Principles of Surgery, McGraw-Hill, New York, 1969, pp. 1776 and 1777. By permission of the publishers.]*

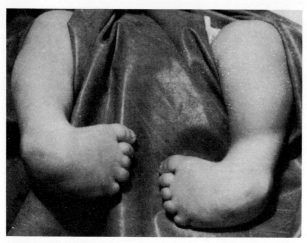

Figure 4-15   Bilateral clubfeet (talipes equinovarus).   [*From R. B. Duthic in S. I. Schwartz (ed.), Principles of Surgery, McGraw-Hill, New York, 1969, p. 1592.   By permission of the publishers.*]

recting and then overcorrecting the deformity, holding the foot at each stage in a plaster cast.   Occasionally surgical therapy such as lengthening of tendons may be necessary.   Most cases respond satisfactorily.

Congenital Dislocation of the Hip

Congenital dislocation of the hip is one of the few anomalies which affects girls more frequently than boys, the ratio being approximately 6:1.   The hip is a ball-and-socket type of joint in which the head of the femur rests in the cuplike acetabulum of the pelvis.   In childhood the acetabulum may be quite shallow, and if the ligaments are inadequate, the pressures of weight bearing may result in the upward displacement of the femoral head.   If a normal relationship cannot be maintained, the acetabulum may not develop properly and the dislocation remains permanent.   The ultimate result is an awkward and waddling gait.   The defect is usually bilateral.   Dislocation of the hip is rare among Negroes and most common in the southern European countries.   The condition should be recognized and treated early, since after the age of 3 years, complete correction is usually not achieved.   After the age of 6 or 7 years, results are generally unsatisfactory.

INCIDENCE OF CONGENITAL ANOMALIES

The previous discussion makes it apparent that attempts to determine the incidence of congenital anomalies depend to a great extent upon the lesions included and the effectiveness of follow-up. Obviously it is necessary to follow a given number of births for a period of time in order to get accurate statistics, since data based on recognized instances may overstate the number due to the losses of healthy individuals from the study. Potter makes some interesting speculations regarding the importance of defective development. First, ovulation occurs at midcycle and—normally—subsequent menstruation is prevented by the presence of an implanted trophoblast. However, errors in the development of the ovum during the first 2 weeks may not be identified as pregnancies because, when these errors lead to failure of implantation, there is no cessation of menses. Hertig and Rock studied eight preimplantation embryos and found that half were so abnormal that they would have died had they not been removed surgically. If this ratio is consistent, then 50 percent of conceptions are lost. Potter takes the figure of 4,200,000 live births for 1958 and estimates that there was failure of implantation due to defective development in an additional 2 million. She estimates further that miscarriages before midpregnancy amounted to another million conceptions, and that perhaps half of these failed due to defective development. Vital statistics data for the United States indicate that not quite 9,000 infants died of malformations in the first 2 weeks of life and another 13,000 died at an older age. To this she adds 5,000 anomalous stillbirths and 2,800 hydatidiform moles.* Thus the total annual loss of life in the United States directly attributable to malformation is about 30,000, with the possibility that more than one out of every three conceptions is defective. It is worth noting that deaths in the first year due to congenital anomalies are several times as great as deaths due to all the common infectious diseases combined. During the same year there were approximately 1,100 deaths due to whooping cough, measles, diptheria, scarlet fever, and poliomyelitis.

Table 4-1 presents a comparison of the frequency of common malformations at birth in Swedish, Japanese, and English studies and compares them with revised estimates at 9 months in Japanese data and 5 years in English data. The total frequencies are remarkably similar, being about 1.3 percent at birth and 2.4 percent at later follow-up. It can be seen from the table that, while the total number of anomalies is comparable in the different areas, there is a great variability of frequency in the individual causes. For example, anencephaly is relatively infrequent in Sweden and Japan but common in England. Spina bifida is infrequent in Japan, intermediate in Sweden, and high in England. However, cardiac malformations are higher in Japan than in England, talipes is three times

---

* The hydatidiform mole is a developmental defect in which the chorion develops a mass of cysts, likened to a bunch of grapes, which usually prevents the development of the fetus.

Table 4-1   Incidence of Malformations (per 1,000 Total Births)

	Estimates soon after birth			Revised estimates	
Type of malformation	Swedish data (44,109)*	Japanese data (64,570)	Birm- ingham (56,760)	Japanese data (to 9 months)	Birm- ingham (to 5 years)
Anencephalus	0.54	0.63	1.96	0.63	1.96
Spina bifida, etc.	1.09–1.45	0.26	2.80	0.32	3.00
Hydrocephalus	1.00	0.32	1.76	0.50	2.57
Down's syndrome	0.48	0.09	1.11	0.87	1.69
Cardiac malformations	0.79	4.21	2.11	6.97	4.18
Cleft lip and/or palate	1.75	2.78	1.76	2.96	1.94
Talipes	2.79	1.10	3.95	1.40	4.44
Dislocation of hip	0.00	0.31	0.02	7.13	0.67
All malformed individuals	11.18	12.22	17.30	24.54	23.08
Individuals excluded	2.27	1.16	0.0	4.81	0.0

* Numbers in parentheses are the populations (total births) in which the malformations were identified.
  SOURCE: Thomas McKeown and R. G. Record, CIBA Foundation Symposium on Congenital Malformations.

as common in England as in Japan, but congenital dislocation of the hip is twelve times more common in Japan. An understanding of these regional differences may be helpful in reducing their frequency. In a New York study reported by McIntosh and Mellin, 16.8 percent of fetal deaths were associated with congenital malformations and 28.9 percent of neonatal deaths were so associated. Malformations were found in 3.5 percent of children at birth, and by the end of 1 year, 6.9 percent were recognized to have malformations. When minor malformations were excluded, there were still 3.3 percent significant defects (Table 4-2).

ETIOLOGY OF CONGENITAL ANOMALIES

Until very recently very little has been known regarding the origin of congenital anomalies. The general attitude has been that the fetus received its genetic endowment and subsequently was quite well protected from the environment until birth. Part of this bias was undoubtedly scientific reaction to folklore belief regarding prenatal influences. However, it was well known that a number of infections could cross the placental barrier, and congenital syphilis in particular was known to produce characteristic effects which were somewhat different from the disease when contracted in adult life. The role of Rh incompatibility,

Table 4-2   Incidence of Congenital Malformations in All Births Over 500 Grams

	Number of births	Diagnosis		
		Malformations, percent	Clinical, percent	Autopsy or 1-year follow-up, percent
Fetal deaths	107	16.8	9.3	7.5
Neonatal deaths	97	28.9	15.5	13.4
Live births	5,531	6.9	3.5	3.4
Adjusted*	5,531	3.3	2.1	1.2
Total	5,735	7.5	3.8	3.7
Adjusted*	5,735	4.0	2.5	1.5

  *Adjusted for major malformations only.
  SOURCE: Mellin in Fishbein, 1963.

first elucidated in the 1940s, demonstrated another specific type of effect on the fetus.   It has been known for some time that women who deliver large infants weighing over 9 pounds very often either have diabetes or subsequently develop that disease.   Down's syndrome and other congenital anomalies have been known to occur more frequently in offspring of older mothers.   Extensive studies have shown that improvement in socioeconomic well-being is associated with decreased fetal wastage from all causes.   Yet surprisingly, the incidence of anomalies is twice as great in Caucasians as Negroes.   It is of interest that increased maternal height up to 5 feet 6 inches improves the fetal outlook in all social classes.   Although the number of abnormalities increases when the mother works during pregnancy, too little exercise and work also appear to be detrimental.

Knowledge of the mode of development of the fetus should make it apparent that the period of greatest vulnerability is during the development of the various organ systems and that therefore the period up to 3 months is the most critical.   It is of interest that despite this knowledge, the general well-being of the mother and the lack of apparent manifestations of pregnancy other than amenorrhea (cessation of menses) in most women has resulted in relatively less concern for this period than for the later and more obvious periods of pregnancy.

It has now become amply apparent that many fetal abnormalities can be attributed to both general and specific causes.   Progress in this area has been most encouraging.   In many instances it is now possible to predict the frequency with which abnormalities can be expected as well as the precise type of abnormality.   Neel estimates that 20 percent of congenital anomalies are due to new mutant genes, 10 percent to newly discovered chromosome abnormalities, 10 percent to virus infections, and 60 percent to unknown causes. However, even this latter category is yielding to further information.

Single-Gene Mutations

This category probably accounts for 20 percent of anomalies. A number of attempts have been made to classify them, but none has been complete. Dominant and sex-linked abnormalities will become immediately apparent, and if the individuals survive, these abnormalities will demonstrate their genetic characteristics and provide data for subsequent predictability. Sporadic lethal mutations may be much more difficult to demonstrate. Sporadic, recessively determined abnormalities can only be identified as such if the sibling frequency is appropriate or if there is recurrence in the offspring of a consanguineous marriage.

   A corollary of these factors is that if there is a dominant mutation in the fetus, the risk of similar abnormalities in the sibship is low; however, 50 percent of the offspring of the affected individual will be similarly involved. The homozygous recessive state implies that the mutation is not new, since it must involve both parents; the risk to the sibship is one in four. The risk to children of the involved individual is very low in marriages to normal, unrelated individuals. One problem in evaluating mutation is the existence of so-called *phenocopies.* It has been demonstrated that individuals with otherwise normal genes may, under certain experimental conditions, produce offspring with abnormalities which resemble specific genetic defects. Proof that the effect is environmental rather than genetic is established by the failure of recurrence of the abnormality when the specific environmental stress is removed. Specific phenocopies have been demonstrated in experimental animals and have been strongly inferred for man. The appropriate environmental factors will have to be identified in each case.

Chromosomal Abnormalities

The role of chromosomal abnormalities was discussed in the last chapter. Three general types have been recognized. The first is the reduction in the total amount of chromosomal material, as demonstrated in Turner's syndrome in which the Y chromosome is missing. No other defect of this type has been recognized, and it seems probable that absence of the X chromosome (in the male) or any of the autosomes is lethal. The second type, associated with an increased number of chromosomes, is characterized by Klinefelter's syndrome, in which there is an extra X chromosome, and by Down's syndrome, in which there is an extra autosome. No other autosomal syndromes are clearly delineated; however, individuals with three, four, and five X chromosomes have been reported, as well as others with up to four X chromosomes and the Y chromosome. All patients with a Y chromosome, regardless of the number of X chromosomes, have male characteristics. In both sexes there seems to be some mental retardation with the increased number of sex chromosomes.

Finally, there are the translocation abnormalities in which part of one chromosome appears to be stuck to another, leaving a normal number of chromosomes but with associated abnormalities of chromosomal structure. Several cases of Down's syndrome have been reported due to this type of abnormality. Down's and Klinefelter's syndromes both show a remarkable direct correlation with the age of the mother. In particular, Down's syndrome appears only once in 2,000 pregnancies of mothers aged 25. This increases to one in 800 if there has been a previous abnormality of this type. On the other hand, the frequency increases to one in 40 births of mothers aged 45, and one in 16 if there has been a previous such abnormality. As the ova age they seem to be more susceptible to nondisjunction during the mitotic cleavages. The expectation of having an infant with Down's syndrome increases fiftyfold for mothers as they age from 25 to 45 years. The frequency of Turner's syndrome, in which there is the loss of a Y chromosome rather than a chromosome gain, is unassociated with maternal aging.

Multiple-gene Abnormalities

Carter has summarized a large number of studies bearing upon the genetic factors relating to pyloric stenosis, talipes equinovarus, harelip, spina bifida, anencephaly, and congenital dislocation of the hip (Table 4-3).

Table 4-3   Increase in Frequency of Common Malformations Relative to the General Population in First-, Second-, and Third-degree Relatives of Affected Individuals

Relationship	Harelip ± cleft palate	Congenital dislocation of hip	Talipes equinovarus	Pyloric stenosis	Anencephalus and spina bifida
Monozygotic twins	500×	500×	325×	150×	
First degree	35×	40×	20×	20×	8×
Second degree	7×	4×	5×	4×	
Third degree	3×	1½×	2×	1½×	2×
Approximate population incidence	0.001	0.001	0.001	0.003	0.005

SOURCE: Carter in Steinberg and Bearn, 1965.

Pyloric stenosis is an obstruction to the outlet of the stomach (pylorus) due to hypertrophy of the smooth muscle at this point. The expected incidence of harelip in the general population is 1 per 1,000. Three separate studies in Copenhagen, Utah, and London showed 49, 46, and 32 cleft lips per 1,000 siblings of propositi (index cases), an increase of fortyfold over the number expected. A similar number were found in the children of propositi with harelip. When second-degree relatives* were examined, the frequency was six to eight times the number expected; and when third-degree relatives were examined, the increase was twofold to fourfold. Ratios of this type are compatible with multiple-gene inheritance acting in conjunction with environmental factors. Remarkably similar data were also obtained for congenital dislocation of the hip, talipes equinovarus, and pyloric stenosis. The data on anencephalus and spina bifida, despite their greater frequency, are less complete and less convincing. However, there is a slight but significantly greater expectation of the disorder in the first-degree relatives.

These socioeconomic and geographic variables strongly suggest that there may be important environmental factors which, when identified, could help to eradicate the defects. For example, anencephaly occurs in 0.09 percent of the children of wives of professional personnel but in 0.36 percent of children born to the wives of unskilled laborers, a fourfold difference. This difference does not seem to be explained by any obvious difference in nutrition. Anencephaly and spina bifida are relatively rare in Negroes, for whom the environmental situation can hardly be considered ideal. There are considerable geographic variations which have not been explained. Anencephaly is twice as frequent in Britain as in Australia, and many other geographic discrepancies have been noted. Birth order is of importance, with a higher frequency of all the above listed anomalies in the firstborn. Some defects, particularly talipes and congenital dislocation of the hip, may be associated with breech delivery, which is most common with the firstborn.

Twins and Twinning

Dizygotic (two-egg) twins do not resemble each other more closely than ordinary siblings and, in fact, are comparable to the siblings in a litter born to an animal that has more than one offspring at a time. Monozygotic (one-egg) twins represent an entirely different mechanism. At some time

---

*First-degree relatives share half the same genes with the propositus, i.e., parents, siblings, and offspring. Second-degree relatives share one-fourth the same genes, i.e., grandparents, grandchildren, uncles, aunts, nephews, and nieces. Third-degree relatives share one-eighth the same genes, i.e., first cousins, etc.

during the early development of the ovum, one of the cells splits off and starts to develop into a separate fetus. Obviously, to be successful, the cell must derive from a cell which has retained the capacity for total differentiation. Both develop in the uterus and, depending upon the time of separation, one or two placentas and sets of fetal membranes may develop. Therefore a single placenta is not a prerequisite for monozygosity. Many fetal monsters are the result of twinning. The most well-known and dramatic are the Siamese twins which presumably result from failure of complete separation of the two embryos (Fig. 4-16). Probably more frequent, but less well known, are unequal twins of the same type in which one member of the pair is smaller or incompletely formed but remains attached to its mate. A final point about twinning is the fact that, although identical twins may start with equal genetic endowment, inequalities in

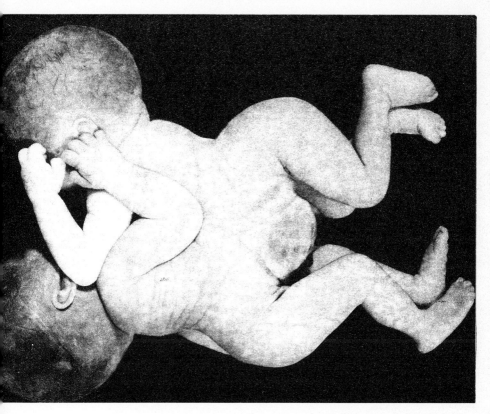

Figure 4-16 Conjoined twins. Many types have been observed; the original Siamese twins represented a coupling compatible with life. *(From R. P. Morehead, Human Pathology, McGraw-Hill, New York, 1965, p. 1467. By permission of the publishers.)*

environmental endowment may develop as early as at the time of implantation, since there may be differences in placental blood flow and subsequent nutrition. Therefore, even at the time of birth, their environmental endowment may already be dissimilar.

Virus Infections

In 1941 there was an extensive epidemic of German measles (rubella) in Australia. Shortly afterward, Gregg, an ophthalmologist, noted an increased incidence of congenital cataracts. Investigation revealed that all the mothers of these infants had had German measles during the first 3 months of their pregnancies. This report aroused great interest and was rapidly confirmed by other studies. The commonest defects caused by rubella are eye defects, especially congenital cataract; heart defects, most commonly patent ductus arteriosus and ventricular septal defect; deafness; microcephaly; and mental retardation. Less frequent defects are harelip, cleft palate, pyloric stenosis, spina bifida, and mongolism (Down's syndrome). The defect is related to the time of the disease; thus cataracts are most frequent following infections during the sixth week and deafness following infections during the ninth week. Heart defects may be produced by disease any time from the fifth to the ninth week.

Rubella is not a particularly common disease in childhood, and as a result large numbers of adults can develop the disease during epidemic years. It is important to evaluate the risk of anomalies following infection. Many studies have been done. One of the best was performed by Bradford Hill and his associates. In this study a group of mothers known to have contracted rubella during their pregnancies were followed and their offspring examined. A prospective study of this type would be expected to give a truer incidence than a retrospective study, which would tend to overrepresent mothers with defective children and miss mothers with normal children. Table 4-4 indicates the frequency of defects observed in this

Table 4-4   Risk of Deformity from Maternal Rubella

Week of pregnancy rubella was manifest	Number of babies	Number with defects	Percent with defects
1–4	12	6	50
5–8	20	5	25
9–12	18	3	17
13–16	18	2	11
17–24	17	1	6
25+	19	0	0

SOURCE: Bradford Hill, *British Journal of Preventive and Social Medicine*, 12:1, 1958.

study. It can be seen that the incidence is very high during the first 3 months, involving one in three infants, whereas no anomalies were noted when infection occurred after the sixth month.

After the recognition of the role of rubella, many studies were initiated to evaluate the possible role of other common viral infections. There is some suggestion that measles may cause anomalies; however, since this disease is common in childhood and rare in adults, its importance is not great. Extensive studies were conducted in respect to the influenza epidemics of the past two decades, but if anomalies have been produced the incidence has not been high. It should be remembered that the first 3 months are critical in the development of the fetus and that maternal disabilities per se may account for the occasional abnormalities noted. Mumps, smallpox, chickenpox, and poliomyelitis may all be transmitted to the fetus and on occasion have been manifest as diseases at birth. However, the production of congenital anomalies by these diseases has not been conclusively demonstrated.

Ionizing Radiation

Ionizing radiation, including x-rays, has been used for the experimental production of mutations since 1927. Radiation may cause three general types of damage. First, there may be breakage or total destruction of an entire chromosome. When this occurs in the parental germ cells, it is usually lethal to the cell and successful pregnancy is rare. Only a relatively small number of defective fetuses will result. This type of damage rarely affects the female. Since there is a rapid turnover of spermatozoa in the male, most of the defective cells will be eliminated if there is an interval of several months between the radiation and procreation.

The second form of radiation damage is due to gene mutation. The commonest effect is the production of a recessive but deleterious gene. This mutation will not manifest itself in the offspring unless the germplasm coincidentally carried the same mutant gene from the other parent. Thus the mutation will not be apparent in most cases for several generations, until an appropriate mating produces an affected offspring. Dominant mutations are less frequent and will, of course, produce an immediately recognizable abnormality. Gene mutations may arise not only in primordial or parental sex cells but also in localized tissues after cellular differentiation. These somatic mutations can then produce localized genetic abnormalities.

The third effect of radiation is a direct one upon the developing embryo. The effect produced will depend, as in all teratogenic agents, upon the time of development and the specific tissue damage. In the mouse, it has been shown that irradiation on the seventh day results in abnormalities of the vertebrae and ribs; on the eighth day it causes harelip and cleft palate; on the ninth day, spina bifida; on the tenth day, abnormalities of the forefeet; and on the eleventh day, abnormalities of the hind feet. Such precise information is not known for humans. More than twenty types of abnormality were recognized in children born after the Japanese atomic bombing. Most of these involved the central nervous system and the most common were microcephaly, already known to be associated with irradiation, and mental retardation. Eye defects were next in frequency.

Man presently receives radiation from a number of natural and artificial sources. Montagu has argued that the amount of radiation received prior to the completion of the reproductive period represents a load affecting the offspring. He estimates that background radiation, including cosmic rays and naturally occurring radioactive substances, create a load of 4.3 roentgens. This may be somewhat higher in individuals living at high altitudes. Medical x-rays may add an additional 3.0 roentgens, while fallout resulting from atomic testing at present levels adds 0.1 roentgens. The total exposure is therefore 7.4 roentgens. While each type of artificial exposure in itself does not increase the load significantly, the number of new abnormalities is appreciable in an entire population. Since the total load has been almost doubled by artificial means, every attempt should be made to keep this load at the minimum possible level. Russell has suggested, in addition, that women of reproductive age not be x-rayed during the 2 weeks prior to the expected onset of menstrual flow. This is the period between ovulation and possible implantation in which an unrecognized pregnancy may occur. It is also the period of maximal vulnerability of the fetus.

Teratogens

A substance which has the capacity to produce an anomaly, or teratoma, is known as a teratogen. It has long been known that some drugs and chemicals have teratogenic properties. This fact was dramatically brought to the public consciousness by the recognition in 1961 that thalidomide, a mild tranquilizer widely distributed in Europe but not in the United States, was the cause of a number of severe and bizarre forms of congenital anomaly. When taken by women during the first 3 months of pregnancy, a large percent of their offspring were born with partial or total absence of one or more extremities, a condition known as *phocomelia* (Fig. 4-17). It is estimated that several thousand defective infants were born. Public attention was drawn dramatically to the possible relationship between drugs and abnormalities because of this tragedy, and it is probable that as a result there will be much less casual medication during pregnancy. In addition, the need for more intensive testing and study of drugs being given to pregnant women was made painfully apparent.

A rather long list of drugs and other substances had been previously known to produce congenital anomalies. Absence of the vitamin folic acid has been demonstrated experimentally to produce a variety of abnormalities, but folic acid deficiency is rare in human beings. However, a group of drugs used to treat acute leukemia can produce severe folic acid deficiency by interfering with the metabolic effects of the vitamin. The most frequently used drug is aminopterin. Because of this property, aminopterin has been used to produce abortion. In the course of such use, a number of anomalous infants have resulted, most frequently with anencephaly. Most of the cancer chemotherapy agents act by their interference with the reproduction of rapidly dividing cells. As this occurs also in the developing embryo, it would be expected that these drugs would also be harmful to the fetus. This has proved to be the case. Since the life of

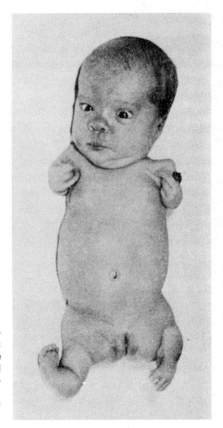

Figure 4-17 Phocomelia. In some instances phocomelia appears to be genetic in origin. In this newborn infant, it was due to intrauterine thalidomide exposure and is an example of the phenocopy mechanism. *(From I. Väänäven and T. Joki, Ann. Paediat. Fenn., 9:65, 1963. By permission of the publishers.)*

the mother with cancer may depend upon adequate treatment, the possibility of teratogenicity does not always represent a contradiction to the use of these agents.

Excess and deficiency of vitamin A have also been observed to produce defects in animals, and the same is inferred for man. Hoet has noted that many women with frequent miscarriages, stillbirths, and children with congenital anomalies have hypothyroidism or an abnormal ability to handle sugar suggestive of potential diabetes. When these women were appropriately treated with thyroid hormone or insulin, their rate of fetal wastage was markedly decreased. There is evidence to suggest that there is some common relationship between vitamin A deficiency and thyroxine and insulin deficiency. Anoxia, or an insufficient amount of oxygen, has been used to produce experimental anomalies in animals, and there are well-documented human cases. The list of chemicals whose presence or absence has been demonstrated to produce anomalies in experimental animals and man is growing rapidly as the study of the subject accelerates.

CONCLUSIONS

With the decline in importance of childhood infectious disease, knowledge regarding congenital anomalies takes on new importance. Significant anomalies are present in probably more than 3 percent of births. Each individual has only one life to live, and there is no greater tragedy than to have to live it with grotesque and irremediable defects. Significant progress is being made in recognizing causes of congenital defects and in devising treatment for those affected. It is obvious that factors affecting the mother between conception and delivery are of extreme importance, especially during the first 3 months of pregnancy. Proper rest, exercise, and nutrition and the avoidance of all medication not specifically indicated are essential. Pregnancy should be discouraged in women over the age of 35 and in those with previous anomalous infants of types known to have a high recurrence rate.

BIBLIOGRAPHY

AREY, L. B.: *Developmental Anatomy,* 7th ed., Philadelphia: W. B. Saunders Company, 1965.

BREMER, J. L.: *Congenital Anomalies of the Viscera: Their Embryological Basis,* Cambridge, Mass.: Harvard University Press, 1957.

CARTER, C. O.: "The Inheritance of Common Congenital Malformation," in A. G. STEINBERG and A. G. BEARN (eds.), *Progress in Medical Genetics,* vol. 4, New York: Grune and Stratton, 1965.

COOPER, L. Z.: "German Measles," *Scientific American,* July, 1966.

FISHBEIN, MORRIS (ed.): *Birth Defects,* Philadelphia: J. B. Lippincott Company, 1963.

MONTAGU, M. F. A.: *Prenatal Influences,* Springfield, Ill.: Charles C Thomas, Publisher, 1962.

PATTEN, B. M.: *Human Embryology,* New York: McGraw-Hill Book Company, 1968.

POTTER, E. L.: *Pathology of the Fetus and the Newborn,* Chicago: The Year Book Publishers, Inc., 1952.

ROBSON, J. M., F. M. SULLIVAN, and R. L. SMITH (eds.): *Embryopathic Activity of Drugs,* London: J. & A. Churchill, Ltd., 1965.

SMITHELLS, R. W.: *The Early Diagnosis of Congenital Abnormalities,* London: Cassell & Co., Ltd., 1963.

WILLIS, R. A.: *The Borderland of Embryology and Pathology,* London: Butterworth & Co. (Publishers), Ltd., 1958.

WOLSTENHOLME, G. E. W. and C. M. O'CONNOR (eds.): *Ciba Foundation Symposium on Congenital Malformations,* London: J. & A. Churchill, Ltd., 1960.

Malnutrition

Throughout history man's greatest preoccupation has been the procurement of adequate food. At first he subsisted by hunting and gathering edible vegetation. The domestication of animals and the establishment of agriculture were revolutionary developments, which allowed the creation of stable societies with improved assurance of nutritional adequacy and reduction in the hazards associated with primitive hunting. As a result of this increased productivity, the population grew but became vulnerable to those natural and man-made disasters (of war and politics) which produced famines. It has only been within the past century that there was developed sufficient precise knowledge of nutrition, food production, transportation, and population regulation to make it possible to conquer the complex problems of malnutrition on a worldwide basis. Those of us who live in North America find it hard to appreciate the impact of famine and its effect on cultures where it is a constant threat.

Little research was done on the nature of food until the middle of the nineteenth century. Liebig then characterized the major organic components of food as carbohydrates, fats, and proteins. Initially, it was thought that only protein was essential. Yet the necessity for specific nutrients had been recognized in the eighteenth century when Lind, a British naval surgeon, found that scurvy could be prevented during long voyages at sea by the addition of citrus fruits to the diet. The provision of limes to British seamen earned them the title of "limeys." The similar addition of the polishings from milled rice to the diet of Japanese seamen a century later resulted in the prevention of beriberi. Definitive strides were taken during the first half of the present century when the necessary nutrients were characterized, deficiency states identified, chemical structures defined, and prophylactic procedures initiated.

The classic method of identifying the necessity for a specific nutrient was to add it to the diet of those suffering from the disease and determine if a cure resulted. This technique was modified by the use of experimental animals or human volunteers for whom test diets were prepared, eliminating the suspect nutrient and determining the effect of its absence and eventual replacement. Finally, it became possible to construct diets with all the known nutrients to determine if they were sufficient to maintain a normal state of health. With this technique it was also possible to observe the effects of varying the relative quantities of individual nutrients.

One important experimental method is the balance study. Using this method, for example, the fate of protein metabolism can be determined by following nitrogen balance. The total nitrogen intake in the diet and the total nitrogen loss from the urine, stool, and skin are determined by analysis over a fixed period of time. If the nitrogen losses equalled the nitrogen input, the patient was said to be in nitrogen balance. If the nitrogen losses were less than the intake, the individual was in positive balance, and protein conservation or growth could be inferred. On the other hand, if the total nitrogen losses exceeded intake, the subject was in negative nitrogen balance and the nitrogen intake was not sufficient to maintain a constant tissue mass. Balance studies indicate the overall pattern, but determination of the precise chemical pathways and mechanisms requires more complex experimental procedures. These have been greatly implemented by the use of radioactive tracers and the development of extremely sensitive analytic methods in the past 25 years.

NUTRITIONAL REQUIREMENTS

Nutrition must fulfill two fundamental needs. First, it must provide the essential components for growth and the replacement of tissues lost or damaged by use. The essential dietary components are listed in Table 5-1. Second, it must provide fuel to produce the energy for metabolic processes and physiological activity.

Table 5-1 Essential Nutritional Components

Chemical elements
  Major: C, H, O, N, S, Ca, P, Na, Cl, K, Mg
  Minor: Fe, I, Mn, Mo, Co, Zn, Cu
  Uncertain: Se, Cr, F
Vitamins
  Water-soluble: Thiamine (B_1)
              Riboflavin (B_2)
              Pyridoxine (B_6)
              Niacin
              Folacin
              Pantothenic acid
              Cobalamine (B_{12})
              Biotin
              Ascorbic acid (C)
  Fat-soluble: Vitamin A
            Vitamin D
            Vitamin E
            Vitamin K
Essential amino acids
  Lysine
  Threonine
  Leucine
  Isoleucine
  Methionine
  Tryptophan
  Valine
  Phenylalanine
  Arginine }
  Histidine } for children only
Essential fatty acids
  Linoleic acid
  Arachidonic acid
Water

Chemical Elements

Eighteen chemical elements have been identified as essential, and three other elements may also be required. *Carbon, hydrogen,* and *oxygen* are present in all organic materials and are readily available in food. *Nitrogen* is an essential component of all amino acids and thus of all proteins. *Sulfur* is a component of three amino acids—methionine, cystine, and cysteine; and inorganic sulfates are produced by the metabolism of these amino acids. *Sodium* and *chloride* are the primary inorganic ions of the extracellular fluid, and *potassium* and *magnesium* are the primary inorganic intracellular ions. Bone is made up primarily of *calcium* and *phosphorus;* in addition, phosphate is widely present as the ion and as a component of creatine phosphate; adenosine mono-, di-, and triphosphates; and phospholipids. Trace elements include *iron,* which is essential for hemoglobin and myoglobin; *iodine,* a component of thyroid hormone; *manganese, copper,* and *zinc,* which are probably necessary components in some enzyme systems; *cobalt,* an essential component of vitamin B_{12}; and *molybdenum,* which may also be an enzyme cofactor. *Fluorine* may not be essential, but when present in small amounts it appears to stabilize teeth and bones, increasing the resistance of the former to decay and of the latter to osteoporosis. *Selenium* and *chromium* have been found in trace amounts, but no essential role has been identified.*

Protein

The essential nature of proteins and the mechanism for their production have been described in Chaps. 2 and 3. Eight of the amino acids cannot be synthesized by the human organism from available materials. These eight are lysine, threonine, leucine, isoleucine, methionine, tryptophan, valine, and phenylalanine. In addition, growing children cannot produce adequate amounts of arginine and histidine. These amino acids have been termed essential amino acids and must be available in the diet. The mechanism for protein synthesis requires that the proper mixture of amino acids must be available or production will be unsuccessful. This follows naturally from the sequential linkage of amino acids along the RNA template.

Vegetable proteins are said to be biologically poor because the amino acid mixture may be deficient in some components. On the other hand, animal proteins are said to be of high quality since their composition more nearly matches the human requirements. Eggs and milk contain particularly high quality proteins because they were specifically designed to serve as nutrients for growing organisms. There is relatively little storage of amino acids or proteins. Some amino acids may be available in the turnover state within cells, particularly in muscle. In the absence of protein intake, amino acids become available primarily through cell breakdown. Ordinarily the protein intake exceeds replacement needs, and the excess amino acids are converted to carbohydrates and burned to provide energy at the rate of 4 calories per gram. The residual nitrogen is excreted in the urine, chiefly as urea.

Carbohydrates

Carbohydrates are derived from plant foods, primarily grains and potatoes. The most common form is starch, which is a polysaccharide made up of a

---

*Recent evidence suggests that silicon, tin, and vanadium may also be required in trace amounts (E. Frieden, *Scientific American,* 227:53, 1972).

long chain of glucose molecules. In digestion, starch is broken down to maltose, a disaccharide composed of two molecules of glucose. Sucrose is a disaccharide composed of glucose and fructose and is the carbohydrate found in table sugar and many fruits. Lactose is milk sugar and is a disaccharide composed of glucose and galactose. Fructose and galactose are converted to glucose by the liver. The liver can store excess glucose as glycogen; when increased glucose is needed, the liver can produce glucose from amino acids and from the glycerol of triglyceride fats. The central nervous system is capable of deriving energy only from the combustion of glucose, and therefore adequate amounts of glucose and oxygen must be delivered to the brain at all times. The body store of carbohydrates is relatively small and sufficient to provide only 12 hours of energy. Carbohydrate produces 4 calories per gram.

Fats

Fats (or lipids) represent the energy reserve of the body. They are an economical storage form and provide 9 calories per gram. Fat is stored as a triglyceride consisting of three long-chain saturated fatty acids linked to a glycerol molecule. Other chemicals considered to be in the same class as fats are the phospholipids, cholesterol, and related compounds. Two unsaturated fatty acids, linoleic and arachidonic, are essential to the diet. In their absence growth is impaired.

Vitamins

Casimir Funk, a Polish scientist, coined the term *vitamine* in 1910. He is credited with characterizing the concept that diseases such as scurvy, pellagra, and beriberi, which responded to specific foods, were due to the absence of specific compounds. This was revolutionary, since it first expressed the possibility that a disease could be the result of the absence, rather than presence, of a causative agent. The vitamins turned out not to be amines, but the concept was sound and the name captured the public fancy. Two general groups of vitamins have been identified. One is fat-soluble and the other water-soluble. The fat-soluble vitamins include vitamin A, vitamin D, vitamin E, and vitamin K. The water-soluble vitamins include thiamine (B_1), riboflavin (B_2), pyridoxine (B_6), niacin, folacin, pantothenic acid, cobalamine (B_{12}), biotin, and ascorbic acid (C).

The human organism is capable of synthesizing thousands of compounds from the available dietary materials. Yet there are only twenty-odd compounds which are necessary for the normal metabolic processes and which cannot be synthesized from other dietary components. Many of them can be synthesized by other species of animals. This inability is probably due to the lack of appropriate enzymes and might be considered analogous to some of the genetic aberrations which result in a failure to properly carry out certain specific metabolic sequences. However, once these metabolic requirements are met, the human is extremely adaptable to a great variety of diets providing the necessary caloric requirements. On one extreme is the typical Oriental farmer whose diet approaches 90 percent carbohydrates and on the other, the African Masai herdsman whose diet consists of almost 90 percent protein and fat (Fig. 5-1). The diets in most developed countries approach a more equal mixture of fats, carbohydrates, and proteins. There seems to be little evidence that these extreme diets in any way affect the health of their adherents. However, the lives of the individuals at the extremes are subject to greater general hazards with a lower longevity and a greater likelihood of specific deficiencies. It is still too early to be certain that any specific diet delays aging or the development of chronic deteriorative diseases.

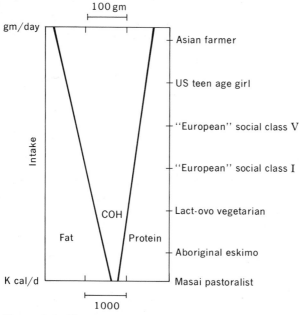

Figure 5-1 The proportions of fat, carbohydrate, and protein compatible with good nutrition provided that essential nutrients are available. The Registrar General of the United Kingdom classes socioeconomic status from class I (professional) to class V (unskilled). *(From G. V. Mann in Harrison's Principles of Internal Medicine, 6th ed., McGraw-Hill, New York, 1970, p. 392. By permission of the publishers.)*

MALNUTRITION

Malnutrition covers a broad spectrum. The usual connotation is that of undernutrition, but in the literal sense it can apply to any inappropriate diet. *Starvation* is a long-continued deprival of food. *Marasmus* is the progressive wasting of infants which may, as one cause, be due to under-nutrition (Fig. 5-2). *Cachexia* means general illness, but the implication is that of weight loss as well. Specific deficiencies, particularly of vitamins, lead to specific diseases. Caloric overnutrition leads to *obesity*. The excess of several vitamins, particularly A and D, may lead to toxic effects.

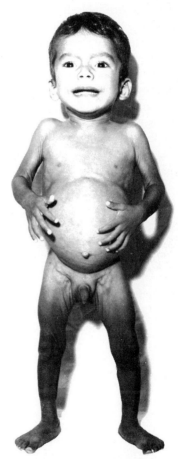

Figure 5-2   Juvenile marasmus. *(From G. V. Mann in Harrison's Principles of Internal Medicine, 6th ed., McGraw-Hill, New York, 1970, p. 401. By permission of the publishers.)*

Rarely, the diet may be adequate in the necessary nutrients but incompatibilities of some of the components may result in malnutrition. The major nutritional disorders are summarized in Table 5-2.

UNDERNUTRITION

The causes of undernutrition may be classified broadly as follows:

1. Inadequate intake. In the past, inadequate intake was most often due to the physical unavailability of food as a result of natural disaster such as drought, flood, locust plague, the depletion of game by over-hunting, and so forth. In more recent times, food may also have been unavailable because of lack of economic resources or political restrictions. In the United States, these primary types of inadequate intake have become progressively less common and now represent a very small fraction of total malnutrition. Inadequate intake may also be due to poor dentition and to disease of the mouth or throat. Oral and pharyngeal pain constitutes an obvious mechanism for the inhibition of swallowing. Anorexia, or lack of appetite, is common in many illnesses. Since a satisfactory

Table 5-2   Major Nutritional Disorders

Undernutrition	Manifestation
Calorie	Wasting (cachexia in adults, marasmus in children)
Protein	Growth failure, kwashiorkor, nutritional edema
Protein-calorie (starvation)	
Acute	Death due to wasting before development of specific deficiencies
Chronic	Cachexia, marasmus, and specific deficiencies
Thiamine (B_1)	Beriberi
Niacin	Pellagra
Ascorbic acid (C)	Scurvy
Folic acid	Magaloblastic anemia
Vitamin A	Xerophthalmia, night blindness
Vitamin D	Rickets
Vitamin K	Hemorrhage (hypoprothrombinemia)
Calcium	Osteomalacia
Iodine	Hypothyroidism, goiter
Iron	Iron-deficiency anemia

Overnutrition	Manifestation
Calorie	Obesity
Vitamin D	Soft-tissue calcification, weakness

diet requires not only appetite satiation but also provision of all of the necessary constituents, a number of factors may contribute to selective malnutrition. One of the most obvious examples of such malnutrition is the alcoholic, who obtains 7 calories from each gram of alcohol to meet energy requirements. When the consumption of alcohol is sufficient to meet all caloric needs and produce satiation, a large number of dietary deficiences may result. Dietetic ignorance may contribute to malnutrition even when food and economic resources are adequate. Societal cultures may result in rigid dietaries which are deficient. Examples are the use of milled rice in the Orient, which gives rise to beriberi, and the former dependence upon corn in the American South, which resulted in pellagra. Psychosis and coma may also lead to inadequate intake, often requiring tube feeding or other drastic measures for treatment.

    2.   Failure of absorption. The failure to absorb food is present in a relatively large number of diseases. Inadequacy of gastric secretion may interfere with the absorption of vitamin B_{12}, calcium, and iron. Deficiency of digestive enzymes is an obvious cause of malabsorption. Carbohydrates are least likely to be affected, but the absorption of proteins and particularly fats may be greatly impaired. The adequate secretion of bile into the intestinal tract is also essential for fat absorption, and there are a number of conditions which can interfere with adequate bile secretion. In these conditions, fat-soluble vitamins as well as fats are not absorbed. The absorptive surfaces of the intestinal tract may be impaired by disease or by surgery. Occasionally, long lengths of bowel may be removed, particularly as the result of occlusion of intestinal blood vessels, extensive intestinal injuries, and cancer. This results in a greatly reduced absorptive surface area and a proportionate decrease in the efficiency of absorption. Diarrheal disease may move food too rapidly past the absorptive sites. Finally, there may be chemical or physical competition as in the case of unabsorbable mineral oil, which traps fat-soluble vitamins. Similarly, phytic acid binds calcium and makes it unavailable for absorption.

    3.   Excessive loss. Nutrients may be lost to the body through a variety of routes. In the entity known as protein-losing enteropathy, blood proteins seep across the gastric mucosa and are lost in large quantities in the stool. Diarrheal diseases not only cause the loss of ingested nutrients but also result in excessive losses of intestinal secretions which are normally reabsorbed. The kidney may be the route of loss of large quantities of protein in nephrosis, of large amounts of glucose (sometimes amounting to several hundred grams a day) in diabetes mellitus, and less frequently of calcium, phosphorus, and amino acids in the relatively rare entities of renal tubular acidosis and Fanconi's syndrome. Proteins may be lost in tremendous quantities through the skin following burns, although this is generally an acute situation. Chronic suppurations also lead to protein loss, especially when combined with such factors as fever and anorexia. Chronic blood loss may be occult, yet after a period of time iron stores of the body may be so depleted that blood replacement is not possible without iron supplementation.

4. Increased nutritional requirements. Pregnancy requires the addition of 200 calories per day and lactation requires the addition of 1000 calories daily. In addition, fetal growth requires large amounts of specific structural components, particularly proteins, calcium, and phosphorus. Hypermetabolic states, such as fevers from any cause and hyperthyroidism, require caloric supplementation. Malignant neoplasia (cancer) also appears to require increased food intake. Malignant cachexia is common, but the mechanism is not known.

5. Impaired utilization. An adequate supply of dietary components may fail to be utilized because of chemical or physiological competition. For example, isoniazid, which is used for treatment of tuberculosis, interferes with the effectiveness of pyridoxine, vitamin B_6. Another example is the deliberate use of dicumarol to interfere with the action of vitamin K and the liver mechanism for producing prothrombin, the precursor of thrombin, which is necessary for normal blood clotting. The tendency of the blood to clot in such diseases as coronary thrombosis and thrombophlebitis can thereby be reduced (see Chap. 10). In diabetes there is failure of the proper utilization of glucose because of inadequate or ineffective insulin, which results in a significant loss of glucose through the kidneys.

Starvation

Extensive studies have been made of starvation, particularly of victims of World War II and volunteers studied at approximately the same time. Starvation is usually accompanied by lethargy, irritability, and a progressive loss of all interest other than the pursuit of food. Tissues are consumed to provide energy, particularly from fat depots; however, various organs, with the major exception of the brain, also decrease significantly in size. The body becomes cooler; spontaneous activity decreases, as does oxygen consumption. In addition, secondary sexual characteristics diminish, sexual interest wanes, women develop amenorrhea, and reproduction becomes impossible. All these factors tend to conserve energy, and the basal caloric expenditure of the normal man drops from 1800 to 1200 calories per day. The available caloric reserves from a normal adult male are sufficient for approximately 2 months' survival. Most of this energy is derived from the normal fat stores, although body protein may be reduced as much as 20 percent.

Women, because of their greater fat reserves, and obese individuals may survive longer. If more than half the normal body weight is lost, recovery is unusual. In acute starvation, the body stores of the essential nutrients are usually sufficient to prevent specific deficiencies prior to death from the exhaustion of caloric reserves (Fig. 5-3).

Protein Deficiency

The minimum protein requirement of a nongrowing adult receiving material of high biological value is on the order of 0.3 grams per kilogram body weight. For a 70-kilogram man, this would be approximately 20 grams of protein. The exact amount is variable and depends upon such factors as activity and amino acid proportions. The generally recommended value is 0.5 to 1.0 grams per kilogram of body weight, with 1.0 to 2.0 grams recommended during growth. Diets deficient in specific essential amino acids result in failure of protein synthesis and

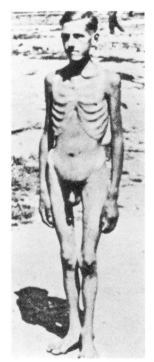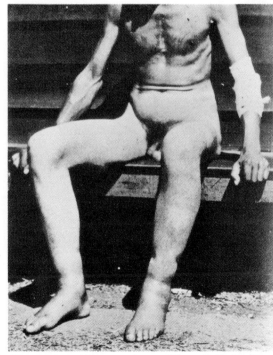

Figure 5-3   Starvation and hunger edema. [*From C. S. Davidson in Beeson and McDermott (eds.), Cecil-Loeb Textbook of Medicine, 12th ed., Saunders, Philadelphia, 1967, p. 1150. By permission of the publishers.*]

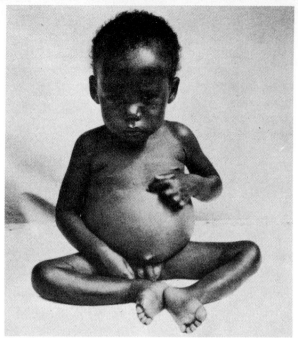

A

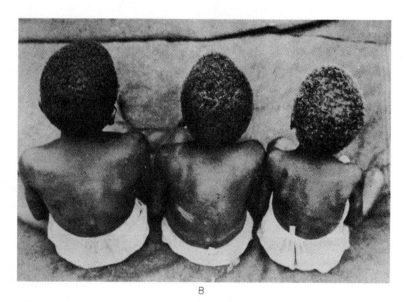

B

Figure 5-4   Kwashiorkor.   *A:* Typical case demonstrating abdominal distension and peripheral edema.   *B:* Note increasing depig-
mentation of hair from left to right.   *(From J. F. Brock and M.
Autret, Kwashiorkor in Africa, World Health Organization, Geneva,
1952.   By permission of the publishers.)*

136

negative nitrogen balance. Diseases characteristic of specific amino acid deficiencies have not been described. This is not surprising, since most peptides contain a variety of amino acids, and an absence of any one would interfere with synthesis of the entire peptide. Prolonged protein undernutrition interferes with growth in children, and the recent increase in stature in most adult populations is undoubtedly the result of better juvenile nutrition. Prolonged protein malnutrition in adults eventually results in reduced serum protein values, particularly albumin. Surprisingly, this is not invariable, and in some studies normal males failed to show change in the serum protein levels after 6 months of protein deprivation. Starvation edema is generally attributed to the low serum proteins. However, this interrelationship does not appear to be firm, and the ultimate explanation for this manifestation has not been established.

During the past two decades a specific form of protein malnutrition in growing children has been delineated and well characterized. It was first identified in Ghana and is known by the local name *kwashiorkor* (Fig. 5-4). It is now recognized that this entity is common in all areas of malnutrition, but it is particularly frequent in the tropics. The history is usually consistent: The child has been nursed for a varied period of time, up to several years, and then suddenly weaned to a diet high in carbohydrates but extremely low in protein. In Ghana, this is a porridge of cassava meal. Growth is poor, edema and potbelly develop, skin lesions resembling pellagra (and possibly due to niacin deficiency) appear, diarrhea is common, and in black children the hair becomes straight and reddish as the black pigment is lost.

Obviously, there is a spectrum extending from pure protein deficiency to total energy deficiency, and the all-inclusive expression "protein-calorie malnutrition" has been used. Recently the public has been made conscious of the appearance of this type of malnutrition through the wide press coverage of the Biafran children during the Nigerian Civil War.

Water-soluble–vitamin Deficiencies

Thiamine (B₁) Beriberi, due to the specific deficiency of thiamine, has been documented in the Orient for many centuries. During the years around the turn of the century, it was demonstrated that beriberi could be prevented by administration of rice polishings. The actual structure of thiamine was finally demonstrated by Williams in 1932. Thiamine serves as a coenzyme in one of the steps in metabolism of carbohydrates. Several forms of beriberi are recognized, the most common is peripheral neuropathy manifested by pain and weakness in the extremities, gradually progressing to paralysis with foot drop and wrist drop (Fig. 5-5A). Occasionally the central nervous system may be involved, with Wernicke's

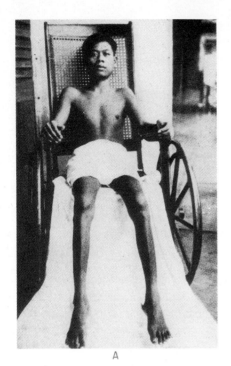
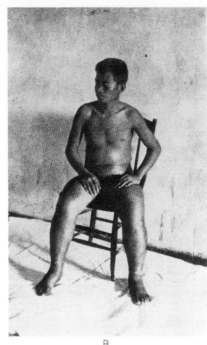

A   B

Figure 5-5   Beriberi.   *A: Dry beriberi, demonstrating peripheral neuropathy.* There is atrophy of muscles of extremities and foot drop.   *B:* Wet beriberi.   Note the resemblance to hunger edema. *(From E. B. Vedder, Beriberi, Wood, Baltimore, 1913, pp. 58 and 304.   By permission of the publishers.)*

disease or Korsakoff's syndrome.   The former is an acute condition characterized by confusion and paralysis of the eye muscles.   The latter is a peculiar disorder in which the patient has a severe memory defect which he often conceals by bizarre confabulation.   There may be heart failure due to dilatation of the heart, and death may occur suddenly. This particular manifestation of thiamine deficiency has been particularly common among alcoholics in Western Europe and the United States. Finally, there is wet beriberi, which is associated with extensive edema (Fig. 5-5 B).   The exact mechanism for edema formation has not been established, and it is possible that it may be due to multiple nutritional deficiencies.   Small doses of thiamine often produce dramatic responses, sometimes with improvement as soon as 12 hours after ingestion.   The normal daily requirement is less than 1 milligram.   Within the past decade, beriberi accounted for 25 percent of all deaths in several Philippine provinces.   The simple addition of thiamine to polished rice almost entirely eliminated the disease.

Riboflavin (B$_2$)   Riboflavin is also a constituent of several enzyme systems, yet despite its extensive chemical importance, very little clinical importance has been demonstrated.   Riboflavin deficiency is associated with fissures at the angles of the mouth (cheilosis), a magenta-colored tongue, and a mild dermatitis that affects primarily the face and the scrotum.

Pyridoxine (B$_6$)   Pyridoxine is also a component of enzymes which are involved in a number of important metabolic processes.   Small amounts of pyridoxine are produced by a bacterial action in the intestinal tract.   There is no specific disease associated with pyridoxine, but it has been established that deficiency will produce a characteristic anemia, and there is a high frequency of convulsions in children and infants on a low-pyridoxine diet.   There is also probably a reduction in growth. Pyridoxine is widely present in food and deficiency is probably extremely rare except in combination with other deficiencies.

Nicotinic Acid (Niacin)   Nicotinic acid, or niacin, is a component of two coenzymes.   Some niacin is available to the individual as a result of bacterial metabolism of dietary tryptophan in the intestinal tract. Pellagra is the characteristic syndrome produced by niacin deficiency. This disease was first recognized in Europe during the eighteenth century and is characterized by the four Ds—dermatitis, diarrhea, dementia, and death (Fig. 5-6).   Dermatitis is usually the first overt manifestation, starting as a reddened area like sunburn in the exposed areas of the hands, face, neck, and occasionally, the feet.   The redness gives way to dark and roughened skin, which led to the original Italian name, *pelle agra* ("skin," "rough").   Frequent small, watery, diarrheal stools are characteristic.   Other gastrointestinal lesions include anorexia, glossitis (inflammation of the tongue) with tenderness and a beefy red appearance, ulcerations at the corners of the mouth, and abdominal discomfort. Neurological manifestations occur late and may present a varied picture of coarse tremors, diminished reflexes, and depression progressing to apathy, confusion, and delirium.

Pellagra was once common in the southern part of the United States and was the apparent cause of death in 3,500 cases in 1935.   It was common where corn was the primary component of the diet.   The protein in corn is deficient in tryptophan and lysine.   Thus the intestinal production of niacin is reduced.   In addition, some mechanism in this diet seems to interfere with the niacin that is present.   The reduction in pellagra is probably the result of multiple factors including the diversification of diet and the availability of the pellagra-preventing factors.

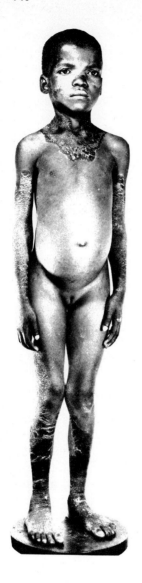

Figure 5-6 Pellagra. Scaling dermatitis is present on the exposed areas of the neck, arms, and legs. The lesion on the neck is known as Casal's collar. *(From G. V. Mann in Harrison's Principles of Internal Medicine, 6th ed., McGraw-Hill, New York, 1970, p. 403. By permission of the publishers.)*

Pantothenic Acid   This important coenzyme is present in all cells and cannot be synthesized by man.   It is widely present in food and it is synthesized by intestinal bacteria.   Specific deficiency manifestations are not known.   Its absence from the diet produced gray hair in black rats; however, attempts to prevent graying in humans by pantothenic acid supplementation have been unsuccessful.

Cobalamine (B_{12})   This vitamin is necessary for the normal manufacture of red blood cells.   It is also essential for the maintenance of the integrity of several sensory tracts in the spinal cord.   The normal requirement for vitamin B_{12} seems to be extremely small, on the order of 0.000001 gram daily.   In addition, it is synthesized by intestinal bacteria.   Vitamin B_{12} cannot be absorbed from the ileum unless "intrinsic factor" is secreted by the cells of the stomach wall near the pylorus.   Therefore, vitamin B_{12} deficiency is rarely seen except in pernicious anemia, where there is atrophy of the stomach wall, or following surgical removal of this portion of the stomach for cancer or peptic ulcer.   Cobalamine contains cobalt and is the only known requirement for this element.

Folic Acid   Folic acid is actually a group of substances which are essential to cell development.   Lack of folic acid produces an anemia which very much resembles that of pernicious anemia.   In fact, folic acid can often correct the anemia of pernicious anemia but is unable to prevent the neurological complications.   Tests recently developed indicate that the frequency of folic acid anemia is of the same order of magnitude as that of pernicious anemia.   Folic acid is also effective in treating the disease called sprue, which is characterized by frequent, fatty stools, failure of intestinal absorption, and anemia.

Biotin   Biotin is found widely in foods of animal origin and deficiency is extremely rare.   However avidin, a protein which is present in raw egg white, binds biotin and prevents its absorption from the intestinal tract.   The deficiency so produced causes dermatitis, depression, nausea, anorexia, and anemia.

Ascorbic Acid (C)   Scurvy is one of the classical deficiency diseases. Manifestations usually appear 6 to 8 months after the initiation of a deficient diet.   In adults the first lesions usually are prominence of the hair follicles, due to plugging with excessive keratin, and perifollicular hemorrhage (Fig. 5-7A).   Later there is extensive bruising of the skin, particularly in the saddle area of the buttocks and on the backs of the thighs.   The gums become swollen, spongy, and bleed easily, and eventually the teeth are lost (Fig. 5-7B).   Leg pain and weakness, postural hypotension (low blood pressure on standing), and fainting are common. As we note from the old log books of long exploratory cruises, death was frequent before modern treatment.   In infants, the disease becomes evident between 8 and 12 months of age in most instances, as reserves derived from the mother are exhausted.   Characteristically, the child

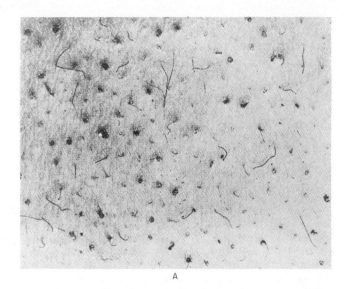

A

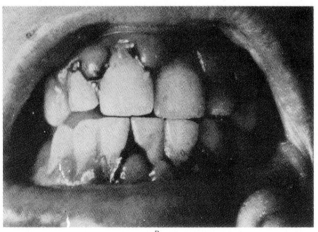

B

Figure 5-7 Scurvy. *A:* Skin lesions. The keratin layer thickens around the hair follicles and causes a coiled ingrowth of the hairs. In advanced cases there is often hemorrhage about the follicles, particularly in pressure areas such as the buttocks and the backs of the legs. [*From C. F. Davidson in Beeson and McDermott (eds.), Cecil-Loeb Textbook of Medicine, Saunders, Philadelphia, 1967, p. 1158. By permission of the publishers.*] B: Gingival lesions associated with advanced scurvy. The gums become thickened and spongy, bleed easily, and eventually there is loss of teeth. Gum thickening may also occur in other disorders, such as leukemia and diphenylhydantoin toxicity. [*From J. Pemberton in F. Bicknell and F. Prescott (eds.), Vitamins in Medicine, Grune and Stratton, New York, 1946, p. 525. By permission of the publishers.*]

142

has extremely painful legs which he maintains in a flexed and guarded position. Slight movement causes screams of pain. Bruises may be present, but other lesions of the skin and gums are not noted unless the teeth have already erupted. On x-ray, there is almost invariably a large hemorrhage between the periosteum (the connective tissue layer enclosing bone) and the bone itself. It is also evident that there is serious impairment of bone development. Healing of wounds is markedly delayed. In both the adult and the child, other tissue hemorrhages are quite frequent and are probably the major cause of the observed anemia. King isolated ascorbic acid in 1932. It was found that in normally nourished individuals, the tissues are saturated and excess ascorbic acid is excreted in the urine. If this store is not replenished, the tissue levels are gradually depleted. Experimentally, clinical scurvy can be prevented by intakes of as little as 10 milligrams a day, even though serum levels cannot be detected. Present evidence suggests that a major role of ascorbic acid is the in vivo conversion of proline to hydroxyproline. The production of collagen requires hydroxproline which has been produced in the body; dietary hydroxproline cannot be utilized. Since it is collagen that gives strength to the connective tissues and makes up most of the matrix of the bone, this defect in collagen production readily explains the manifestations of scurvy.

Fat-soluble–vitamin Deficiencies

Vitamin A Vitamin A deficiency results in night blindness and xerophthalmia. Between 1930 and 1940, carotene was demonstrated to be provitamin A, and the vitamin itself was characterized and synthesized. Vitamin A deficiency is said to be the most common cause of blindness occurring in the tropical areas where carotenes are plentiful and nutritional education could greatly reduce the incidence. Night blindness is the inability to adapt to vision under reduced light. Vitamin A is essential for the replenishment of rhodopsin, which breaks down to initiate the nerve impulses essential for dark vision.

In the discussion of epithelium, we have noted that the outer layer of the skin consists of a horny substance called keratin. Modifications of keratin make up the hair and nails of man as well as the feathers, horns, and other modified skin structures in animals. In the absence of vitamin A, a number of epithelial structures undergo metaplasia, and dry keratinized surfaces form where previously unprotected mucosal epithelium had been present. Xerophthalmia is a manifestation of this type of change in the conjunctiva. As a result, the cornea is subject to deterioration, and ulceration and loss of the lens may be the ultimate outcome (Fig. 5-8).

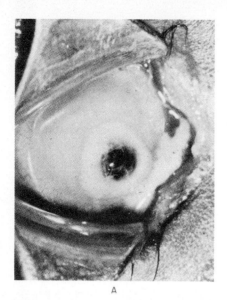

A

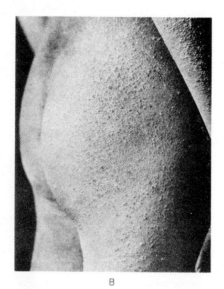

B

Figure 5-8 Vitamin-A deficiency. A: Advanced keratomalacia with probable early loss of the eye. [*From C. S. Davidson in Beeson and McDermott (eds.), Cecil-Loeb Textbook of Medicine, Saunders, Philadelphia, 1967, p. 1160. By permission of the publishers.*] B: Hyperkeratosis. As in scurvy, thickened plugs of keratin form about the openings of the hair follicles. *(From R. L. Sutton, Jr., Diseases of the Skin, 11th ed., Mosby, St. Louis, 1956, p. 728. By permission of the author.)*

Vitamin D Provitamin D is actually synthesized by the body, but in order to be effective it must be irradiated by ultraviolet light. This normally occurs by the exposure of blood supplying the skin to the sun. Increased clothing, indoor occupations, and the atmospheric conditions in most cities combine to reduce the level of active vitamin D below that needed to prevent rickets. Vitamin-D enrichment of milk has made rickets extremely rare in North America. Rickets usually becomes manifest during the growing period. Due to the failure to absorb calcium and phosphorus, the bones do not develop normal rigidity and a variety of deformities may appear. The skull may take on a peculiar and characteristic shape known as craniotabes. The ribs tend to enlarge at their free ends where they join the cartilage going to the breastbone. This visible deformity is known as the rachitic rosary. Leg deformities, either bowed legs or knock-knees, are common (Fig. 5-9). If the blood calcium drops too low, the patient may have tetany, a form of muscle spasms, and occasionally even convulsions. X-rays of the bones show characteristic findings with irregularities, retardation of bone development, and deformity. In adults, the only finding may be a characteristic type of pseudo-fracture. Pelvic deformities are common in girls with rickets and become manifest in adult women as defects in the birth canal, which may interfere with normal delivery. The actions of vitamin D are to facilitate the absorption of calcium and phosphorus in the intestinal tract, to maintain the blood calcium and phosphorus levels, to condition the osteoid (uncalcified bone protein matrix) for calcium and phosphorus deposition in bone growth and repair, and to inhibit the urinary loss of calcium.

Vitamin E Vitamin E, or alpha-tocopherol, is widely distributed throughout the tissues, cannot be synthesized by the body, and yet no unequivocal essential function has been found for it in man. In some animals it is necessary for normal fertility.

Vitamin K Vitamin K is essential for the hepatic synthesis of prothrombin, a component in the blood clotting mechanism which is the precursor of thrombin. Deficiency results in cutaneous bruising, urinary- and intestinal-tract bleeding, and frequent internal hemorrhage, often with minimal trauma. Severe hemorrhage, especially into the brain, can be fatal. Deficiency is infrequent because there are many dietary sources and because there is production of vitamin K by intestinal bacteria. In the newborn, deficiency may occur until intestinal bacteria become implanted and vitamin K production results. For this reason it is customary to give pregnant women supplemental vitamin K prior to delivery. Anything which interferes with the absorption of fat-soluble substances will

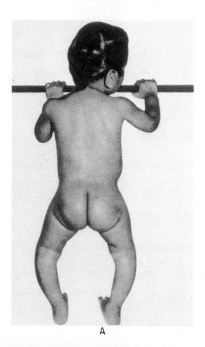

A

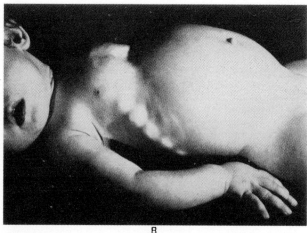

B

Figure 5-9   Rickets. *A:* Bony deformity of legs.   Bowlegs result
from standing on weakened bones after the second year.   Earlier
rickets produces a combination of bowed thighs and knock-knees.
B: Rachitic rosary.   This is one of the earliest signs of rickets and
is due to enlargement of the junction between the bony portion of
the rib and rib cartilage.   [*From R. L. Nemir in B. A. Thomas (ed.),*
Scope Manual on Nutrition, The Upjohn Company, Kalamazoo,
Mich., 1970, pp. 82 and 86.   By permission of the publishers.]

cause vitamin K deficiency. The situation often arises in which there is an obstruction to the biliary tract, blocking the delivery of bile and interfering with vitamin K absorption. Surgery is then hazardous unless supplementary vitamin K is administered by injection in order to bypass the ineffective intestinal absorption.

Electrolyte and Trace Element Deficiencies

The normal individual is capable of severe *sodium* conservation so that, with most dietary sources, sodium depletion is extremely rare. The chief exception in a normal individual is during the brief period of acclimatization in hot climates. Salt depletion may, however, occur in a variety of disease conditions, most prominently through the intestines and through the urine. Cholera is characterized by the loss of sodium chloride into a profuse diarrhea, often leading to staggering losses of salt and water which are fatal unless there is intravenous replacement. Some forms of kidney disease are associated with the specific loss of sodium into the urine, and the intensive use of drugs called diuretics, which enhance sodium loss through the kidneys in edema states, may also result in excessive salt depletion.

Chloride tends to follow the pattern of sodium. *Potassium* is not as well guarded as sodium, and urinary losses will continue even though there is evident body depletion. Fortunately, it is almost impossible to contrive a diet which does not have large amounts of potassium, and dietary inadequacy is rare. *Calcium*-poor diets can result in osteoporosis and, when associated with the inadequate intake of vitamin D, may demonstrate combined osteoporosis and osteomalacia.* Various deformities can result; one of the most common and important is distortion of the pelvic inlet with subsequent problems in childbirth. *Phosphorus* is extremely widespread in food and inadequate intake is unusual; low blood and tissue values are almost invariably due to excessive phosphorus losses. *Magnesium* deficiency rarely occurs as a result of inadequate intake. Exceptions to this include chronic alcoholism and kwashiorkor. Hypomagnesemia (low blood magnesium) is a vague syndrome which may manifest weakness, muscle twitching, and convulsions. Some of the characteristics of acute alcoholism have been attributed to magnesium losses. The administration of magnesium will promptly relieve the manifestations of hypomagnesemia. Calcium administration to these patients may magnify the signs and symptoms.

Iron deficiency leads to a characteristic anemia. The usual cause of

---

* Osteoporosis is the reduced density of bone due to a decrease in both protein matrix and calcium; osteomalacia is the reduced calcification of the normal protein matrix.

iron deficiency is chronic blood loss rather than inadequate intake. However, the amount of iron available in the normal diet may not be sufficient to cause optimal blood regeneration, and iron supplements are advisable. This is particularly true in women, who may lose excessive blood with the menstrual flow. *Iodine* intake may be inadequate, particularly in mountain and glacial areas in which drainage has leached the soil of an adequate iodine content. Inadequate iodine causes incompletely synthesized thyroid hormone to be stored in the glands, which enlarge to form a colloid goiter (Fig. 5-10). Marine and Kimball demonstrated in 1917 that colloid goiter could be prevented by the administration of iodine and introduced the use of iodized salt for this purpose. Iodized salt contains a hundred parts per million of iodine. This type of goiter is now rare where adequate iodine is used. *Fluoride,* in the concentration of one part per million in drinking water, will drastically reduce the rate of dental caries. Despite several decades of education, political pressures continue to block the

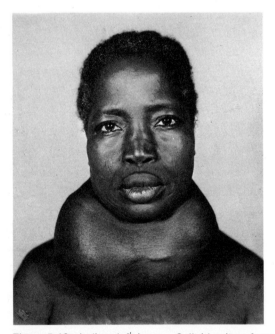

Figure 5-10 Iodine deficiency. Colloid goiters form where there is insufficient iodine in the soil or water to provide dietary iodine for the completion of the thyroid hormone molecule. The incomplete thyroid hormone is stored in the thyroid gland, causing it to enlarge. [*From A. O. Adesola in S. I. Schwartz (ed.), Tropical Surgery, McGraw-Hill, New York, 1971, p. 261. By permission of the publishers.*]

fluoridation of water in many communities. The rest of the elements are present in such small amounts that deficiency has probably not been a significant problem.

The Prevention of Nutritional Deficiency

For the first time, man has the knowledge and the technology to prevent diseases due to dietary insufficiency provided, of course, that population growth does not outstrip the potential for food production. The isolation, chemical identification, and in many cases, the synthesis of most of the vitamins by the end of the 1930s led to food enrichment programs in the 1940s. Thus milk is required to contain 400 units of vitamin D per quart, and white flour has been enriched with thiamine, riboflavin, nicotinic acid, and iron. It is now estimated that 90 percent of the white bread sold in the United States is enriched. Iodized salt is widely available although not universally used.

As a result of these measures, nutritional diseases which were once commonplace have become extremely rare in the United States and other technologically developed countries. Even in public hospitals, cases that were frequently seen three decades ago are no longer available for teaching purposes. The cases seen are rarely due to primary malnutrition, that is, unavailability of food, but are usually due to ignorance, faulty dietary habits, and disease. The elimination of malnutrition due to primary causes and ignorance should continue to be one of our major goals, but the limited nature of the problem should make this relatively easy.

By 1940, there was sufficient dietary and nutritional knowledge so that it was possible to prepare complete diets in which the content of each component was exactly known. These diets contained adequate calories, essential amino acids, essential fats, vitamins, and minerals. With these diets there was normal growth in children, maintenance of weight in adults, and the absence of any signs of nutritional deficiency. Experience in the past 30 years has failed to demonstrate any further unknown components. As a result, it was then possible to formulate absolute dietary requirements. The first of these was presented by the United States Food and Drug Administration in 1941 and is known as the Minimum Daily Requirement (MDR). This is the minimum *safe* amount of various components which will prevent the specific conditions and diseases which would be produced by lack of the specific component. The MDR has been widely quoted by manufacturers of vitamin pills and manufacturers of prepared foods. It does not follow that intakes of less than the MDR will necessarily produce deficiency manifestations, but recognizing that variations in diet will occur, this minimum level should be maintained.

In 1943, the Food and Nutrition Board of the National Research Coun-

Table 5-3 Recommended Daily Dietary Allowances, Food and Nutrition Board, National Academy of Sciences, National Research Council

	Age,[a] years	Weight, kg	Height, cm	Kcal[b]	Protein, gm	Fat-soluble vitamins			Water-soluble vitamins							Minerals				
						A,[e] IU	D, IU	E, IU	Ascorbic acid, mg	Folic acid, mg	Nicotinic acid,[c] mg eq.	Riboflavin, mg	Thiamine, mg	Vitamin B$_6$, mg	Vitamin B$_{12}$, μg	Ca, gm	P, gm	I$_2$, μg	Fe, mg	Mg, mg
Infants[d]	0–1	4–9	55–72	kg × 120	kg × 2	1,500	400	5	35	0.05	6	0.4	0.3	0.3	1.5	0.6	0.5	40	10	100
Children	1–10	12–28	81–131	1100–2200	25–40	2,500	400	10	40	0.2	10	1.0	0.7	1.0	4	0.8	0.8	80	10	200
Adolescent																				
Male	10–18	35–59	140–170	2500–3000	45–60	5,000	400	20	50	0.4	18	1.4	1.2	1.8	5	1.4	1.4	135	18	350
Female	10–18	35–54	142–160	2250–2300	50–55	5,000	400	20	50	0.4	15	1.4	0.9	1.8	5	1.3	1.3	115	18	350
Adult[f]																				
Male	18 up	67–70	175 up	2800	60 up	5,000	—	30	60	0.4	17	1.7	1.0	2.0	5	0.8	0.8	130	10	350
Female	18 up	58 up	163 up	2000	55 up	5,000	—	25	55	0.4	12	1.7	0.8	2.0	5	0.8	0.8	100	18	300
Pregnant	—	—	—	+200	65	6,000	400	30	60	0.8	15	1.8	1.0	2.5	8	+0.4	+0.4	125	18	450
Lactating	—	—	—	+1000	75	8,000	400	30	60	0.5	20	2.0	1.2	2.5	6	+0.5	+0.5	150	18	450

[a] The age ranges are more abridged here than in the original table.
[b] Calorie adjustment must be made for size and expenditure.
[c] Nicotinic acid equivalents include preformed nicotinic acid and tryptophane. 60 mg eq. to 1 mg nicotinic acid.
[d] Allowances for calcium, thiamine, riboflavin, and nicotinic acid are proportional to calorie requirement.
[e] Assuming one-fifth from preformed vitamin A and four-fifths from beta-carotene.
[f] These allowances will include a range of individual requirements for individuals living in the United States under usual environmental conditions. They can be achieved with a variety of common foods which will also supply other nutrients for which human requirements are uncertain.

SOURCE: Harrison's Principles of Internal Medicine, 6th ed., McGraw-Hill, New York, 1970, adapted from the more detailed table of the "Recommended Dietary Allowances" of the National Research Council, Food and Nutrition Board, 7th ed. Publication 1694 Price $1, NAS Printing and Publications Office, 2101 Constitution Ave. N.W., Washington, D.C. 20418.

cil of the United States put forth a Recommended Daily Allowance (RDA). In preparing these recommendations it was assumed that toxic levels of vitamins and minerals were not likely to be approached by the consumption of ordinary foods, but that all possibility of deficiencies should be excluded. Thus, the RDA exceeds by several fold the amount of each of these components necessary to prevent deficiency manifestations. On the other hand, an attempt was made to recommend caloric intakes which would be optimal. It is obvious that many individuals may fall below these recommendations in some individual components of the diet yet may not manifest evidences of deficiency. Therefore caution should be used in equating a diet inadequate in some components with actual malnutrition. Nevertheless, with exceptions to be noted in the next section, these recommendations are useful guides and represent major milestones. Table 5-3 is a modified presentation of the currently accepted Recommended Dietary Allowance.

OVERNUTRITION

It is ironic that the major dietary problem in the United States today is overnutrition. Extensive statistics, particularly by the insurance industry, indicate that weight more than 10 percent in excess of the mean is associated with a progressively increasing mortality rate. With the elimination of diseases due to undernutrition and infection, most individuals survive long enough to run the risks of arteriosclerosis, hypertension, diabetes, and a number of other metabolic and degenerative diseases, many of which appear to be aggravated by overnutrition.

Obesity

Obesity is due to the accumulation of fat, which represents the storage of unused energy. Therefore, ultimately all obesity is due to an excessive caloric intake and can be reversed by the proper regulation of that intake. Normally, the caloric intake is carefully adjusted by the appetite, and the precision of this mechanism must be appreciated. The normal caloric needs depend upon the sex, age, and activity of the individual, upon the environmental temperature (more calories are needed for heat in cold weather than in hot), and upon the size of the individual. The excess input of only one pat of butter or one slice of bread daily would theoretically result in a 10-pound weight gain in the course of a year. This would be slightly compensated by the increased energy requirements for the same level of activity in a larger individual. Yet with all these variables, the day-to-day and year-to-year weight changes are ordinarily remarkably small.

As the individual ages, the cell mass decreases and physical activity becomes less, reducing the caloric needs. However, for reasons of habit or otherwise, the caloric intake is insufficiently reduced and most aging individuals tend to maintain the same weight or even to gain weight, replacing cell loss with adipose tissue.

The etiology of obesity is not at all clear and undoubtedly many factors are involved. Much of what passes for hereditary factors may in fact be cultural. A family of hearty eaters may have the appetite level set higher than the average, and this conditioning is transmitted to the children, who are brought up in the same environment. Recently Hirsch has proposed that there are two types of obesity: one in which the normal number of fat cells are overloaded by fat storage, and the other in which there is an excessive number of fat cells. His investigations suggest that the number of fat cells is not hereditary but is conditioned early in life by overfeeding. The patients with a normal number of overstuffed fat cells are relatively amenable to weight reduction, whereas those who have an increased number of fat cells may have altered fat metabolism and are extremely refractory to treatment. Although intriguing, this hypothesis has not yet been established.

Undoubtedly, modern life, with its reduced physical activity on one hand and the increased use of refined foods with high calories and low bulk on the other, contributes to the difficulty in maintaining an optimal weight. Certainly, psychological factors are important in obesity. It has been thought that for some individuals eating provides gratifications which cannot be fulfilled in any other way. The common supposition that metabolic defects account for obesity is rarely demonstrable. Patients with hypothyroidism are not outstandingly obese, and much of their increase in weight is due to retention of fluid in the tissues. It has been demonstrated that in experimental animals damage to the appetite control center in the brain can produce compulsive eating and grotesque obesity which is ordinarily rare in animals not subject to forced feeding. There is little evidence that this is the cause of obesity in any but rare human instances. For the present, at least, the reasons for the failure of appetite control are obscure.

There is little doubt that obesity is associated with early mortality from the major current causes of death. As we saw in the previous section, the major nutritional preoccupation has been with undernutrition and minimum standards have been established. There is some suspicion that the zeal in this direction may have been excessive and that some level that is now considered caloric undernutrition and results in relative physical underdevelopment may in fact be optimal for longevity. Some work along these lines was conducted by McCay over 40 years ago. He demonstrated that if rats were sufficiently calorically undernourished to prevent normal maturation and then eventually allowed a sufficient diet, the experimental animals would survive an average of approximately 1,500 days as opposed to the normal average for the strain of 900 days. This type of experiment has been repeated a number of times on a variety of animals and has been essentially confirmed. Its applicability to humans is not known, but there is evidence to suggest that populations that have been calorically undernourished by our standards and that have succeeded in avoiding early mortality may, in fact, have a greater average longevity than more "optimally" nourished populations.

The treatment of obesity has been less than satisfactory, and it has been commented that the prognosis for a 5-year cure of obesity is less than that of a 5-year cure of cancer! Appetite suppressants are of only temporary value. Obviously, in order to maintain an optimum weight, there must be a permanent readjustment of the caloric intake and expenditure. The essence of weight control is that a continued program is required which includes both decreased food intake and increased physical exercise.

Other Forms of Nutritional Excess

Excesses of other nutrients infrequently produce toxic manifestations, although there are specific exceptions. Ingestion of vitamin A in doses of 75,000 to 500,000 international units (IU) daily has produced a wide variety of symptoms which are reversed on withdrawal of the drug. Intakes of this level could only result from the use of concentrates and not of natural foods. An exception is polar bear liver, which contains tremendous amounts of vitamin A, and death has resulted from its ingestion. Hypervitaminosis D is more serious. At one time large doses of vitamin D were used in an attempt to treat a variety of diseases, particularly arthritis. Doses in excess of 50,000 units per day produced an abnormal elevation of calcium in the blood and the characteristic symptoms of hypercalcemia as well as neurological signs and soft-tissue calcifications. Deposition of calcium in the kidney can cause kidney failure and death. A few years ago a bizarre syndrome was noted in England in which children developed elevated blood calcium and a peculiar "elfin" appearance. This was found to be due to the excessive addition of vitamin D to fortified milk. Since the recognition of hypervitaminosis D, the frequency of its occurrence has decreased abruptly.

Excess fluoride at the level of five parts per million in water will produce mottling of the teeth. A number of the elements such as magnesium, manganese, iron, and even sodium or potassium can be toxic if taken in large quantities, normally many times beyond those possible in any natural combination of foods.

REMAINING PROBLEMS IN NUTRITION

The focus of research in nutrition is shifting now that metabolic diseases and diseases of aging are becoming more prevalent. New approaches are being explored regarding the quantitative interrelationships of various dietary substances. This is particularly applicable to the development of atherosclerosis (Chap. 10), which contributes to nearly 50 percent of all deaths. For example, it has been found that there are genetic factors which control the concentration of the blood lipids, which in turn may have some effect upon the development of arteriosclerosis. In most people the concentration of blood fats is sensitive to the total caloric intake; however, in some individuals hyperlipemia (excessive fat in the blood) is stimulated particularly by a diet high in carbohydrate, while in others it is enhanced by a diet high in fats or cholesterol. Other studies show that the replacement of some of the long-chain saturated fatty acids, which are the usual components of the triglycerides, with unsaturated fatty acids has resulted in a reduction in the concentration of the blood lipids and may impede the development of arteriosclerosis.

A moderately extensive list of similar examples could be presented. It should be apparent, however, that a complex interrelationship of dietary intake, individual variation, and possibly specific chemical intervention may be involved. It is probable that there will not be all-inclusive generalizations. Yet the potential for intricate and rational diet manipulation is virtually unexplored and challenging. (It may be, in fact, that one man's meat is another man's poison.)

In conclusion, the minimum dietary requirements are now well established, and deficiency disorders have been identified and are reasonably well understood. There is little reason for the persistence of overt deficiences, and these are in fact becoming quite rare. The optimum quantities and ratios of the constituents have been less well established and will be subject to continuing investigation.

BIBLIOGRAPHY

DAVIDSON, L. S. P. and R. PASSMORE: *Human Nutrition and Dietetics,* 4th ed., Baltimore: The Williams & Wilkins Company, 1969.

KEYS, A., J. BROZEK, A. HENSCHEL, O. MICKELSEN, and H. L. TAYLOR: *The Biology of Human Starvation,* Minneapolis: The University of Minnesota Press, 1950.

WILLIAMS, S. R.: *Nutrition and Diet Therapy,* St. Louis: The C. V. Mosby Company, 1969.

WOHL, M. G. and R. S. GOODHART (eds.): *Modern Nutrition in Health and Disease,* 4th ed., Philadelphia: Lea and Febiger, 1968.

THOMAS, B. A. (ed.): *Scope Manual on Nutrition,* Kalamazoo: The Upjohn Company, 1970.

Trauma

Trauma is defined as injury. Although other causes are often included, such as bacteriological, immunological, and even psychological causes, the present discussion will be limited to physical and chemical injuries. Trauma, as a cause of disability and death, has been frequent throughout man's history. Minor degrees of trauma may occur almost daily; in the past, severe and often lethal trauma was associated with falls, hunting accidents, attacks by dangerous animals, and human combat. Today, the list is probably similar, although with markedly different emphases; automobile and industrial accidents have become increasingly important and have replaced hunting accidents and animal attacks. To ancient man the immediate cause of injury was undoubtedly obvious. However, it is only with modern scientific techniques that the indirect effects of injury could be determined and effective therapy instituted. At the same time, there are a number of types of tissue injury caused by physical and chemical agents whose actions are not as evident as those of direct physical trauma. Many of these have resulted from modern technology, such as the production of electricity and ionizing radiation. However, since the tissue injury results and healing responses are similar, they are all appropriately discussed as a group.

MECHANICAL INJURY

Mechanical injuries are subject to the physical laws of force and to the nature of the tissues involved. It is well to remember that force is related linearly to mass and to the square of the velocity. Thus, doubling the weight of the missile, whether it be a bullet or a passenger in a car, doubles the force which can be expressed by the missile, whereas doubling its speed quadruples the force. In addition, a missile may have additional energy due to rotation or torque. The mode of application of the energy is important; a force applied to a large area will have less effect than the same force applied to a smaller area. The duration of the period of deceleration is also of great importance, and a cushioning effect will reduce the severity of injury.

Wounds

A wound is a mechanically produced disruption of tissue. If injury is superficial and results only in the frictional loss of surface cells, it is called an *abrasion;* if it is linear, it is a *scratch.* These injuries, of themselves, are usually minor and heal without difficulty. A *contusion* results from injury to deep tissues without disruption of the surface epithelium. In a contusion blood vessels are ruptured, resulting in extravasation of blood (leakage of blood outside of the vessels), which causes pain and swelling of the tissues and some interference with function. Extravasation of blood under the skin results in a bruise or ecchymosis, which is initially red but turns blue and then green as blood pigment is metabolized. If the contusion is deep, there may be a period of delay before the blood pigments are visible under the skin, or they may not appear at all.

A *laceration* is a tear in the tissue, resulting from stretching forces greater than the tensile strength of the tissue (Fig. 6-1). Oblique forces produce linear or curved lacerations, whereas vertical forces more frequently have ragged margins and a stellate (star-shaped) configuration. Compressive forces on internal organs may cause lacerations with or without external evidence. This may involve such organs as the liver; hollow, gas-filled viscera; and blood vessels. An *incised wound* is caused by a sharp instrument, perhaps most frequently a knife, and commonly in the deliberate production of surgical incisions.

Penetrating injuries may result from missiles and pointed weapons. Occasionally the broken ends of bones, such as fractured ribs, may cause

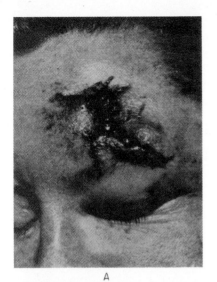 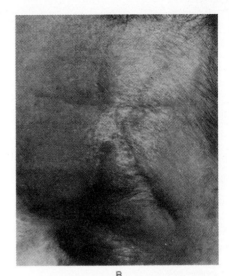

A B

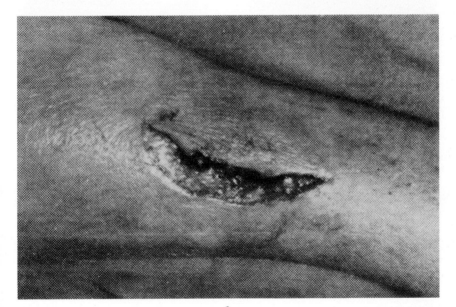

C

Figure 6-1 Lacerations. *A:* A stellate lesion caused by a direct blow with a relatively blunt object. *B:* The stellate nature of the lesion is more readily evident after healing. *C:* A semilunar laceration produced by an oblique blow. *(From R. V. S. Thompson, Primary Repair of Soft Tissue Injuries, Melbourne University Press, Carlton, Victoria, 1969, pp. 100 and 218. By permission of the publishers.)*

penetrating injuries unrelated to the site of surface trauma. Wounds produced by missiles, especially gunshot wounds, are associated with specific characteristics. The entry wound usually conforms to the shape of the missile and, in the case of a bullet, is generally round and slightly smaller than the size of the bullet itself (Fig. 6-2A). On impact the tissue is set in motion and acts as a secondary missile, creating injury in an enlarging cone. Fragments of bone or metal may also act as secondary missiles and may go in a different path than the bullet. Any rotational force of the missile will also be taken up by the tissues, and this component will be enhanced if the missile is irregular in shape, such as a piece of shrapnel or an irregular fragment from an explosion. If sufficient energy remains in the missile to enable it to leave the tissues, the exit wound will, as a result of these processes, be considerably larger and more irregular than was the entry wound (Fig. 6-2B). The path of a missile in the body

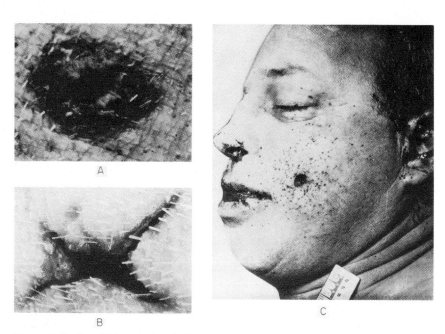

Figure 6-2   Gunshot wounds. *A:* Entry wound showing punched out margins. *B:* Exit wound with irregular lacerations and larger tissue defect. [*From A. R. Moritz and L. Adelson in W. A. D. Anderson (ed.), Pathology, 6th ed., Mosby, St. Louis, 1971, p. 150. By permission of the publishers.*] *C:* Entry wound in which there was a moderate distance between the gun muzzle and the face (6 to 12 inches), producing powder burns. [*From A. R. Moritz in W. A. D. Anderson (ed.), Pathology, 5th ed., Mosby, St. Louis, 1966, p. 122. By permission of the publishers.*]

may not be direct because of the varying densities of tissue, and often the missile is found at a great distance from the anticipated track. If the gun is fired at short range, the skin may be impregnated with gunpowder and there may be flashburns from the muzzle (Fig. 6-2C). Stellate entry wounds may result from the expansion of muzzle gases when the muzzle is pressed directly against the skin. Obviously, information regarding gunshot wounds must be collected carefully and in great detail because of its possible medicolegal significance.

Fractures

A *fracture* is a discontinuity in bone from any cause (Fig. 6-3). If the fracture is not complicated by a disruption in the skin, the fracture is a *closed fracture*. If, on the other hand, the tissues have been lacerated either by the bone fragments or the trauma which produced the fracture, then it is an *open fracture*. These terms are preferable to the previously used terms of *simple* and *compound* fractures. The loss of skin continuity introduces the possibility of infection to the problems proposed by the presence of the fracture itself. A *linear fracture* is one in which the bone discontinuity can be seen as a line in the x-ray but in which the bone components retain their normal position. A *displaced fracture* is one in which

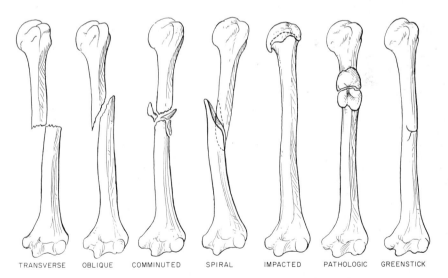

TRANSVERSE   OBLIQUE   COMMINUTED   SPIRAL   IMPACTED   PATHOLOGIC   GREENSTICK

Figure 6-3 Fractures of long bones. [*Modified from O. P. Hampton, Jr., and W. T. Fitts, Jr., in J. G. Allen et al. (eds.), Surgery, Principles and Practice, Lippincott, Philadelphia, 1957, p. 311. By permission of the publishers.*]

the bones no longer lie in their proper relationship to each other. An *impacted fracture* is one in which one part of the bone has been telescoped into the other at the site of the break. *Spiral fractures* are most frequently seen in the leg bones and are due to a shearing force such as might occur when a ski is caught and the body goes on to a twisting fall. *Greenstick fractures* are seen in young children in whom there is a large cartilaginous component to the bone. The bone may be bent with some disruption of tissue but without a complete fracture, such as occurs in the greenstick from which it derives its name.

Occasionally bones undergo pathological processes, such as infection, tumor, or metabolic change, in which the bone is markedly weakened. Under these circumstances a relatively small amount of trauma may result in a fracture at the disease site. These are *pathological fractures* and are often the first evidence of the underlying disease process. A particularly complex type of fracture is the *comminuted fracture,* in which there is a shattering of bone with a production of multiple fragments. This is most likely to occur in severe accidents and in missile injuries. It is often difficult to reassemble the multiple fragments into a pattern resembling the normal state, and the frequent association with open wounds increases the possibility of serious infection.

Dislocation refers to the disruption of joint alignment without fracture of the bones. Ligaments, tendons, and joint capsules may be torn and this complicates healing. In the *fracture-dislocation* there is not only dislocation of the joint but also an associated fracture.

Certain types of accidental forces are so common that they are associated with specific fracture patterns. For example, a fall in which the outflung arm is used to break the impact characteristically results in a fracture of the wrist which involves the radius and ulna and is known as a Colle's fracture. It is especially common in young children and aged individuals. Such a fall may produce an impacted fracture of the humerus at the shoulder, especially in older individuals. The shoulder is also a relatively frequent site of pathological fractures, especially due to a spreading cancer of the breast in women. Fractures of the metacarpal bones (the long bones in the hand) are frequently the result of blows with the unprotected fist, as in street fights. Fractures of the toes often result from dropping heavy objects on them. An extremely common fracture of the leg results from a twisting fall and involves the tibia and fibula just above the ankle joint. The tibia at or just below the knee is often fractured as a result of being struck by an automobile bumper, and common causes for fractures of the shaft of the femur are automobile and especially motorcycle accidents. Aging is associated with a loss of calcium from the bones, which increases their brittleness. For this reason fractures of the femur

at the hip are extremely common in elderly individuals and constitute a
serious threat to life in this group. Reduction in bone calcium or osteoporosis may affect the bodies of the vertebrae, and compression or impacted fractures may occur as a result of lifting heavy weights or even of bend-
ing forward under stress. Fracture of the mandible most frequently results
from fistfights and automobile accidents.

Skull fractures are of two types: explosive and penetrating. The skull
is an extremely rigid sphere and compressive forces may result in explosive
fractures at a distance from the site of maximal applied force. Penetrating
injuries may be produced by missiles, pointed weapons, or other forms of
locally applied force. The danger of skull fractures lies more in injury
to the brain tissue than to the bone. Indirect explosive fractures may be
linear. The most common types are basal skull fractures and fractures to
the temporal bone. Direct injury may cause immediate destruction of
brain tissue and may, in the case of an open wound, create a pathway for
infection. The outer portion of the skull is made up of a double layer, and
a blow which causes only a small depression of the outer table may cause a
much larger depression of the inner table (see Fig. 6-4).

The amount of tissue damage caused by the injury may be sufficient to
make the injured part functionless or may even lead to death. However,
injury also leads to certain secondary effects which may compromise the
function and even the survival of the individual. Important immediate
effects are shock and hemorrhage, and later effects are often associated

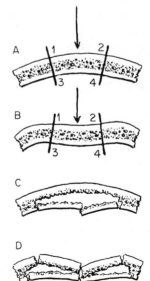

Figure 6-4 Skull fractures demonstrating how damage
to the inner table of the skull can be extensive and
cause damage to the brain without proportionate damage to the outer table. *(From B. J. Anson and W. G.
Maddock, Callander's Surgical Anatomy, 4th ed.,
Saunders, Philadelphia, 1958, p. 11. By permission
of the publishers.)*

with secondary infection. When there is interference with a vital function, it may be necessary to substitute for that function, as with a respirator or an artificial kidney. The success of measures to combat these complications has been so great that if the individual does not die immediately from the injury, his chance of survival is extremely good, although the processes of repair may be inadequate for the complete restoration of function of the injured tissues.

ATMOSPHERIC PRESSURE INJURY

Exposure to extreme variations in atmospheric pressure is increasingly frequent as a result of high-altitude flying, space exploration, mountain climbing, deep-sea diving, underwater construction, and related activities. The number of participants in recreational deep-sea diving and mountain climbing, and especially those uninstructed in pressure techniques, is so great that injuries resulting from atmospheric pressure changes are not uncommon.

High Environmental Pressure

Rapid increases in atmospheric pressure in general are not harmful, and pressure several times that of the atmosphere can be tolerated without difficulty. Such problems as may arise are related to the gas mixtures rather than the pressures. Above 3 atmospheres the usual proportions of nitrogen result in a narcotic effect with decreased ability to work, changes in mood, and impaired judgment in motor performance. The pressure of carbon dioxide must be kept within normal limits in order to prevent acidosis. Even oxygen in high concentrations has been associated with problems. Many of the difficulties are now being surmounted by the use of helium in place of nitrogen. If the passageway of the eustachian tube is not freely open to the middle ear, increases in pressure may result in a painful inward pressure on the eardrum. This is a common experience for all who holiday in the mountains or who travel by air.

Decompression

Pressure injury is most frequently encountered in association with a too rapid decrease in environmental pressure. According to Behnke, at atmospheric pressure there are about 9 milliliters of nitrogen dissolved in each kilogram of body water and about 55 milliliters in each kilogram of body fat. A 70-kilogram man with 7 kilograms of fat contains about 400 milliliters of nitrogen in his body fluids, 100 milliliters in bone and spinal cord, and 400 milliliters in his adipose tissue. Presumably a comparable amount of nitrogen can be held in the tissues with each additional atmosphere of pressure. Largely as a result of the poor circulation through fatty tissue, the nitrogen is not released all at one time upon decompression. Thus, if decompression has been performed too rapidly, bubbles of nitrogen may gradually form in the blood vessels over a period of several hours.

Three types of organ involvement and associated symptoms have been described. The most common of these has long been known as the *bends* and is characterized by slowly developing, throbbing pain most frequently felt in the bones and joints. Late complications include areas of bone and joint destruction. A more life-threatening type of complication has been known since early caisson* work as the *chokes.* This is due to the gradual accumulation of nitrogen bubbles in the right side of the heart and pulmonary vessels, resulting in anoxia (inadequate oxygenation of the blood) and dyspnea (shortness of breath). This syndrome may require several hours after decompression for its full manifestation. The early symptoms include substernal distress made worse by deep inspiration, which is frequently followed by severe coughing. Sensitivity to tobacco smoke may be an early symptom. The third group includes central nervous system findings which are much less frequent than would be expected. A relatively common and serious complication is paralysis of spinal cord origin. Almost all these findings can be reversed if treated early by recompression and more gradual decompression. The presence of large gas emboli (bubbles in the blood vessels) can be fatal if a major vessel remains obstructed or if the heartbeat is unable to force the gas out of the ventricles.

Another form of disability resulting from decompression is due to the expansion of gas in natural body cavities. For example, air trapped in the stomach may expand upon the reduction of external pressure, and rupture may result. Similarly, gases trapped in the intestines, in the sinuses, and in the middle ear may, with their expansion, result in acute local symptoms. Rapid ascent in scuba diving (in which air is breathed under pressure) without allowing excess pulmonary gas to be released may cause great intrapulmonary pressure, laceration of veins, and accidental air embolism.

Low Environmental Pressure

The body can tolerate reduced pressure considerably less well than increased pressure chiefly because there is reduction in the pressure of oxygen and consequent failure to oxygenate the tissues adequately. In

---

*The caisson is a diving bell which is used in underwater construction. The bottom is open, but water is kept out by maintaining an adequate air pressure.

altitudes under 10,000 feet, or 0.60 atmosphere, the normal individual experiences very little difficulty. It is possible to work at altitudes as high as 15,000 feet, but this requires adaptation. An important component of adaptation is an increase in the hemoglobin so that more oxygen can be transported to the tissues. It is not possible to maintain permanent residence above 18,000 feet, or 0.05 atmosphere, and supplementary oxygen is necessary. At the present time commercial airplanes are pressurized to 10,000 feet or lower, and there are few individuals capable of traveling for whom this altitude represents any specific hazard.

Blast

Blast is a sudden change in pressure due to an explosion. Air blast affects the side toward the blast most severely. Immersion blast occurs when the individual is partially or completely in the water and the pressure is evenly distributed. Solid blast is transmitted through the parts of the individual in contact with the solid, such as the deck of a ship, the wall of a shelter, or the floor of a building. Characteristically, air blast produces multiple lacerations of the lung with intra-alveolar bleeding and air embolism into the veins through vascular ruptures. Immersion blast results in frequent visceral ruptures. In both air and immersion blasts there may be no external injury, and the internal injuries may be obscure. Solid blast produces injuries similar to those of a simple mechanical injury acting through the area of contact. A blast may be so severe that the body is completely demolished by the explosion. In addition to the direct blast injuries caused by the change in pressure, there may also be secondary injuries from objects set into motion by the blast, burns, asphyxia from combustion products, and in the case of the atom bomb, ionizing radiation injury as well.

SONIC INJURY

Relatively little injury has been attributed to sound waves. Excessive audible sound may affect hearing acuity after long periods of exposure. The classical examples have generally been those of boilermakers and jackhammer operators. Single episodes of intense sound have also been reported to cause hearing loss. Most commonly, this claim is made in association with either blast injury or close proximity to the firing of large cannon. High-frequency sound waves above 20,000 cycles per second are known as ultrasonic waves and have increased penetrating ability. The energy of these waves is dissipated by frictional heat, and these properties are useful in the production of local and deep heating of tissues. Excessive energy produces gas-filled tissue cavities which can cause increased local heating, electrical discharges, mechanical movement, and certain types of chemical reactions. By using special focusing equipment, ultrasonic waves can be used for several types of operative procedures without actually cutting into the tissues. For example, nerve tissue can be destroyed without affecting the blood vessels. Pain from heat usually precedes tissue damage and serves as some protection from overexposure.

THERMAL INJURY

Burns

Cellular damage results if the tissue temperature is maintained $5°C$ or more above normal. Tissue may, of course, be destroyed immediately by incineration. Tissues not immediately killed respond with dilation of capillaries and small blood vessels. This is associated with increased blood vessel permeability, the production of local edema, cell injury, and cell death. These responses decrease with the increasing depth of the tissues away from the surface.

Burns are generally classified as follows: *First-degree burns* are associated with erythema, or redness, due to dilation of the superficial blood vessels; the epidermis is injured but not destroyed, and healing is prompt. *Second-degree burns* are associated with epidermal cell death; blisters frequently form separating the epidermis from the dermis (Fig. 6-5). However, since the dermis is intact, there is rapid replacement of epidermal cells from hair follicles and glands within the dermis and there is no scar formation. *Third-degree burns* are associated with irreversible injury to the dermis. The wound fills with scar tissue and is covered by a thin layer of epithelium which grows in from the normal tissue at the edges of the burn. Severe burns can produce incapacitating and disfiguring scars. Healing can be accelerated and deformity reduced by the effective use of skin grafts.

Burns involving large areas of skin are frequently fatal. The extensive destruction of epithelium results in excessive loss of fluids and protein from the denuded surface. This, in turn, causes dehydration, blood concentration, and shock. The protein-rich serum on the surface of the wound becomes an ideal culture medium for bacteria, and infections are common and serious. Digestion of dead tissues by proteolytic (protein-dissolving) enzymes may release toxic substances and add to the critical situation. Blood concentration and shock predispose to phlebothrombosis (clotting of blood in the veins). In the past, degenerative changes in the

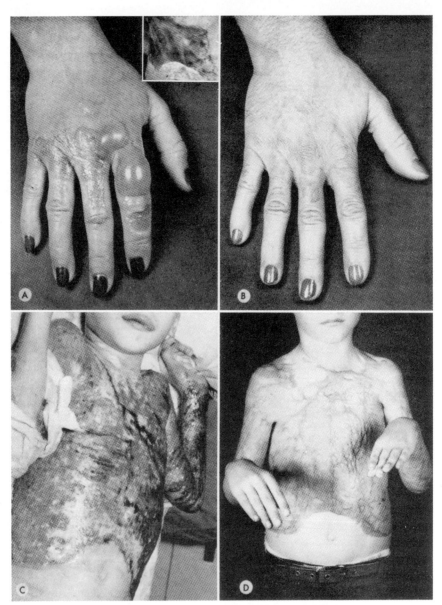

Figure 6-5   Burns.   A: Second-degree burns from ignited cooking
fat.   B: Healing, showing lack of scar formation because dermis
was undamaged.   C: Third-degree burn from ignited clothing.
D: Healing, with massive scar formation requiring skin grafts.
(From R. P. Morehead, Human Pathology, McGraw-Hill, New York,
1965, p. 309.   By permission of the publishers.)

kidney, adrenals, and liver were attributed directly to the burn. It is now believed that the kidney changes may be due to shock; the adrenal changes to the stress response with depletion of adrenal hormones; and the liver changes to absorption of tannic acid, which at one time was though to be an effective way of covering the exposed area of the burn but which, for this reason, has now been abandoned.

The prognosis with burns depends largely upon the amount of surface which has been involved. A simple rule has been devised: The head and arms each represent 9 percent of the body surface and the legs and front and back of the torso are each 18 percent of the body surface; the perineal region represents 1 percent. Age is an important factor in the prognosis of burn injury. Almost all patients over the age of 65 with 25 percent body surface involvement will die, whereas only 10 percent of individuals under 45 years of age will die with this much body surface involvement. Therapy is aimed at treatment of shock by fluid replacement, prevention of infection, eventual skin replacement by grafting, and restoration of function.

Environmental Heat Injury

Except under extreme stress, the normal individual is able to maintain a normal body temperature by insensible perspiration. Some individuals, especially the aged and those with brain damage, may lose this capacity for heat regulation. Systemic hyperthermia results when the blood temperature exceeds 45.2°C and leads to the condition known as *heat stroke.* Such high levels of body temperature may result from fever, but they are more likely to occur with elevated environmental temperatures. There is vasodilatation with an effective decrease in the blood volume, tachycardia and cardiac dilatation, and erratic stimulation of the respiratory centers. In experimental animals, the blood-potassium concentration has been reported to be elevated; if this is true in humans, lethal levels may be reached. Immediate cooling is essential since the mortality is extremely high. The most common response to environmental heat is *heat exhaustion,* characterized by peripheral vascular failure with cold, clammy skin, dilated pupils, decreased blood pressure and temperature. The cause of heat exhaustion is not known, and it does not appear to be due to depletion of fluids or salts. This response is usually seen early on exposure and responds quickly to rest and shading. *Heat cramps* are well known and are due to salt depletion. They are characterized by painful spasm of voluntary muscles and respond quickly to salt replacement. They almost invariably occur in unacclimatized persons in good physical condition. Salt adaptation occurs in a few days, and extended salt replacement is usually not necessary.

Cold Injury

Cold injury can be divided into three major classifications: first, very low temperatures with actual tissue freezing; second, cold beyond temperature defenses but not to freezing; and third, environmental cold within temperature defenses. Actual freezing injury is termed *frostbite*. Frostbite (Fig. 6-6) results in severe and often irreparable injury to the blood vessels. Skin injury may or may not be reversible. Because of blood vessel injury, tissue is often lost by ischemic necrosis (tissue death due to inadequate circulating blood). Treatment consists of rapid rewarming, avoidance of trauma, and conservative surgery. No treatment as yet seems to alter the course. Fifty percent of frostbite patients will have serious sequelae (residual complications) consisting of painful cold feet, numbness, excessive sweating, abnormal color, and limitation of motion; scars, tissue loss, abnormal nails, and cystlike bone defects near the digital joints persist as objective find-

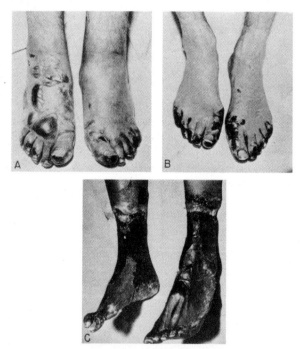

Figure 6-6   *A* and *B:* Trench foot. There is evidence of considerable healing.   *C:* Gangrenous frostbite. The blood vessels have been destroyed and there is a clear line of demarcation between the living and dead tissues. *(From D. M. Pillsbury, W. B. Shelly, and A. M. Kligman, Dermatology, Saunders, Philadelphia, 1956, p. 1261. By permission of the publishers.)*

ings. Prevention of frostbite requires proper equipment, training, and acclimatization.

The largest recent American experience with cold injury was in Korea in 1951. In additon to frostbite, a nonfreezing injury was recognized which has been termed *immersion foot* or *trench foot.* This condition has also been seen in survivors of shipwreck adrift for long periods in open boats. Although there is no actual freezing, the difference from frostbite is more of degree than kind. Injury to muscle and nerve is relatively permanent, whereas injury to blood vessels and skin appears to be reversible. The sensation of "burning feet" may persist for several years after recovery from the acute episode.

Environmental Cold Adaptation

In general, man can tolerate a greater degree of lowering of the environmental temperature below the blood temperature than he can elevation above it. Even so, modern man's tolerance is less than generally imagined. In one study a lean man was unable to stay in water of 16°C (60°F) for 2 hours, although an obese man was able to do so. At temperatures below 10°C (50°F), the unprotected normal individual appears unable to maintain his normal body temperature. In another experiment, three subjects clad only in shorts were exposed to an atmospheric temperature of 8°C (46°F) for 4 days. Their metabolism was greatly accelerated and pulse rate and respirations were elevated. Weight loss was marked. Surprisingly, there was an immersion-foot syndrome which appeared several days after the test and consisted of swelling, pain, tingling, and numbness of the feet which persisted for 2 months. There is evidence that some cold adaptation is possible and genetic selection may be a factor, since Arctic peoples such as Eskimos are capable of performing functions which even adapted but nonresident individuals are unable to duplicate at the same temperatures.

Hypothermia

Until recently it was believed that cells could not withstand hypothermia (temperature lowering) more than 15° below the normal level. Recent studies indicate that it is possible to produce reversible hypothermia to temperatures of 10°C or even lower. Apparently, the principal problem has been that cooling of tissues does not progress equally. Tissues with delayed cooling have continued to produce metabolic products which, on rewarming, have flooded the system. The load has been aggravated by the inadequate response of the organism to the stress. The use of techniques to continuously cool the blood outside the body by circulating it through a refrigerating unit makes it possible to cool the tissues more uniformly, and chemical measures designed to counteract the metabolic imbalances have made the recent achievements possible. Hypothermia is important because the body metabolism slows down with the lowering of the temperature. This has made hypothermia especially valuable in the treatment of a number of infections and as an adjunct to heart surgery, where reduced metabolic needs are helpful because the circulation must be temporarily impaired during the course of the procedure. Another use for cold is the recent development of cryosurgery. By this technique, the tissues to be removed are first frozen. This has provided promising technical advantages for handling some tissues.

ELECTRICAL INJURY

A complete circuit is necessary to produce electrical injury. Since interposition between two electrodes is rare, this means that the individual must be grounded before electricity from a live wire will pass through his body. In general, the effects depend upon the kind, amount, pathway, and duration of the current flow. Alternating current has approximately five times the effect of direct current. In accordance with Ohm's law, the amount of current which passes through the tissues depends directly upon voltage and inversely upon resistance. Water and sweat will decrease the resistance and increase the current. If the heart or the respiratory center (in the brain stem) is in the pathway of the current, as little as 100 milliamperes may be effective in stopping the heart or respiration. A 60-cycle alternating current appears to be particularly effective in producing cardiac arrest. In general, low voltage tends to produce ventricular fibrillation, an ineffective quivering of the heart muscle, whereas high voltage produces respiratory arrest as well as cardiac standstill during the current flow. However, the respiratory arrest is more likely to persist than cardiac arrest after the current has been discontinued. The duration of current flow is obviously important.

In addition to interference with cardiac and respiratory rhythmicity, electric current can cause direct cellular destruction by heat and electrolysis (chemical decomposition as a result of the passage of a electrical current) and may produce indirect results by stimulation of strong muscular contractions. Heat production increases with the square of the current. Therefore, linear increases in voltage and decreases in resistance produce a geometric increase in heat. If a contact is large, the current in any particular area may be insufficient to cause injury, while the same current in a small area may be capable of producing a burn. Since most resistance is at the point of contact between the source and the skin, skin burns are the most common. No consistent pathological change has been noted. An arc may produce local pitting and alternating current may cause small amounts of electrode metal to be deposited at the site. Voltages up to 110 rarely cause a large electrothermal injury. Burns also may be caused by contact with an electrically heated conductor. However, these should be considered as thermal burns, since they are caused by the heat in the conductor rather than by the electric current.

The stimulation of strong muscular contractions by an electrical current has practical implications. For example, many individuals are unable to release the wire or other source of electrical current which is the cause of the shock. As a result, current continues to flow and shock persists. Muscular contractions may be quite violent, and actual convulsions are common. These injuries frequently result in compression fractures of the vertebrae. At one time vertebral fractures were frequently seen following electroshock therapy for various psychoses. The use of curarelike drugs to block muscle spasm has almost completely eliminated this hazard of electroshock therapy.

Electroshock can cause cardiac arrest and ventricular fibrillation, both fatal if untreated. However, Lown has shown that properly timed direct current can be extremely effective in treating cardiac arrest and in converting a number of types of irregularity of the heartbeat, including ventricular fibrillation, into a normal rhythm. Cardiac arrest and ventricular fibrillation are particularly common following a "heart attack," which is usually due to coronary occlusion and myocardial infarction (see Chap. 10). In many instances the heart is not sufficiently damaged to be unable to support life, but the sudden injury interrupts the mechanism for rhythmic contraction and the heart "stalls." New instruments have been developed for cardiac monitoring and for safely shocking the heart back into a normal rhythm, and a significant number of lives are being prolonged.

CHEMICAL INJURY

All the body functions are ultimately chemical, and it is at times difficult to separate chemical from other types of injury. A *poison* has been defined as an injurious substance which acts in small amounts, usually less than 50 grams if a solid or a liquid. It must have an external origin and act by chemical rather than physical means. Remote systemic and protoplasmic effects of chemicals are more easily discussed in the context of metabolic disorders, and unique sensitivities to certain chemicals are more appropriately discussed in the section on allergy and hypersensitivity. Our attention will be focused on direct local chemical effects. Irritation implies that there is an active tissue response to the offending chemical.

Corrosive effects are due to the direct local chemical action on the tissues. These effects generally cause tissue death, thus precluding an active tissue response.

Irritant Poisons

Irritant poisons most generally act on the skin, respiratory system, or gastrointestinal tract. The usual response is a swelling of the tissues and an exudation of fluids. In the respiratory system these responses result in obstruction of the flow of oxygen into the lungs, and in the lung tissue they block the absorption of oxygen into the blood. The patient often dies of asphyxiation, literally drowning in his own fluids. Characteristically, there is a delay of several hours as the exudates form. For reasons unknown, various chemicals act at different levels of the respiratory tract. Ammonia affects the eyes, nose, and pharynx and produces early effects which are generally fairly quickly reversible and rarely fatal. Chlorine affects the tracheobronchial tree and may cause death by obstruction after 12 to 24 hours. Phosgene, ozone, and nitrous oxide affect the alveoli and cause death by exudation after the usual lag period. The common sources of irritant gases are riot and military gases, industrial accidents, fires, and smog. Intestinal irritants may cause nausea, vomiting, and diarrhea. If fluid losses are excessive, serious complications and even death may result. Many gastrointestinal irritants also have systemic effects. For example, acute arsenic poisoning generally causes death by its systemic effect, although gastrointestinal irritation is a prominent part of the clinical picture.

Corrosive Poisons

Corrosive poisons include (1) mineral (inorganic) acids and alkalis, (2) fluorides and oxalates, (3) phenol and other organic corrosives, (4) inorganic oxidizing agents, and (5) alkaloidal reagents. Inorganic acids and alkalis act chiefly through their properties as strong acids and bases. Similar effects are produced by strong acid and base salts and by strong organic acids. These strong chemicals act both by direct dissolution of tissue and by protein coagulation. Acid injuries tend to remain localized, but alkali injuries tend to extend. The mortality rate of skin burns from acid is relatively high. Corneal damage and resulting blindness is an especially important complication of this type of injury.

Ingestion of strong acids and alkalis results in burns with tissue necrosis in the mouth, esophagus, and stomach. Peculiarly, acids are more likely to affect the stomach, whereas alkalis seem to produce their maximum damage in the esophagus. Delayed deaths are more common with alkali burns, and scar contracture is more common in the survivors. Alkali burns are most common in young children who obtain and swallow lye from the laundry closet. These esophageal burns are associated with much scar formation which results in a stricture producing a marked stenosis (narrowing) of the esophageal passageway. Repeated mechanical dilatation may be necessary to maintain the patency (mechanical continuity) of the esophagus. When death occurs early, characteristic tissue changes may be visible. Alkalis tend to produce a gray-white gelatinous and edematous tissue. Hydrochloric acid produces a whitening of the tissue which gradually gives way to a gray-brown color. Nitric acid results in the deposition of yellow xanthoproteins. Sulfuric acid may leave the tissues charred and black. Phenol produces a grayish discoloration. Iodine leaves its characteristic brownish stain. As with the irritants, corrosives may also produce effects due to metabolic actions. For example, phenol produces central nervous system depression, and the absorption of tannic acid may lead to hepatic necrosis.

LIGHT INJURY

Solar energy is delivered to this planet largely in the form of infrared, visible (light) and ultraviolet rays (Fig. 6-7). Most of the solar heat is delivered by the infrared rays, which are longer than visible light waves. These waves produce immediate sensations of heat and prompt transient reddening of the skin. Visible light seems to have a very minimal effect.

The ultraviolet rays, which have a shorter wavelength than visible light, produce most of the cutaneous injury.* These rays have no penetrating power and relatively little energy. This energy is insufficient to produce ionization; however, energy is dissipated as heat, fluorescence, and the induction of photochemical reactions. The latent period is 2 to 12 hours, and for this reason the fiery red erythema does not usually appear until after sundown. The cause of this latent period is intriguing but unknown, as is the actual mechanism of the response. It is thought that the ultraviolet rays produce photochemical changes in proteins and nucleic acids. Dead cells may be found after 2 to 3 days in the basal cell layers of the skin. The toxemia may be due to the absorption of protein breakdown products, and the degree of toxemia appears to be related to the degree and area of exposure. Systemic symptoms include fever, headache, nausea, and prostration. Eventually there is an increase in the deposition of melanin pigments in the epidermis resulting in a "tan." There is also a thickening of the stratum corneum, the dead cell layer on the skin surface. These two factors, but chiefly the latter, result in increased

*Sunburn.

WAVELENGTH IN CM   TYPE OF RADIATION   FREQUENCY

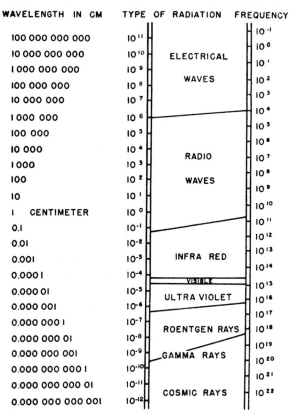

Figure 6-7   The electromagnetic spectrum. The slope of the lines between the various types of waves indicates that there is some overlap in the nomenclature. [*From O. Glasser (ed.), Medical Physics, Year Book, Chicago, 1944, p. 1164. By permission of the publishers.*]

tolerance to ultraviolet light.   Excessive and prolong exposure accelerates the aging changes in the skin.

The photodynamic actions of ultraviolet rays may produce unusually excessive reactions in some individuals.   Photosensitivity may be a manifestation of certain disease states, such as pellagra, lupus erythematosus, porphyria, and xeroderma pigmentosum.   Photosensitivity has also been noted in individuals receiving therapeutic administration of a variety of drugs, but this reaction most commonly occurs with the antibiotic tetracyclines, sulfonamide derivatives, and phenothiazine tranquilizers.   On the other hand, the action of sunlight is necessary to convert the normal steroid precursors into vitamin D.   The absence of adequate sunlight probably accounts for the prevalence of rickets in some northern climates, notably Great Britain. Extensive exposure to sunlight also predisposes to hyperkeratoses (areas of thickened, keratin-containing epidermis) and skin cancer. Sunlight is of benefit in some skin conditions, including psoriasis, pityriasis rosea, and acne vulgaris.

IONIZING RADIATION INJURY

Ionizing radiation comes from two different energy sources, electromagnetic radiation and particulate radiation. *Electromagnetic radiation* includes a continuous range from electrical waves of very long wavelengths to gamma and cosmic waves of extremely short wavelengths. The various bands were given individual names before it was realized that they were different parts of the same spectrum. In order of decreasing wavelength, they include electrical, radio, infrared, visible, ultraviolet, roentgen, and gamma rays. Injuries due to electrical, infrared, and ultraviolet rays have already been discussed. Roentgen (x-rays) rays and gamma rays (including cosmic rays) are the only ones with sufficient energy to produce ionization. *Particulate radiation* is produced by alpha and beta particles, protons, and neutrons.

Ionizing radiation can be produced by natural or artificially made isotopes, which are unstable atoms, or by such equipment as x-ray tubes, cyclotrons, and linear accelerators. *Alpha particles* are the central nuclei of helium atoms. The penetrating ability of alpha particles is extremely short, and their effect is limited almost to the cells with which they are in immediate contact. *Beta particles* are electrons, and their penetration may be up to a centimeter or more. Electromagnetic waves have greater capacity for penetration which, in general, is proportional to the energy of the wave. This, in turn, is inversely proportional to the wavelength.

A number of units have been established in order to measure the amount of radiation produced. The unit for roentgen rays, which has also been adopted for gamma rays, is the *roentgen*. This is a practical unit since it is a measure of the number of ionizations produced by the energy source and thus of the energy imparted. A similar unit for particulate radiation is termed a *rad,* which is almost equivalent in energy to the roentgen. The *curie* is equal to the number of particles emitted by 1 gram of pure radium per second, a value which has been determined to be 3.7×10^{10} emissions. In order to relate the curie to the rad, it is necessary to indicate the duration of exposure. It should be appreciated that 1 curie of radium with a long half-life will produce much more total energy as well as more energy per unit time than will 1 curie of radioactive phosphorus, which has a much shorter half-life.

The precise mechanism by which ionizing radiation produces its effects is not known, although many theories have been proposed. Ionization is the splitting of a molecule into two oppositely charged particles. This is generally associated with the loss of energy and the production of heat. The following facts appear to be fairly well established. The cellular nuclei are far more susceptible to injury than are the cellular cytoplasms. Rapidly multiplying cells are more susceptible than are cells which multiply infrequently. Genetic effects have been demonstrated both by altering nucleoprotein chains and by producing chromosomal abnormalities. No specific chemical changes have been noted. These observations all suggest that the relatively few ionizing radiations hit a target in the cell where maximal damage is produced. It seems quite likely that the energy generated by the ionization results in disruption of the DNA particle, which, in turn, causes either cell death or mutation.

The effects of radiation exposure depend upon a number of factors. There is a great variability in specific tissue susceptibility to irradiation. Irradiation of one organ or of one part of the body is generally much better tolerated than is total body irradiation. Although the point is not completely resolved, there is evidence that the more rapidly a dose of radiation is given, the more marked will be the resultant injury. Radiation causes not only immediate but also late effects. Thus the cumulative effect of the many small doses may, over a period of time, result in as much disability as a few large but not lethal doses.

Acute Radiation Injury

Acute radiation injury is now a major public threat not only because of the existence of the atom bomb but also because radiation energy is being used increasingly for industrial and scientific purposes. It is generally accepted that acute exposure of the entire body to between 300 and 700 roentgens will result in death to 50 percent of the exposed individuals. Exposures below this level usually result in recovery, whereas exposures to higher doses are almost always fatal.

A rather predictable sequence follows acute radiation exposure. The *central nervous system syndrome* is seen if the exposure is extremely large. There is a brief latent period of up to 3 hours followed by lethargy, convulsions, ataxia, coma, and death, generally within 36 to 48 hours. Tissue changes are found only within the brain. The *gastrointestinal syndrome* is usually due to a smaller exposure averaging about 500 roentgens. The patient is usually well for 3 to 5 days and then has a sudden onset of malaise, anorexia, nausea, retching and vomiting, diarrhea with watery stools progressing to bloody stools, and high fever. Death, if it occurs, is usually during the second week. The *hematopoietic syndrome* is due to injury of the bone marrow with reduction in the ability to produce blood cells. A minimum dose of 100 roentgens is necessary for this syndrome. Since it is the blood-producing organs which are affected, the blood manifestations depend upon the rate of replacement required for the various blood elements. Thus depletion of lymphocytes appears within a few days, of leukocytes in the second week, of platelets in the third week, and of red cells in the fourth week. Symptoms usually occur in the second or third week and are usually due either to infections subsequent to the reduced body protection offered by the reduced number of leukocytes or to hemorrhages into the skin and mucous membranes due to the depletion of platelets. Death usually occurs within 2 months and depends upon the extent of the destruction of blood-producing organs. If fatal hemorrhages and infections can be prevented, it is rare that ultimate regeneration of the bone marrow fails to occur. Promising work has been done with marrow transplantation, and it is well established that if marrow cells of an animal are stored, the animal can withstand an otherwise lethal dose of radiation by reimplanting its own cells.

It should be pointed out that, within a few hours after an acute radiation exposure, nausea, vomiting, and malaise are quite common. This generally subsides within 36 hours and may not by itself indicate the severity of the radiation exposure. This type of radiation sickness has long been known in association with the x-ray treatment of tumors in which radiation is given locally and no more dangerous side effects are observed. Therefore, after a radiation accident, it may be difficult to differentiate severe from mild exposure on the basis of the initial symptoms.

It is of interest that acute radiation injury does not result in permanent sterility for most of those exposed. Approximately 500 roentgens are required to completely sterilize the ovaries and testes. Most people exposed to total-body, as opposed to organ, radiation of this level would die a radiation death. Although experimental data unequivocally indicate that radiation exposure creates an unfavorable genetic burden, as yet there has been no direct confirmation of this expectation in man.

Chronic Radiation Effects

Chronic radiation effects have been previously noted. Excessive exposure of the skin to ionizing radiation eventually results in scarring, thinning of the surface epithelium, and atrophy of the glands and hair follicles. Patches of skin thickening may appear and skin cancer is often seen (Fig. 6-8). Over 20 years may elapse from the time of exposure until the full pattern of change is observed. Many of the changes in the skin and elsewhere suggest the aging process, and in fact there seems to be a correlation

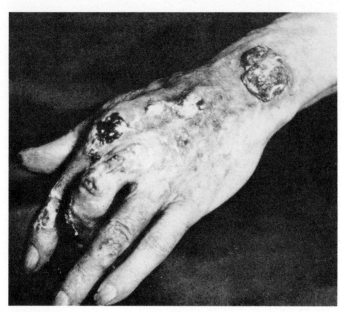

Figure 6-8   Radiation dermatitis and carcinoma. The skin atrophy and thinning as well as the hyperkeratoses and multiple foci of carcinoma are typical. The patient was a physician who had many years of repeated small exposures to x-ray irradiation. [*From W. A. Meissner and S. Warren in W. A. D. Anderson (ed.), Pathology, 6th ed., Mosby, St. Louis, 1971, p. 555. By permission of the publishers.*]

between the amount of exposure and the total length of life.   In addition to effects on the skin, chronic exposure may lead to malignant neoplasms in other organ systems.   The frequency of leukemia has been noted to be increased in survivors of the Japanese atomic bombing, radiologists exposed to x-rays in the course of their work, and patients with arthritis who were given x-ray treatment of the spine.   The evidence for this increase appears fairly convincing.   The increase in leukemia in Japan continued for several years but subsequently has declined to the normally expected rate.   At one time it was considered good therapy to radiate the enlarged lymph nodes of the neck which were associated with chronic respiratory infections in children.   Subsequently it was found that many of these individuals developed carcinoma of the thyroid; fortunately, this was a very slow-growing tumor and most of the patients were successfully treated.

One of the potential hazards of the increased use of isotopes is the entrapment of radioactive isotopes within the body.   Under these conditions even nonpenetrating alpha particles can become dangerous.   During World War I a number of women were exposed to radium while painting luminous watch dials.   The radium concentrated in their bones, and an average of 23 years later many of them developed malignant tumors of bone.   Inhalation of radioactive uranium dust by miners in the Bohemian mines has given rise to cancer of the lung.   Several other such examples have been observed.

Atomic Explosion Effects

The explosion of an atom bomb immediately releases energy in the form of electromagnetic and particulate radiations, blast, and heat.   In Hiroshima and Nagasaki, the blast and heat totally destroyed all life within a radius of several thousand yards from the center of explosion.   Beyond this area injuries were due not only to the direct effects of the blast but more frequently to objects hurled by the blast and by the collapse of walls and other structures.   Despite the intensity of the heat, its duration was so brief that often the burns were extremely superficial and much protection was offered by even the lightest of clothing.   Secondary burns occurred, however, as a result of exposure to burning rubble.   The importance of ionizing radiation during the initial stage was minimized by the fact that lethal blast and heat injury extended beyond the range of lethal radiation injury.   The later injuries due to radiation were largely due to fallout.   Of the deaths in Hiroshima and Nagasaki, 85 percent were due to mechanical and thermal injuries while only 15 percent were due to radiation.

After the blast, with its outward pressure, a vacuum develops in the epicenter, and there is a sudden suction drawing debris into the fireball. It is this debris which contains the particulate radiation which later produces danger by fallout.   In the air it can be widely dispersed, and concentrations in any one area may be relatively low.   Since this matter is particulate, much of it can be filtered out of the inspired air.   The usual bomb will be exploded in air and dangerous local levels of radioactivity will be dissipated within 2 weeks.   If the fireball touches the ground, or if the radioactivity is trapped by rain or deposited by a tidal wave after an underwater explosion, the local concentration is greatly increased. Atomic war or accident would be catastrophic, yet it seems probable that the resultant disability and death could be greatly reduced by adequate preparation.

BIBLIOGRAPHY

ANDERSON, W.A.D.: *Pathology,* 5th ed., St. Louis: The C. V. Mosby Company, 1966.
CRONKITE, E. P. and V. P. BOND: *Radiation Injury in Man,* Springfield, Ill.: Charles C Thomas, Publisher, 1960.
DAVIS, L. E., (ed.): *Christopher's Textbook of Surgery,* 9th ed., Philadelphia: W. B. Saunders Company, 1968.

FALLIS, B. D.: *Textbook of Pathology,* New York: McGraw-Hill Book Company, 1964.
FLOREY, SIR H.: *General Pathology,* 4th ed., Philadelphia: W. B. Saunders Company, 1970.
"Ionizing Radiation," *Scientific American,* September, 1959.
LOWN, B.: "Intensive Heart Care," *Scientific American,* July, 1968.
SCHWARTZ, S. I.: *Principles of Surgery,* New York: McGraw-Hill Book Company, 1970.
WINTROBE, M. W., et al. (eds.): *Harrison's Principles of Internal Medicine,* 6th ed., New York: McGraw-Hill Book Company, 1970.

Inflammation and Healing

Inflammation is the tissue response to injury. The characteristic responses of local heat, swelling, redness, and pain are well known to everyone. Celsus in the first century was the first to characterize these four findings in the language of the day: *calor, tumor, rubor,* and *dolor.* A century later Galen added the fifth major characteristic of inflammation to the description when he included limitation of function. It was not, however, until the eighteenth century that John Hunter introduced the important concept that the inflammatory reaction was a mechanism of body defense and not the disease itself. One of the major contributions of the past century was the demonstration by Metchnikoff of the phenomenon of phagocytosis, which shall be discussed later in this chapter. During the same period the immunological mechanisms were first recognized. Inflammation of a specific organ or tissue is indicated by the suffix *itis* (e.g., *appendicitis, sinusitis,* etc.).

   The general outline of the inflammatory process has been well defined and there is relatively little disagreement, although many details continue to be under active investigation.   The etiology of the inflammatory reaction includes all causes of tissue trauma: The physical and chemical mechanisms described in the previous chapter, the allergic responses to be examined in Chap. 8, and the living agents to be discussed in Chap. 9.

Injury and the subsequent inflammatory reaction cause cellular damage and cellular death, which result in disruption of tissue and impairment of function.   *Repair* and *healing* are general terms for the processes leading to restoration of tissue structure and function.   This process may not be perfect, and the healed tissue may not be completely normal. *Regeneration* is a more specific term; it implies that lost tissue is replaced by tissue which is structurally and functionally the same as the original. Many invertebrates can regenerate major portions of the organism.   For example, hydra and planaria will regenerate the severed half when the organism is cut in two.   Some amphibia can regenerate portions of limbs, and lizards are well known to regenerate their tails.   These powers of regeneration are extremely limited in mammals.   Nevertheless, mammalian repair is quite effective, and with present methods of treatment extensive areas of injury of all sorts can often be made to heal satisfactorily.

THE INFLAMMATORY REACTION

The first response to injury is a change in the pattern of vascular flow.   It was originally believed that these changes were initiated by foreign substances; however, it is now generally agreed that the process is initiated by the release of specific chemicals into the area as a result of cellular damage.   Normally the capillaries and venules are of uniform character, and in suitable preparations the blood can be seen flowing through these vessels in a characteristic fashion.   There is streamlining of the flow, with the cells in the center of the column and relatively clear plasma in contact with the vessel walls, an arrangement which reduces the friction.   When the capillary lies in an area of tissue injury, the vessels initially dilate and the blood flow increases.   Shortly afterward white cells, which could not have been identified in the normally flowing stream, become adherent to the inner walls of the capillaries and venules.   The number of these white cells increases until there is literally a "pavementing" of the vessel wall. At about this time the white cells put out pseudopodia (false feet) and by amoeboid movement work their way between the cells lining the blood vessel into the tissues, a process known as *emigration* (see Fig. 7-1).   An occasional red cell may be passively forced between the cells of the blood vessel wall.   However, in this instance the process is known as *diapedesis*.

At the same time that the white cells can be seen actively emigrating through the blood vessel walls, somewhat more indirect methods demon-

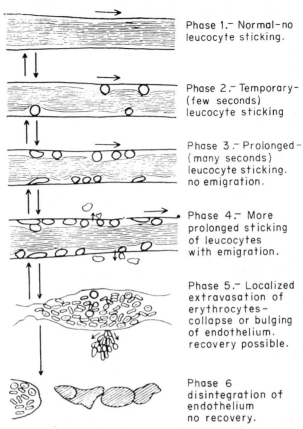

Phase 1.– Normal–no leucocyte sticking.

Phase 2.– Temporary– (few seconds) leucocyte sticking

Phase 3.– Prolonged– (many seconds) leucocyte sticking. no emigration.

Phase 4.– More prolonged sticking of leucocytes with emigration.

Phase 5.– Localized extravasation of erythrocytes– collapse or bulging of endothelium. recovery possible.

Phase 6 disintegration of endothelium no recovery.

Figure 7-1   Vascular response to inflammation. The adhesion of leukocytes and their subsequent emigration, the diapedesis of red blood cells, and the eventual disintegration of the blood vessels themselves are characterized. The initial increase in blood flow is not shown. *(From H. W. Florey, General Pathology, 4th ed., Saunders, Philadelphia, 1970, p. 75. By permission of the publishers.)*

strate that significant amounts of blood plasma are also going into the tissues. These two components, the cellular and the fluid, make up a defensive contribution to the inflammatory exudate. By this time the blood vessels in the inflamed area, which initially manifested an increased blood flow, have become stagnant pools of blood, and there are irregularities in the configuration of the vessel walls. These vessels are still capable of restoration to normal function. However, if the inflammatory reaction is not stopped at this point, the process proceeds to irreversible vascular destruction.

The lymphatic vessels are ordinarily extremely inconspicuous. Structurally they resemble the venous end of the vascular circuit in many respects. They originate as closed-ended capillaries which drain into lymphatic channels and proceed to the regional lymph nodes. They then pass on into larger lymphatic channels and eventually drain into the venous circulation, primarily at the junction of the jugular and subclavian veins in the neck. The lymphatic flow participates in a continuous cycling of fluids which pass out of the blood capillaries into the tissues, are picked up by the lymphatic system, and eventually return to the circulation. Initially the lymph contains no cells and only a very small amount of protein. Normally lymphocytes are discharged from lymph nodes into the lymph, and it is probably in this manner that most of the lymphocytes enter the blood circulation. The important role of the lymphatics in inflammation is manifest by the evidence that the flow of lymph increases seven- to eightfold during an active inflammatory process. The lymphatic system thus joins the blood circulation as a route whereby toxic substances and infectious agents may be dispersed widely from a local inflammatory site.

The dilatation of the blood vessels, slowing of flow, pavementing of white blood cells, emigration of leukocytes, and escape of blood plasma are all well documented. The mechanism which initiates these changes is not as certain. Many years ago Lewis demonstrated that when the skin is stroked firmly with a blunted point, a characteristic sequence of reactions can be observed. First, a dull red line indicates the path of the stroke, followed by a brighter red halo surrounding the immediate injury. The red line then begins to fade and is replaced by an area of slight swelling which becomes paler than the surrounding flare. The swelling then becomes a small weal. This phenomenon can be duplicated by the injection of a minute amount of histamine, a chemical which is present in adequate amounts in the tissues to produce this response if it is liberated from an injured cell. It seems probable that the vascular phase of the inflammatory response is caused either by the release of histamine or by some other compound which behaves in a similar manner.

The Cellular Exudate

The white cells which emigrate from the circulation manifest two interesting and important phenomena, chemotaxis and phagocytosis. *Chemotaxis* means literally "chemical direction." Upon leaving the blood vessels, the cells migrate through the tissues by amoeboid movement. This movement is not random but is directed toward areas of tissue injury, and it appears to be in response to the diffusion of specific chemicals from the injured cells. In addition to the chemotactic effects of injured tissue, some

bacteria exhibit varying degrees of chemotaxis, one of the most notable
being *Staphylococcus* (Chap. 9), which is a common resident of the skin
and therefore is frequently introduced into the tissues by local injury.

The second phenomenon is that of phagocytosis, which was elucidated
by Metchnikoff during the last years of the nineteenth century. *Phagocy-*
tosis refers to the process by which certain cells engulf and digest foreign
particulate material in the tissues. The word derives from *phagein,* "to
eat," and *cyte,* "cell." A number of different cells are capable of phagocytosis and will be discussed subsequently in some detail. The process can
be observed in a number of different ways. Perhaps one of the simplest is
to place white blood cells and bacteria together on a slide and to examine
the preparation under the microscope. When this is done, the white blood
cell can be observed sending out a protoplasmic extension known as a
pseudopod which envelops the bacteria, eventually forming a vacuole
within the cell itself (see Fig. 7-2). Another mechanism for the ingestion of
foreign substances has been recently demonstrated by the electron microscope and is termed *pinocytosis.* In this process small, inwardly directed
pouches form in the outer membrane of the cell. These are subsequently
pinched off and migrate within the substance of the cell. A number of
factors appear to determine the effectiveness of phagocytosis. One of the
most important is the presence of substances known as *opsonins.* These

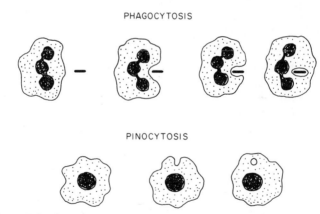

Figure 7-2 Phagocytosis and pinocytosis. *A:* Phagocytosis. A
neutrophilic polymorphonuclear leukocyte is demonstrated ap-
proaching a bacterium by ameboid movement, flowing around the
organism and eventually engulfing it. *B:* Pinocytosis. Small in-
vaginations have been observed by electron microscopy to form
on the surface of cells and eventually to be pinched off as intracellular vesicles. While phagocytosis can be seen by light microscopy, pinocytosis is a finer process which can only be discerned
by electron microscopy.

are protein antibodies (Chap. 8) and are a component of the immune mechanism. They are specific for the infecting microorganism and make it easier for the phagocytes to "grab hold" of the bacteria. If the material to be phagocytosed can be backed against a firm structure, phagocytosis is more effective than if both the phagocytes and the bacteria or debris are floating free in a liquid medium. Phagocytosis is not always successful and the phagocytes may be destroyed, resulting in a release of digestive enzymes from the cells into the tissues. Some organisms may survive and persist in the phagocytes, thus perpetuating the infection.

The *polymorphonuclear neutrophilic leukocyte* is the most numerous white cell; when it enters the inflammatory exudate it is known as a pus cell (Fig. 7-3A, B, C). Since it is a small phagocyte, it is occasionally termed a *microphage*. In the early stages of an inflammatory reaction, large numbers of polymorphonuclear neutrophils enter the inflammatory area. In addition, many inflammations, especially those caused by bacteria, stimulate the production of polymorphonuclear neutrophils; the most common manifestation is the increase in their number in the blood-stream where they can be easily counted. This phenomenon is termed *leukocytosis* and is an important indicator of inflammation. It is presently believed that the factors causing emigration, chemotaxis, and leukocytosis are all different and distinct.

There are several situations in which the polymorphonuclear neutrophils are decreased in number, a condition termed *leukopenia.* A moderate leukopenia is frequently seen with some viral infections, and more severe degrees of leukopenia are seen after an exposure to a variety of chemicals and to moderately high doses of radiation. The defensive importance of the polymorphonuclear neutrophil is seen in the fact that prolonged and persistent leukopenia is almost inevitably associated with severe and frequently fatal bacterial infections. Very little is known about the role of the polymorphonuclear eosinophils and the polymorphonuclear basophils in the inflammatory reaction. The eosinophils are often very much increased in both the blood and tissues in individuals undergoing an allergic reaction, such as asthma and hay fever. They may also be increased to rather large numbers during active infestation with various types of worms; an increase in the number of the eosinophils in the blood may on occasion be the first clue to the presence of this type of infection. They may also be increased in diseases such as periarteritis nodosa and Hodgkin's disease. The role of the polymorphonuclear basophil is even less well understood. However, it is of interest and possible significance that the granules in this cell contain large amounts of histamine and heparin. Cells resembling the basophil, called *mast* cells, are found in small numbers in the connective tissue. It may be that the breakdown of the basophils and

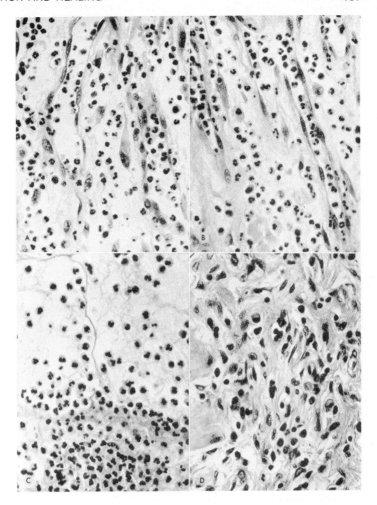

Figure 7-3 Inflammation. *A, B,* and *C* represent acute inflammation. The predominant inflammatory cells are the polymorphonuclear leukocytes, which can be identified by their small, lobular, or horseshoe-shaped nuclei. In *A* and *B,* the cells are relatively widely separated by exudate. Capillaries can be seen running from the lower right to the upper left-hand corner of the illustrations. There are many leukocytes in the capillaries, and some can be seen to be passing through the capillary walls. *C:* The exudate in the upper portion is composed primarily of fibrin with leukocytes, but the lower portion is purulent with necrotic tissue, dead and active neutrophils, and fibrin. *D:* This is a characteristic chronic inflammatory response with predominantly mononuclear cells and fibroblasts. *(From R. P. Morehead, Human Pathology, McGraw-Hill, New York, 1965, p. 102. By permission of the publishers.)*

mast cells by injury releases histamine, which initiates the inflammatory response. The polymorphonuclear neutrophils are frequently referred to as neutrophils, polys, or PMNs when reports of blood counts are given.

The *macrophages* or "large eaters" are made up of a number of cells of different origins. In the bloodstream they are derived from the monocytes. These cells exist in considerably fewer numbers than the polymorphonuclear white cells. However, they emigrate from the bloodstream and move toward the inflammatory area in much the same way. In the tissues they are capable of considerable enlargement and may attain diameters of 2½ to 3 times that of the pus cells. Unlike the latter, they are capable of reproduction in the tissues. Occasionally, and especially in chronic inflammation, the nuclei may divide while the cytoplasm remains intact, producing what are termed multinucleated giant cells. These cells are much more resistant to destruction than are the pus cells and become more important as the inflammation persists and the pus cells are destroyed. When inert particulate matter such as carbon (india ink) is injected into the tissues, the particles are ingested by the macrophages and may remain there indefinitely. This is the phenomenon observed in tattoos, for example, which survive the lifetime of the subject although the outlines may become indistinct. The relative proportion of macrophages to microphages increases with time in most inflammatory reactions. Eventually a rim of macrophages may surround the area of active inflammation, forming a layer of "epithelioid" cells, so called because of their supposed resemblance to epithelium.

The macrophages arise not only from the monocytes but also from cells in the connective tissue. The exact origin of these cells is not certain. Tissue macrophages are called histiocytes. Another extremely important source of macrophages is the reticuloendothelial system, usually called the RE system. These cells lie in the lining of the circulatory system but are not true lining cells. They are present in large numbers in the lymph nodes, liver, spleen, and bone marrow, where they are very effective in clearing the lymph and blood of all particulate matter, including bacteria, which has escaped the local defenses at the portal of entry. These cells are incapable of movement and are also called fixed macrophages.

The *lymphocytes* are the most common white cells in the blood after the polymorphonuclear neutrophils. It was originally thought that they were relatively nonmotile in the tissues; however since, with time, they appear in increasing numbers in the inflammatory area, they undoubtedly must have some motility. The role of the lymphocytes is not as clear as that of the phagocytes. It is now generally believed that they contribute in some way to the local immune reaction. Two very suggestive observations can be presented: first, techniques which selectively destroy the lymphocyte result in demonstrable impairment of the immune mechanisms; second, the immunological rejection of transplanted tissues is associated with the infiltration of the graft by host lymphocytes. On the other hand, antibodies cannot be demonstrated in or near the lymphocytes. The role of the lymphocyte in relation to immunity will be discussed further in Chap. 8.

The *plasma cell* is a very characteristic cell. Its nucleus is about the same size as that of the lymphocyte, but it has considerably more cytoplasm. Plasma cells are rarely seen in the circulation, but they are common in inflammatory areas, especially those with any degree of chronicity. Normally, they are found in largest numbers in the lymph nodes. It is now generally believed that the plasma cell is the primary source of antibodies.

Chronic inflammations are frequently associated with the presence of many small round cells with relatively large nuclei lying at the periphery of the inflammatory reaction (Fig. 7-3D). These cells have the general appearance of lymphocytes in the tissues, but pathologists were reluctant to make such a specific identification. It had been proposed that these cells might be plasma cells, undifferentiated connective tissue cells, polymorphonuclear cells with fused nuclei, or lymphocytes. In order to remain noncommittal, observers usually described their accumulation as an infiltration of small round cells. It is now fairly definite that these cells are lymphocytes in the tissues.

The Fluid Exudate

The fluid portion of the inflammatory exudate results from filtration of a large amount of plasma through the damaged lining of the capillaries and small veins. It is relatively deficient in the larger protein molecules; however, fibrinogen, which is converted to fibrin, is present. It is fibrin which forms the basis of the blood clot when it is precipitated at the site of a hemorrhage, and in the tissue it produces a protein network throughout the inflammatory area. The role of the fibrin has been subject to much dispute. A popular theory is that it forms an actual mechanical barrier which is particularly important in impeding the spread of bacteria. Mencken has pointed out that streptococcal infections, characteristically associated with very little fibrin formation, often have an early local and systemic bacterial spread, while staphylococcal infections, associated with large amounts of fibrin, are generally well localized. The presence of firm strands of fibrin may enhance the ability of the phagocytes to trap bacteria against a solid surface, as was previously mentioned.

The fluid exudate undoubtedly serves as a vehicle for the transportation of circulating antibodies to the inflamed area and probably of nutrients to the surviving tissues and phagocytes. The lymphatic flow from an inflamed area may be almost tenfold the normal volume, and probably this circulation of fluid also serves as a vehicle for the removal of inflammatory end products. It should be noted, however, that this increased flow may also serve to carry bacteria from the area into the lymphatics, to the lymph nodes, and occasionally into the general circulation as well. Perhaps the most important contribution of the fluid exudate is the delivery of specific antibodies, which will be discussed in the next chapter.

SYSTEMIC MANIFESTATIONS OF THE INFLAMMATORY REACTION

Although the inflammatory reaction is an attempt to isolate and localize the area of injury, obviously this localization cannot be complete. The blood and lymphatic circulations through the inflamed area bring to other parts of the body the breakdown products of the tissues and foreign materials, particularly bacteria, present in the inflammatory area, and these materials may include the organisms themselves if they are successful in evading all the inflammatory barriers. The release into the circulation of large amounts of incompletely broken down proteins of almost any source generally results in a toxic reaction. The presence of *toxins* (poisons of bacterial, plant, or animal origin) in the blood is termed *toxemia* and is characterized by the symptoms of malaise, lassitude, and weakness. There may be headache and muscle weakness, loss of appetite, and central nervous system manifestations varying in degree from mental sluggishness and sleepiness to delirium and convulsions. Fever may result either as a direct response to the toxemia or as a response to the increased metabolic needs imposed by the inflammatory process.

Some inflamatory reactions produce an initial chill which is characterized by a sensation of coldness, shivering, and chattering teeth. This is due to the reduction in dermal circulation which allows the skin to cool toward the lower environmental temperature. As a result, there is a sensation of coldness and the physiological response of shivering ensues. Because less heat is lost in maintaining the skin temperature, the body temperature goes up, and fever follows the chill. Convulsions in children are often the equivalent of chill in the adult. The characteristic increase in the heart rate is usually a response to the fever; there is a direct relationship between the metabolic needs of the body and heart rate. This is normally seen in the cardiac acceleration associated with exercise. A severe and persistent inflammation may result in cellular changes in remote organs. Often these can be recognized by microscopic examination of the tissues involved. Although the systemic responses so far enumerated are generally ascribed to the nonspecific flooding of the circulation with the products of inflammation, it is quite possible that they are caused by specific chemical compounds.

Leukocytosis, or the increase in the number of circulating white cells, appears to be a response to such a specific metabolite. It has been established that the factor producing leukocytosis is different from that which prompts emigration or produces chemotaxis. One of the current theories is that the breakdown of the white cells produces the material which can cause this stimulus. The presence of leukocytosis is of great importance in evaluating an inflammatory reaction. Generally the white cells increase from the normal value of 5,000 to 10,000 per cubic millimeter of blood to a range between 12,000 and 30,000, although higher values are not infrequently observed.

The characteristic leukocytosis associated with inflammation is due to a specific increase in the polymorphonuclear neutrophils. The tremendous number of these cells which may be required results in the release of immature leukocytes from the bone marrow. This characteristic helps to differentiate the leukocytosis of inflammation from that due to other causes. The presence of a leukocytosis may be extremely helpful in establishing the presence of an occult inflammation. For example, it may help differentiate the pain of appendicitis, which is inflammatory in origin, from that of mechanical or traumatic origin. In general, leukopenia is produced by viral infections and a few bacterial infections, such as typhoid fever. Leukopenia in other bacterial infections is often of ominous significance, since it is usually associated with a toxic depression of the bone marrow. As a result of the reduced phagocytosis, the infection is often fatal.

An important systemic response to the inflammatory stimulus is the production of various antibodies. Since these are produced only after stimulation by specific foreign proteins, it is apparent that these intact molecules must have escaped from the site of the inflammation to that of antibody production. The effects of specific inflammatory agents which cause characteristic toxic or infectious manifestations, and therefore can be characterized as specific disease entities, will be discussed in relation to the appropriate diseases.

THE RELATIONSHIP OF SYMPTOMS TO LESIONS

The initial bright redness of the inflammatory area is due to the increased local blood supply. As the lesion progresses, the flow through the area of active inflammation decreases and takes on the purple color of stagnant, unoxygenated blood. However, on the periphery of the lesion, where injury is less, the circulation continues at its previous accelerated rate and provides a bright halo around the inflamed area. The swelling is due chiefly to the formation of the inflammatory exudate, although vascular dilatation contributes. The increased local heat is also due to the increased blood supply. The inflamed area is never hotter than blood temperature. Ordinarily the skin is cooled several degrees below that of blood. However, when the circulation increases, the warm blood from the interior increases the temperature on the surface. Pain is due to several factors, the most important of which is the swelling of the tissues due to the inflammatory exudate. This is dramatically demonstrated by the great relief of pain upon the drainage of an abscess. Undoubtedly direct inflammatory injury and specific toxic substances add to the discomfort. Finally, reduction in function is an obvious sequel to local tissue damage and limitation of motion by pain and swelling. Besides being a symptom, pain serves a useful purpose by encouraging the limitation of motion of the affected part. It is well established that motion interferes with the normal inflammatory and reparative processes and encourages dissemination of infection. It should be remembered, however, that inhibition of activity beyond that which is necessary increases disability and prolongs recovery.

VARIATIONS IN THE INFLAMMATORY RESPONSE

Duration of Inflammation

It is customary to divide inflammatory responses into acute, subacute, and chronic varieties. In general, the course of an *acute inflammation* rarely exceeds 1 to 2 weeks. The *chronic inflammation* persists months to years. Usually there is little difficulty in differentiating between the two. In some instances it is appropriate to designate as *subacute* a type of inflammation which lasts from one to several months. In general, the duration of the inflammatory response can be fairly accurately estimated from its etiology. However a streptococcal inflammation, for example, which is usually acute, can become chronic if complications such as mastoiditis develop. Tuberculosis, which is usually a chronic, local inflammatory disease, may become relatively acute when it is manifest in the miliary form, the rapid, blood-borne dissemination of "galloping consumption."

As the inflammation persists, the inflammatory exudate becomes less important. The macrophages become more prominent and, in turn, the small round cells become increasingly numerous. There is increasing evidence of connective tissue activity, with fibroblasts producing scar tissue. This is known as a productive reaction. The *chronic inflammation* is due to a relative equilibrium between the inflammatory agent and the patient. However, a persistence of the reaction, the progressive extension of the inflammatory destruction of tissue, and the increasing amount of scar tissue ultimately results in death unless there is favorable intervention to alter the balance.

The *granuloma* is a specialized form of chronic inflammatory reaction. It may be caused by the bacteria of tuberculosis, leprosy, brucellosis, and syphilis; the fungi of actinomycosis, coccidioidomycosis, and related diseases; and the virus of lymphogranuloma venereum. Many foreign bodies — including splinters, sutures, small projectiles, silica, asbestos, carbon, and some oils and fatty substances, such as cholesterol and fatty acids — may also produce a granulomatous response. Sarcoidosis is a granuloma of unknown etiology.

The granuloma is quite characteristic (Figs. 7-4 and 7-5). The central area contains the inflammatory agent. In the case of tuberculosis, the organism appears to be extremely resistant, probably because of the presence of a fatty shell. As a result there is an area of necrosis which, because of its cheesy consistency, is called *caseous* (Fig 7-6). The central area is surrounded by a dense layer of macrophages with epithelioid characteristics. This layer, in turn, is surrounded by a dense layer of small round cells. Surrounding the entire granuloma is a shell of fibrous tissue. Giant cells form either by the incomplete division of macrophages or by

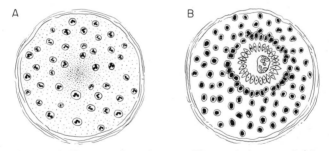

Figure 7-4 *A:* Diagram of an abscess. The central area consists of dead and partially liquefied tissue and inflammatory cells. Surrounding this is a dense infiltrate of active inflammatory cells, predominantly polymorphonuclear leukocytes. On the periphery may be fibroblasts and a fibrous capsule if the process has been of sufficient duration. *B:* Diagram of a granuloma. The granuloma is characteristic of chronic inflammation. There may or may not be a central core of necrotic tissue. The central cells are relatively large mononuclear phagocytes which look like epithelial cells. There may be giant cells with multiple nuclei; these cells have a variable appearance depending upon the etiology of the granuloma. The epithelioid cells are surrounded by a relatively dense layer of small round cells, and there may be an enclosing fibrous capsule.

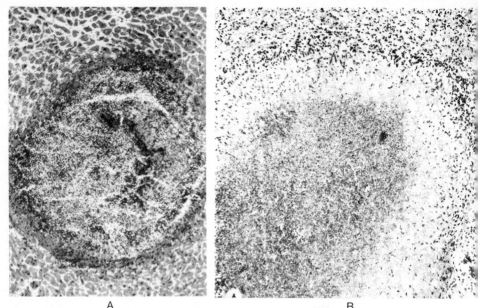

A   B

Figure 7-5   *A:* Abscess.   This is an acute abscess in heart muscle.
The center consists primarily of necrotic pus cells and tissue with
a rim of active cells.   The outer border shows very little fibrous
reaction because of the relatively short duration of the lesion.
[*From H. C. Hopps in W. A. D. Anderson (ed.), Pathology, 6th ed.,
Mosby, St. Louis, 1971, p. 280.   By permission of the publishers.*]
B: Granuloma.   This granulomatous inflammation was tuberculous
in origin.   The central dark necrotic area is surrounded by a light
zone of epithelioid cells.   Beyond this, there is again a darker
layer of small round cells.   *(From R. P. Morehead, Human Pathology, McGraw-Hill, New York, 1965, p. 115.   By permission of the
publishers.)*

the fusion of a number of macrophages and are characteristically found in
the central areas of many granulomas.   The granuloma of tuberculosis,
or the tubercle, measures 0.5 to 2.0 millimeters in diameter.   However, as
the process continues, the tubercles enlarge and coalesce with adjacent
tubercles, destroying increasing amounts of tissue and running the increasing risk of perforation into blood vessels, bronchi, and other structures.

Type of Exudate

The inflammatory response can also be classified by the type of exudate
produced.   If the exudate is composed predominantly of pus cells and
necrotic material, it is said to be *purulent.*   *Suppuration* is the formation of a purulent exudate.   One of the commonest causes of purulent

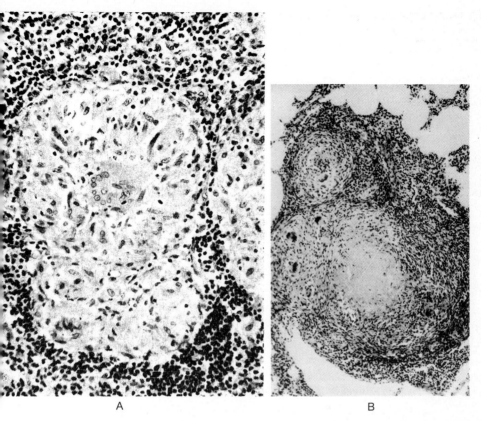

A   B

Figure 7-6   *A:* A granuloma without central necrosis, due to sar-
coidosis. *(From R. P. Morehead, Human Pathology, McGraw-Hill,
New York, 1965, p. 114. By permission of the publishers.)   B: A*
granuloma with central caseation, due to tuberculosis. [*From
F. D. Gunn in W. A. D. Anderson (ed.), Pathology, 6th ed., Mosby,
St. Louis, 1971, p. 248. By permission of the publishers.*]

inflammation is the *Staphylococcus,* a bacterium that is present on the
skin.   When it produces an inflammation in a sebaceous gland, a pimple
or furuncle results.   Localized accumulations of pus are called *abscesses*
(Figs. 7-4 and 7-5).   The common boil is an abscess due to an inflammation usually arising at the base of a hair follicle.   An abscess may arise
in any tissue, however, as the result of infection and inflammation due
to pyogenic (pus forming) bacteria.

Much of the pain of the abcess is due to the pressure and tension of
the purulent exudate.   This pressure causes damage to adjacent tissues,
which gradually erode along the line of least resistance.   The throbbing
pain of an abscess is due to the increased pressure with each pulsation of

blood. Superficial abscesses erode to the skin and spontaneous or surgical drainage usually results in subsequent healing. However, deep abscesses may erode into areas which are favorable for the further dissemination of infection or may cause critical tissue damage.

The eroded tract may not always provide adequate drainage and the infection may persist. Such a tract is known as a *sinus* (Fig 7-7). Sometimes an abscess discharges into two separate areas. For example, an abdominal abscess may discharge into the intestinal tract as well as through the abdominal wall and skin. Such a tract is known as a *fistula*. Sinuses and fistulae rarely heal without surgical intervention. If an abscess is small and relatively stable, it may be gradually absorbed without drainage, leaving only an area of scar tissue. Others become quiescent, leaving a fibrous sac containing residual exudate. Occasionally some such abscesses become impregnated with calcium and form a bony structure, at which time they are said to be calcified. This is frequent following tuberculous infections.

A *serous exudate* is one which is made up primarily of fluid and which contains very little fibrin or cells. Streptococci frequently produce such an infection, and because streptococci contain enzymes which dissolve extracellular cement, these inflammations may spread rapidly. The serous exudate takes its name from the fact that the fluid resembles blood serum. The heart, lungs, and abdominal viscera lie respectively in the pericardial, pleural, and peritoneal cavities. These cavities are lined by mesothelial

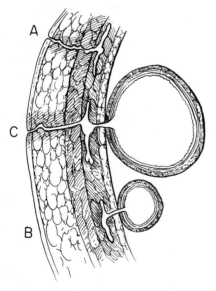

Figure 7-7 Sinuses and fistula. Cross-section of abdomen, showing sinuses and fistula of abdominal wall and bowel. *A:* External, cutaneous sinus. *B:* Internal sinus. *C:* Enterocutaneous fistula.

epithelia which are called serous membranes. The identity of the names is only coincidental, but the serous cavities are frequent sites for the collection of serous exudates. Normally these cavities are only potential cavities. A thin layer of serous membrane covers the organs and their vascular and functional connections, and then it doubles back over the chest and abdominal walls. Thus, there is a *visceral* pericardium, pleura, and peritoneum covering the organs which is in contact with the *parietal* pericardium, pleura, and peritoneum lining the chest and abdominal walls (Fig. 7-8). These serous membranes normally produce a small amount of fluid which makes it possible for the organs to slide smoothly with the heartbeat, respiration, and intestinal peristalsis. It is of practical

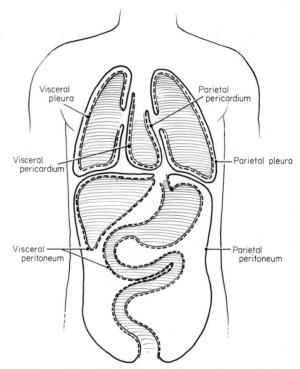

Figure 7-8 The relationship of the serous membranes to the heart, lungs, and abdominal viscera. The visceral pericardium is in direct contact with the heart, and lies within the parietal pericardium, with which it has no attachment except at the base of the heart. Normally, there is only a potential space between the two pericardial layers. A true space forms when the space is filled with air, fluid, or blood. Only the parietal layer contains nerve fibers capable of transmitting pain. The same principles apply to the pleura and peritoneum, and to the potential pleural and peritoneal spaces.

importance that there are pain fibers only in the parietal serous membranes.

The *fibrinous exudate* is one in which the principal component is fibrin. It is also most commonly seen in inflammations of the serous membranes. As fibrin forms, the serous surface is no longer smooth and there is friction as it rubs against the opposite side. This produces a pulling on the parietal membrane and pain results. Very often a rubbing sensation can be felt if the hand is placed over the painful area. This is called a friction rub. A stethoscope placed over this area will detect an abnormal sound like the squeaking of leather. If the reaction is examined during an early stage, the two surfaces will look like the buttered sides of two slices of bread that have suddenly been pulled apart. As the reaction proceeds, the fibrin becomes firmer and may eventually be replaced with fibrous tissue forming a permanent adhesion.

Inflammation of the mucous membranes initially produces a serous exudate, followed later by a *mucus* and then a *mucopurulent exudate.* This is the well-known sequence observed during a respiratory infection, frequently termed a catarrhal inflammation, and is generally quite superficial. A similar pattern occurs in a number of infections of the intestinal tract associated with diarrhea. Necrosis of the mucous epithelium may result from the toxins of diphtheria bacilli in the respiratory mucous membranes and of staphylococci in the bowel. Subsequently, plasma leaks from the injured cells and coagulates on the surface, producing a *pseudomembrane* (false membrane). The resultant process is termed a pseudomembranous inflammation.

GENERAL PROCESSES OF HEALING

Healing is generally not initiated until the acute inflammatory process has subsided to a relatively quiescent level. It is now recognized that complete eradication of infection is not necessary. If there has been no preceding inflammatory response, the first phase of repair is the entry of phagocytes into the injured area. The polymorphonuclear leukocytes appear to undergo lysis, and their released enzymes probably act to digest the necrotic tissue. They are followed shortly by the macrophages, which ingest particulate matter. An important component of the phagocytic activity is disposition of blood within the wound. Disintegration of red blood cells releases hemoglobin which, in turn, breaks down to a brown, iron-containing pigment called *hemosiderin* and a yellow pigment called *hematoidin.* Most of these two pigments are taken up by the macrophages, where the hemosiderin may very slowly release iron as it is needed by the body and the hematoidin is converted to bile pigments which are eventually excreted by the liver.

Shortly after the entry of macrophages, capillaries can be seen to develop small buds which penetrate into the injured area. At first these buds are solid cords of cells, but shortly a lumen, or cavity, develops. These capillaries proceed a short distance and then arch. If this new arching vessel comes into contact with another such bud, they join, and a complete channel develops through which blood can be seen to course. If contact is not made, the bud atrophies (becomes smaller) and eventually disappears. As the process continues, the vessels model into a more mature blood supply. Larger vessels form as needed and the arterioles (small arteries) develop a coat of smooth muscle cells which can contract and relax to regulate the blood flow. The origin of the smooth muscle cells has not been established, although it is believed that they arise from fibroblasts. The lymphatics probably form in essentially the same way although, since the lymphatic system is independent of arterial supply, fusion of loops may not be the initial step. The ingrowth of the circulatory system not only supplies nutrients for repair but also increases the efficiency of removal of the nonparticulate components of the necrotic tissue and the inflammatory exudate.

Concurrent with the ingrowth of the vascular system is the entrance of fibroblasts. The fibroblasts produce collagen, a protein which is deposited between cells to give fibrous tissue its strength. Collagen is generally laid down in long strands which are arranged along the lines of stress. These strands gradually collect into bundles, markedly increasing the strength of the tissue. As the injured tissue fills in, the collagenous "scar tissue" eventually bridges the entire area. If the collection of blood (hematoma) or of exudate (abscess) is too large to be completely reabsorbed or if a low-grade chronic inflammatory process (granuloma) persists, complete resolution of the lesion may not be possible. Under these circumstances the residual exudate or lesion produces a tension which aligns the collagen fibers in a surrounding sphere. The lesion is then said to be encapsulated.

An *ulcer* is a surface injury which has destroyed the overlying epithelium, exposing the deeper tissues. The initial healing of a surface injury is essentially the same as for a deep injury. If the ulcer is due to an infection, the inflammatory action with exudate formation will be prominent. Healing will not start until the lesion has been adequately drained, infection is well controlled, and most of the necrotic tissue has been removed. Often the necrotic tissue will separate spontaneously, or slough; sometimes the physician will find it helpful to remove portions of the necrotic tissue, a process known as debridement. If the lesion is due to physical trauma and the wound is occluded only by a blood clot, healing will proceed normally. Examination of the wound, once healing has started, reveals a velvety red, finely granular surface called *granulation tissue* (Fig. 7-9) (not to be confused with an infection granuloma). This tissue consists of the capillary loops, fibroblasts, and phagocytes. It bleeds extremely freely, as when the dressings are changed, and is relatively resistant to infection.

The final stage in the healing of an ulcer is epithelialization or the

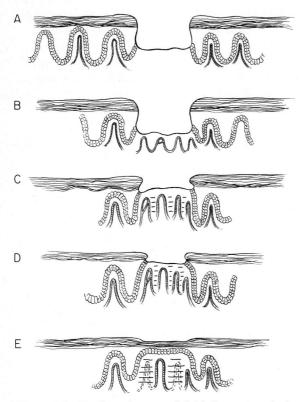

Figure 7-9 Healing of a superficial inflammatory lesion. *A:* As soon as the destructive inflammatory processes cease, healing begins. The wavy row of cells represents the basal cell layer of the epithelium and the loops beneath the epithelium are capillaries. *B:* Capillaries form at the base of the ulcer and epithelial ingrowth has been initiated. The capillary mounds create a granular surface and give rise to the concept of granulation tissue. *C:* The process is continued. Fibroblasts are also activated in the area beneath the ulcer and begin to produce collagen, indicated by the wavy horizontal lines adjacent to the capillaries. *D:* The defect has been almost completely filled in with connective tissue and capillaries and the epithelium almost completely covers the lesion. *E:* The epithelial covering is complete but thinner than normal and no secondary structures are present. The scar tissue has increased. A number of the unnecessary capillaries are undergoing atrophy and the initially red scar is beginning to fade.

ingrowth of an epithelial covering. This can only occur on a solid base of tissue and therefore must await the filling in of deeper defects by the granulation tissue. The epithelial defect is closed by two processes: a thinning and contraction of the adjacent surrounding epithelium, with a resultant sliding over the wound, and an actual increase in epithelial cells. If a plasma clot is present, the epithelium invades between the granulation tissue and the clot, and this "scab" eventually sloughs off. The cutaneous epithelium covering a defect is usually quite thin, and specialized structures such as hair follicles, sebaceous glands, and sweat glands do not develop. However, mucous membranes are more capable of regeneration, and repair of large defects in the gastrointestinal mucosa usually results in the normal formation of crypts and villi (Fig. 7-10).

The ultimate result of wound healing is *scarring*. Initially the scar is highly vascular and stands out as a bright red area. However, with time the vascularity decreases and, since the tissue is relatively inactive, it is less well supplied with blood than adjacent tissues and assumes its characteristically white color. The macrophages leave, the fibroblasts become inert, and the collagen becomes the principal component. Characteristically a scar contracts with time; these *contractures* may lead to late complications, or sequelae. Contractures may result in limitation of motion or marked deformity. This is especially true following burns. Contractures in the hands may make them useless, burns of the neck may pull the head forward, and contractures on the face may distort the mouth or interfere with proper closure of the eyes. Contractures around hollow organs are called *strictures* and may interfere with the normal flow through these organs. Esophageal strictures often follow lye burns; pyloric strictures follow peptic ulcers; strictures of the fallopian tubes follow local inflammation, such as gonorrhea, and may interfere with normal passage of the ovum into the uterus; and strictures of the urethra may also follow gonorrheal infection in the male and interfere with the urinary flow.

The amount of scar formation can be reduced by shortening the period of infection and by reducing the size of the defect. The former can be achieved by the use of antibiotics and other anti-infective treatment; the latter can often be reduced by the use of skin grafts. The proper use of adrenal steroids, cortisone and its related compounds, may also reduce the amount of scar formation. In situations where scars are subject to repeated stress, the inelasticity of the scar may result in its stretching and weakening. Such weaknesses in the abdominal wall may result in hernia (rupture) formation. Other sites where this weakness may be important are the heart, following a myocardial infarction, and the major arteries. Aneurysms, which are localized dilatations of the heart or arterial wall, may form in both of these situations. Finally, there may be an excessive production of scar tissue with the formation of a *keloid*. This

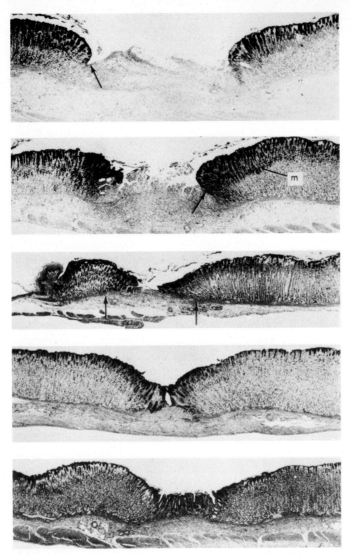

Figure 7-10   Healing of intestinal epithelium.   A superficial ulcer has been created in the epithelium of the small intestine.   By the fifth day, there has been a significant ingrowth of epithelium to cover the defect, and by the tenth day, the epithelial overgrowth is almost in apposition.   The lesion is completely covered over by the eighteenth day, and by the thirty-sixth day there is further restoration of the epithelium toward normal; however, it is still less than half as high as the adjacent normal tissue.   *(From R. M. H. McMinn, Tissue Rapair, Academic Press, New York, 1969, pp. 240–241.   By permission of the publishers.)*

scar may be extremely large and unsightly. Keloids often follow burns and are frequently seen after otherwise normal healing in Negroes.

Healing by first intention, or primary healing, is the ideal response (Fig. 7-11). This usually follows an incised wound and is the desired result after surgery. Under these circumstances there is relatively little tissue damage. If the edges of the wound can be brought into close approximation and held by adhesive tape or sutures, the healing process is much less complex and little granulation tissue need be formed. Blood plasma exudes into the wound and clots, holding the tissues together and making a framework through which blood vessels and fibroblasts can pass. This process is quite rapid, and within 2 weeks the tensile strength of the wound approaches that of normal tissue. Fibrosis is minimal and subsequent contraction of the scar results in an exceedingly small visible defect as well as one that is less likely to undergo the late complications described in the preceding paragraph. In areas where the tissues are relatively loose, a complicated wound can often be converted into a more simple wound by trimming away the irregular tissues and bringing the remaining tissue together in a simplified closure. This can only be done, of course, when there are no foreign bodies or microorganisms in the wound. Much of the work of a plastic surgeon consists of removing scar tissue for functional or cosmetic reasons and, by means of skin grafts and other techniques, achieving a better final result through primary healing.

Factors Affecting Healing

It is apparent that a number of local factors may affect healing. It has been noted that repeated trauma delays healing and increases the likeli-

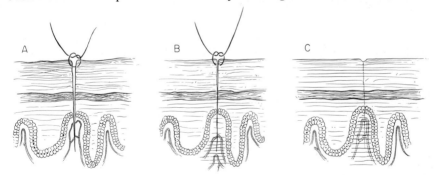

Figure 7-11   Primary healing of an incision. *A:* The edges of the incision are approximated and held together by tape or sutures. *B:* Capillaries and fibroblasts cross the incision line and collagen fibers are laid down. The epithelium bridges the lesion. *C:* With healing, only a minimal collagen bridge is necessary and the scar may be almost invisible.

hood of fibrosis. Inadequate local circulation is an obvious cause of poor healing. Old and debilitated individuals often develop ulcers over bony prominences due to interference with circulation. These are known as decubitus ulcers, or bedsores. These lesions are extremely difficult to heal and require the utmost care to prevent further impairment of the circulation. In fact, susceptible persons should be protected prior to ulceration by frequent moving and proper padding of the most vulnerable sites. Patients with vascular diseases in general, especially arteriosclerosis, are subject to difficulties in wound healing. Comparison of primary and secondary healing indicates that proper apposition of tissues promotes healing, whereas a break in continuity delays it. The immobilization of the affected tissue is often important in order to avoid disruption until the development of adequate tensile strength allows safe movement.

Surprisingly few general factors have been conclusively shown to affect healing. The process is essentially the same at all ages; however, most data indicate that the speed of repair decreases with age. Adequate quantities of vitamin C have been found to be essential for collagen formation. However, there is little evidence that in humans this is a significant factor unless actual scurvy is present. Depletion of protein reserves may also interfere with healing, although extreme degrees of experimental depletion are necessary to demonstrate this phenomenon. Apparently the sulfur-containing amino acids are the most important; these include methionine, cystine, and cysteine. Despite the failure of mildly subclinical deficiencies of both vitamin C and protein to cause delayed wound healing, prudence and general considerations indicate that nutrition should be adequate. The adrenal corticosteroids, specifically the glucocorticoids, have been shown to inhibit both the inflammatory reaction and fibroplasia; thus, healing is slowed and the scar is weaker than normal. Fortunately, the dose of cortisone used for most appropriate indications is generally insufficient to cause major effects. The feared complications are that infection may spread and that the wound may disrupt as a result of steroid administration, and a careful watch must be maintained in order to prevent these developments. However, steroids are useful in the treatment of allergic inflammations, where the inflammatory reaction itself produces the damage. In addition, steroids have been useful in preventing scar formation in certain selected situations, as in inflammation of the eye.

All the factors which are known to affect healing time result in its prolongation. Obviously, the discovery of factors which would shorten healing time would be of great theoretical and practical value. In fact, the mechanism controlling normal healing is still not known. Various "wound hormones" and "chemical organizers" have been suggested but have not had significant experimental support.

REPARATIVE PROCESSES IN SPECIFIC TISSUES

Bone

The healing of bone represents a specialized example of connective tissue healing (Fig. 7-12). Three stages are generally recognized. During the first stage the area of injury is the site of relatively extensive bleeding, with subsequent conversion of the blood into a clot. Macrophages, blood vessels, and cells then invade this mass in the same way that granulation tissue enters wounds in other areas. However, there is one significant difference. Most of the cells accompanying the phagocytes and blood vessels are derived from the bone and the periosteum, which is a dense fibrous layer of tissue immediately surrounding the bone. These cells

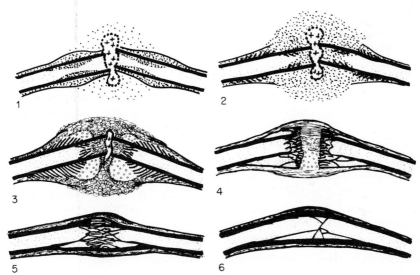

Figure 7-12 Healing of bone. 1. The fracture is shown in cross-section. The two heavy black lines represent the bone and the thinner black lines represent periosteum. At the fracture site, there is debris (crosses), a number of macrophages (large dots), and blood (fine dots.). 2. The callus is beginning to form. Note the new bone growth (slanting lines under the periosteum and in the walls of the marrow cavity). 3. Organization of the callus with replacement of hemorrhage by fibrous tissue, development of cartilage (small circles), and increased new bone. 4. Further organization with enclosure of healing area by completed periosteal sheath and apposition of broken bone ends across fibrous tissue and cartilage. 5. Bony union. 6. Remodeling of cortex and attempt at restitution to near-normal structure. *(From R. M. H. McMinn, Tissue Repair, Academic Press, New York, 1969, pp. 150–151. By permission of the publishers.)*

are known as osteoblasts and are capable of producing collagen and a substance called osseomucin, which can be calcified and converted into bone. During the second phase calcification does occur, and the healing mass is known as a *callus*. The callus forms a rigid bridge between the separated portions of bone. However, this new bone is greater in quantity than will eventually be required and at the same time it lacks strength and normal bone structure. During the third stage of healing the callus is modeled. Osteoclasts ("bone breakers") arise from the same source of cells that produces the osteoblasts. These cells remove the extra bone formed around the fracture site and in the medullary cavity. At the same time the dynamics of stress on the bone, such as muscle pull and weight bearing, cause the osteoblasts to lay down increasingly dense bone in essentially the normal pattern.

The degree of perfection of healing achieved depends upon many factors. Probably the most important is proper alignment and adequate immobilization of the bone fragments. Excessive displacement delays healing and results in deformity. Adequate calcium and vitamin D are, of course, necessary, in addition to vitamin C and protein. Infection delays and jeopardizes the result. It is of interest that cartilage may be formed during the process of bone repair and later replaced by true bone in a manner similar to that displayed during the course of bone development. Occasionally, calcification does not proceed properly, and the bones are joined only by fibrous tissue. This is spoken of as nonunion or fibrous union. This type of failure can be critical, especially in the extremities, where great impairment of function can result. Nonunion usually requires surgery in order to reinitiate a normal healing process. It is of interest that the intact periosteum can form osteoblasts and initiate bone production. A number of operative procedures require the removal of bone, but a careful replacement of periosteum often results in appropriate bone formation to replace the defect.

Tendons, Ligaments, and Cartilage

Tendons and ligaments are fibrous structures containing large amounts of collagen and thus normally have much the same structure as scar tissue. Therefore healing is extremely effective when the severed ends are brought into apposition and sutured. Cartilage is a specialized connective tissue structure and normally does not regenerate in the adult. Arthritis is often the result of aging or injury of cartilage covering the joint surfaces. Eventually, the less satisfactory movement of bone on bone causes the characteristic symptoms of pain and limitation of motion. The failure of cartilage replacement is surprising in view of the fact that it is often produced during the healing of bone.

Muscle

In general, muscle cells do not regenerate and defects are replaced with fibrous tissue. If the cut ends of voluntary or striated muscle are carefully approximated, the muscle cells may enlarge to bridge the gap, but no new cells are formed. If the muscular stresses are great, the remaining cells may hypertrophy (grow larger) in response to the demand. Cardiac muscle responds in essentially the same manner. There is evidence that some new myocardial cells may be formed in response to injury prior to maturity. Subsequently, myocardial cells can respond to stress only by hypertrophy. This limitation in response is an important factor in characterizing heart disease. The evidence for the failure of regeneration of smooth muscle is less absolute. Destructive injuries to the uterus, bladder, and other muscular viscera usually heal by fibrous scars. However, the development of new blood vessels has already been seen to be associated with replacement of the muscular coat, and operations on the gastrointestinal tract rarely result in evidences of subsequent smooth muscle defect.

Nerve

Nerve cells do not multiply and therefore cannot be replaced when destroyed. The restoration of nerve tracts in the central nervous system is extremely limited. However, peripheral nerve fibers may be repaired if the cell body remains intact (Fig. 7-13). The axons of peripheral nerves are surrounded by a fatty coat called the myelin sheath. The myelin, in turn, is held in place by the sheath of Schwann, which is a tube of extremely thin cells. When the nerve fiber is severed, the myelin in both portions undergoes changes known as Wallerian degeneration. The Schwann cells multiply and attempt to form a bridge across the defect. The nerve fiber separated from the cell body degenerates, but the fiber still attached to the cell body sends out numerous shoots. If one of these shoots enters a sheath of Schwann, it then follows this pathway to its normal ending and the other shoots atrophy and disappear.

The rate of regeneration of a nerve fiber is relatively fast and may average about 2 millimeters per day. The severance of a nerve usually involves many nerve fibers going to different structures. The reconstitution of the nerve may lead the individual fibers to follow different sheaths than they did originally. This is often of no importance. However, occasional anomalies result. For example, injury to the seventh cranial nerve may cause fibers which originally innervated the salivary gland to be diverted to the lacrimal gland. This produces the syndrome of "crocodile" tears, since tears appear every time the individual is normally

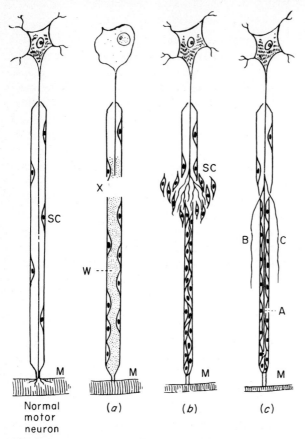

Figure 7-13   Healing of nerve.   Diagram showing the regeneration of a peripheral motor-nerve fiber.   SC, Schwann cells; M,
muscle fiber; W, Wallerian degeneration of myelin.   The normal
motor neuron at the left is cut at point X, resulting in changes in
the cell body, Wallerian degeneration of myelin, and proliferation
of Schwann cells.   Subsequently the nerve cell recovers and a
number of regeneration sprouts appear at the cell end of the axon.
If one of these axons (A) finds a regenerating myelin sheath, it will
continue on down to the motor end plate.   Unsuccessful axon B
and C will eventually atrophy and disappear.   Viability of the muscle depends upon reestablishment of nerve contact.   The successful axon may not be derived from the cell which originally inhabited
the sheath.   *(From R. A. Willis, The Principles of Pathology, Butterworth, London, 1950, p. 32.   By permission of the publishers.)*

stimulated to salivate.   Several other such bizarre syndromes have been
reported.

Muscle cells eventually atrophy if they are not provided with a nerve
supply.   If the motor nerve does not reach the muscle within 2 years after

injury, the muscle cell is replaced by fibrous tissue. Healing of nerves can be facilitated by careful approximation of the cut ends by the surgeon. If regeneration does not occur, the central end of the nerve often develops into a tangled mass of nerve fibers, Schwann cells, and fibroblasts called an amputation neuroma. Such a neuroma may become exceedingly painful and require excision.

Vascular Endothelium

Blood vessels are lined with thin, flattened cells which, because of their mesodermal origin and their function as a lining, are termed endothelial cells rather than epithelial cells. The recent success of various types of blood vessel grafts has prompted examination of these cells. Blood vessel grafts, whether of preserved normal blood vessels or of synthetic material, act only as supporting structures and do not become vital parts of the recipient. The endothelial cells enter the graft from the adjacent host vessels and provide a covering for the vascular surface. Synthetic grafts of dacron are dipped in blood plasma so that a thin film of fibrin will coat the inner surface and increase the success of endothelialization. Experimentally, a segment of graft over an inch in length was found to have a complete endothelium and a subendothelial layer within 10 weeks.

Liver

In many experimental animals 90 percent of the liver tissue can be excised without producing evidence of liver deficiency. However, within a period of time, practically the entire mass of liver will be found to have regenerated with tissue that is functionally normal and shows only a small amount of structural abnormality. Regeneration of this type proceeds by hyperplasia, that is, an increase in the number of cells. In some diseases, such as cirrhosis of the liver, the normal anatomical restoration is prevented by the presence of large amounts of scar tissue.

Kidney

The functional unit of the kidney is called the *nephron*. Nephrons are not capable of regeneration. However, if one kidney is seriously damaged or is removed, the opposite kidney enlarges, and within 3 weeks the single kidney has the functional capacity of 75 percent of the two normal kidneys. Examination of this hypertrophied or enlarged kidney reveals that the increase in function is achieved by hypertrophy of the individual nephrons. This, in turn, is a result of a combination of hyperplasia and hypertrophy of the individual cells. The stimulus to hypertrophy and hyperplasia in organs such as the liver and kidney is not known. This is of special interest, since the residual liver and kidney tissue may be entirely adequate to perform the necessary physiological function without detectable evidence of systemic abnormality.

SUMMARY

Inflammation is the defensive response of living tissues to injury. Although various types of injury may produce specific modifications, the response tends to follow a generalized pattern. Initially there is a vascular response, supplying increased amounts of blood to the injured tissues. Subsequently there is the formation of an exudate made up of cellular and fluid components. The cells act by phagocytosis to destroy and remove residual injuring agents and dead tissue. The fluid provides antibodies and fibrin, which also act to destroy or to localize the injurious agents, most specifically microorganisms. If the inflammatory reaction is successful, there is healing. If it is unsuccessful, the individual may die or a chronic process may ensue.

In healing, macrophages, capillaries, and fibroblasts fill the damaged area. The collagen produced creates the scar. Body surface injuries are covered by epithelium. Most specialized structures do not regenerate. Hypertrophy and hyperplasia may occur to make up for functional defects.

BIBLIOGRAPHY

ALLISON, A.: "Lysosomes and Disease," *Scientific American,* November, 1967.
ANDERSON, W. A. D.: *Pathology,* 5th ed., St. Louis: The C. V. Mosby Company, 1966.
BOYD, W.: *Introduction to Pathology,* 8th ed., Philadelphia: Lea & Febiger, 1970.
DUNPHY, J. E., and W. VAN WINKLE, JR.: *Repair and Regeneration: The Scientific Basis for Surgical Practice,* New York: McGraw-Hill Book Company, 1969.
FLOREY, SIR HOWARD: *General Pathology,* 4th ed., Philadelphia: W. B. Saunders Company, 1970.
MAYERSON, H. S.: "The Lymphatic System," *Scientific American,* June, 1963.
ROSS, R.: "Wound Healing," *Scientific American,* June, 1969.
WILLIS, R. A.: *The Principles of Pathology,* 2d ed., London: Butterworth & Co. (Publishers), Ltd., 1961.
WOOD, W. B., JR.: "White Blood Cells vs. Bacteria," *Scientific American,* February, 1951.

Mature blood cells drawn from a smear of normal human blood stained with Wright's stain. In the center are adult red blood cells, a mature polymorphonuclear neutrophil, and a number of platelets. At the upper left are two polymorphonuclear basophils and two polymorphonuclear eosinophils. At the upper right are three large and four small lymphocytes. At the lower left are five mature polymorphonuclear neutrophils and, below them, one slightly immature band form. At the lower right are six monocytes. [*From L. Weiss in R. O. Greep (ed.), Histology, McGraw-Hill, New York, 1966. By permission of the publishers.*]

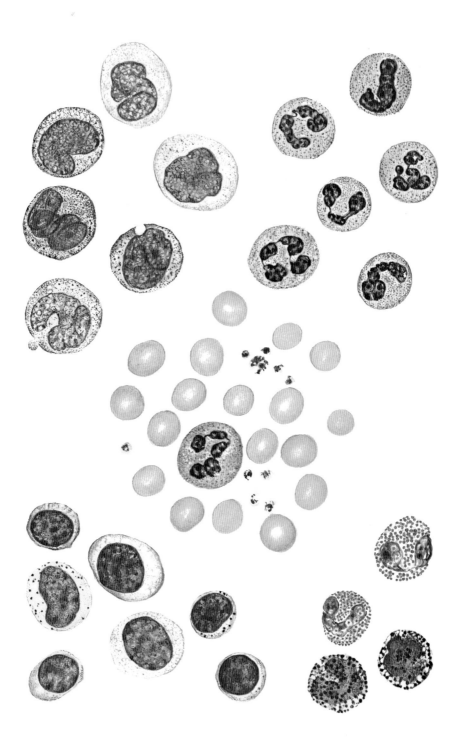

Immunity and Hypersensitivity

The Latin word *immunis* means "not liable for duty" and was applied to the exemption of certain young Roman men from the obligations of military service. Immunity thus implied protection from certain risks. At present the most frequent connotation of *immunity* is protection from disease, and it applies particularly to those factors which protect an individual from a specific infection. Although nonspecific factors of protection against disease could be included, the present usage of the word *immunology* refers to a specific process. This process is characterized by the entry into the body of certain types of foreign chemicals known as *antigens* to which the organism responds by producing *antibodies* which, in turn, modify the effects of the antigens. It is the *antigen-antibody* reaction which characterizes this specific immune process (Fig. 8-1).

ANTIGENS

An antigen, by definition, is a substance capable of producing an immune response. In order to qualify as an antigen, a chemical must have certain

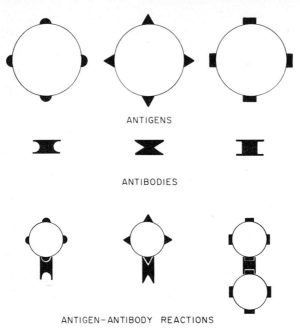

ANTIGENS

ANTIBODIES

ANTIGEN–ANTIBODY REACTIONS

Figure 8-1   Antigens, antibodies, and antigen-antibody reactions.
Paul Ehrlich introduced lock-in-key symbols for antigen-antibody
reactions before the turn of the century. The concepts which he
introduced have now been verified by more precise knowledge of
the antigen-antibody mechanism.

specific characteristics. First, it must be foreign to the individual producing the antibody. Under certain specific conditions this requirement
may appear to have been violated; however, further examination reveals
that this is never the case. Second, antigens are always macromolecules.
Most have a molecular weight of over 10,000 although, under special conditions, smaller molecules, such as glucagon with a molecular weight of
3,800 and insulin with a molecular weight of 6,000, have been effective as
antigens.

Because of the requirements of size, antigens are generally proteins or
long-chain polysaccharides. Some polypeptides are also capable of antigenic activity. Lipids and nucleic acids cannot, by themselves, act as
antigens. However, when coupled with protein, they are capable of doing
so. Most compounds of low molecular weight are incapable of provoking
the formation of antibodies. Often these small molecules can couple
with macromolecules to become complete antigens. For example, this
condition can be satisfied when a drug or drug residue combines with a
normal protein to create a new molecule capable of provoking antibody

production. These small molecules capable of activating a specific antibody response when coupled to macromolecules are termed *haptens*.

An important characteristic of the antigen is that it possesses a high degree of specificity. The exact nature of this specificity is not known at present. The antigenic capabilities of the macromolecule are apparently contained in the sequence and configuration of a very small number of component units (amino acids, simple sugars). Nevertheless, remarkably small changes in these units result in the production of an entirely different antibody. Despite a remarkable degree of specificity, there is evidence that some cross-reactions do occur. In general, these cross-reactions are produced by antigens almost identical in structure with the original one to which the antibody was directed.

It is probable that the most common source of alien macromolecules results from infection with microorganisms and that many of the processes of immunology were developed in response to the selective evolutionary pressure produced by this invasion. It must be remembered that macromolecules taken in the diet must be "digested," that is, broken down into nonantigenic components before they can be absorbed from the intestinal tract. As a result there is normally no antibody response to nutrients.

Bacterial antigens represent a broad and interesting spectrum. One group of bacteria produce extremely potent toxins as part of their normal metabolic processes. Since these toxins are produced by normally functioning organisms, they are known as *exotoxins*. They include the toxins of diphtheria, tetanus, botulism, and gas gangrene; the rash-producing toxin of scarlet fever; and a number of others. In all these diseases the morbidity and mortality are caused mainly by the toxin rather than by the other bacterial activities. For example, the toxin of botulism is produced by the organisms in food which has been improperly canned. The toxin can then exert its lethal effect following ingestion of the food, even though no living organisms are present. Perhaps the most important bacterial antigens are related to the capsule. It is evident that in order to be most effective, the antibody must be capable of reacting with the intact cell wall, since initially the internal components will be inaccessible. However, once the cell wall is broken down, either as a result of antibody action or by phagocytosis, many other antigens are released. The broken-down cell walls and cell contents are termed *endotoxins*, since they come from within the cell. These endotoxins are responsible, at least in part, for the symptoms of infection, including the toxic appearance, malaise, fever, leukocytosis, increased phagocytosis, and the stimulation of antibody production. All foreign cells are capable of acting as antigens.

There is evidence, which shall be expanded later, that most antigens possess two or more sites on the molecule or cell which have antigenic properties. Further, these multiple antigenic loci stimulate the production of only one type of antibody. Two factors have facilitated the use of certain bacterial antigens in the production of antibodies against specific diseases. The first of these is the fact that even when separated from the bacteria, the various compounds retain their antigenic capacity. Second, many antigens, particularly exotoxins, can be modified in such a way as to eliminate the toxic activity but at the same time not interfere with the ability to stimulate the production of a specific and effective antibody.

ANTIBODIES

The ability to produce antibodies appears to be a vertebrate phenomenon. Ordinarily, this capacity does not appear in the individual until about the time of birth, although it may occur a little earlier in some species and a little later in others. The human infant receives an initial set of antibodies from the mother via the placenta. These antibodies have a half-life of approximately 28 days, and the maternal protection continues to be effective for 4 to 6 months. Subsequently, the infant must manufacture its own antibodies.

In some species of mammals the transfer of maternal antibodies is through the colostrum (the fluid produced during the first few days of lactation). In these species the newborn are capable of absorbing relatively large proteins through the intestinal tract, a capacity which, of course, is lost within a few weeks. This is particularly true of calves. Occasionally, a calf fails to nurse for the first few days and as a result does not receive its maternal antibodies. In all animals bacterial invasion of the gastrointestinal tract occurs early and normally confers no risk to the individual. However, these calves, deficient in antibodies, develop diarrhea due to coliform organisms and frequently die. This disease is known as calf scours.

During the period prior to the development of the capacity to produce antibodies, the individual appears to be learning by an as yet unexplained mechanism which compounds are "self," are legitimate body components, and are not to act as antigens. All other compounds are "not self" and are necessarily capable of antigenic activity. Evidence for this phenomenon has come from a number of sources. The most dramatic was the demonstration by Medawar that the injection of foreign antigens and even of foreign cells during this period not only failed to provoke an immediate antibody response but made it impossible for these substances to act as antigens later in life. This observation and the concept which it confirms represent one of the major recent advances in immunology.

Much has been learned about the actual mechanism for the production of antibodies. Three types of cells have been suspected of participation and extensively studied. It now seems quite certain that the most important cell is the *plasma cell*. Electron microscopy shows that this cell contains a cytoplasm which is structurally capable of producing large amounts of protein. Its structure is very much like that of the typical undifferentiated mesodermal cell described in Chap. 2. It is well supplied with endoplasmic reticulum, ribosomes, mitochondria, and Golgi apparatus. The most convincing evidence, established by techniques to be described later, is that it is the only cell in which large amounts of intracellular antibodies can be demonstrated. Finally, plasma cells in tissue culture have been demonstrated to kill appropriate bacteria without coming in direct contact with the organisms, as would occur with phagocytosis.

The role of the *macrophage* is less clear. Particulate antigens can be observed to be cleared from the blood and lymph by the fixed macrophages of the lymph nodes, spleen, and bone marrow. No significant amount of antibody has been demonstrated within these cells. Yet, if phagocytosis is interfered with by prior overloading, as by injection of India ink, the antibody response is much reduced.

There is much evidence to implicate the *lymphocyte* as an immunologically competent cell. Procedures which destroy most of the body lymphocytes impair antibody formation. The presence of the lymphocytes in the exudates surrounding chronic inflammations suggests a role for the lymphocytes; yet the lymphocyte has very little cytoplasm, and this cytoplasm shows little capacity for protein synthesis.

The route of antigen entry determines the site of antibody production. Antigens entering the bloodstream produce maximal stimulation of antibody production in the spleen. Entry into the tissues results in antibody production in the regional lymph nodes. There is some evidence that suggests that in chronic granulomatous infection, the antibodies are produced by the appropriate cells in the granulomatous mass.

We have previously seen that the blood *plasma* contains a significant amount of circulating protein. If the plasma is allowed to clot, the fibrinogen becomes fibrin, and the remaining *serum* contains two general types of proteins: albumin, which is of relatively low molecular weight, and the globulins, which are considerably heavier. The globulins in turn can be broken into three components, alpha, beta, and gamma. The antibodies make up the gamma component; therefore, they are called *gammaglobulins* or *immunoglobulins*. About 80 percent of the immunoglobulins have molecular weight of 160,000. The remainder are heavier and may have molecular weights up to 1,000,000.

The basic structure of the immunoglobulin is Y-shaped (Fig. 8-2). Each immunoglobulin is made up of two long protein molecules—the

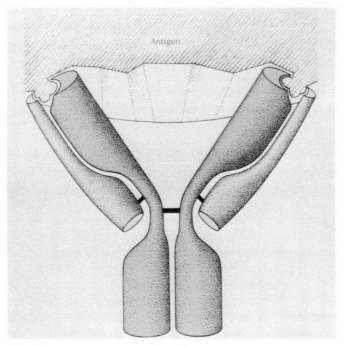

Figure 8-2   Present concept of antibody structure.   The figure is a representation of an antibody linked to two specific areas on the same antigen.   Each antibody is composed of two long protein molecules and two shorter molecules, linked to each other as indicated and termed heavy and light chains respectively.   One end of each paired light and heavy chain has a specific configuration for a specific antigen.   The remainder of each of the chains contains the same sequence of amino acids regardless of specificity.   It should be noted that both the light and heavy chains participate in this antibody specificity.   [*From A. Nisonoff in R. A. Good and D. W. Fisher (eds.), Immunobiology, The Sinauer Associates, Inc., Stamford, Conn., 1971, p. 66.   By permission of the publishers.*]

heavy chains, and two shorter protein molecules—the light chains. These four chains are bound together by relatively weak chemical linkages. The points of specific attachment to the antigen are the tips of the two arms of the Y.   Both the heavy and light chains participate in forming the specific linkage site.   The base of the Y appears to be the point of attachment to complement (see below).   By appropriate chemical treatment, the antibody can be broken into three components.   The two arms of the Y each contain a light chain and half a heavy chain and are still capable of combining with antigen.   Thus each complete antibody is said to be bivalent.   The third portion of the antibody contains the remaining fragments of the two heavy chains.

At the present time, five types of immunoglobulins have been identified in each normal individual (Fig. 8-3).   The fundamental differences lie
in the sequence of the amino acids in the heavy chains.   Immunoglobulin
G (IgG) makes up about 65 percent and is found chiefly in the serum.
IgM comprises about 20 percent.   It is composed of five basic units linked
together and is also found in the serum.   Although there is much overlap,
the specificities of IgG and IgM are somewhat different.   IgA may exist in
single, double, or triple units and makes up about 10 percent of the serum
immunoglobulin.   The importance of IgA lies in the fact that it can enter
mucosal cells, where a "secretory piece" is added.   It then passes into the
tears and secretions of the respiratory and intestinal tracts, where it forms

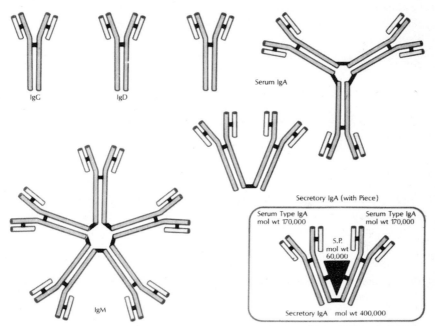

Figure 8-3   The structure of immunoglobulins.   Quantitatively,
the most important immunoglobulin is IgG, which is found largely
in the serum.   IgD and IgA may also have the same approximate
structure; however, IgA may be combined in double or triple units.
IgA may pass through various secretory cells where a so-called
secretory piece is added which binds two of the basic units together.   This type of IgA is then included in the secretions of the
respiratory and gastrointestinal tract, where it forms a line of defense against organisms prior to their entry into epithelial cells.
IgM appears to be a five-component immunoglobulin which is
present in the serum in considerably less quantity than IgG.   [*From
T. B. Tomasi in R. A. Good and D. W. Fisher (eds.), Immunobiology,
The Sinauer Associates, Inc., Stamford, Conn., 1971, p. 79.   By
permission of the publishers.*]

a first line of immunological defense. IgD is present in only small amounts and its specific characteristics are unknown. IgE, a recently recognized immunoglobulin, is normally present in only trace amounts but is found to be markedly increased in allergic individuals and their relatives. This immunoglobulin is capable of fixation within tissues.

Analyses show that the amino acid sequences are identical for most of the length of the chain in all the immunoglobulins of a given group (IgG, IgM, etc.). However, the specific attachment ends vary in the amino acid sequence. Both the heavy and light chains participate in having invariable and variable amino acid sequence segments and thus in the antibody specificity.

Much information regarding the nature and role of the antibody can be clarified by examination of the clinical condition known as *hypogammaglobulinemia,* in which there is a deficiency in the immunoglobulins. This disorder may be hereditary or it may be acquired. At least three hereditary forms have been identified. The acquired forms are found in those diseases which affect the plasma cells and lymphocytes, such as multiple myeloma and lymphatic leukemia, which presumably interfere with the normal immunoglobulin production of these cells. Hypogammaglobulinemia is also found in protein-wasting diseases such as nephrosis, in which most of the gammaglobulin is lost in the urine; and in burns, where much protein is lost through the injured surface. In all these conditions there is a serious loss of resistance to bacterial infection. However, the common virus infections of childhood are handled normally, and permanent immunity develops. In addition, the so-called "delayed" immune reaction of the type seen in tuberculosis and in the ability to reject transplanted tissues, although sometimes delayed, is not fundamentally impaired. This type of reaction will be discussed in greater detail later.

Effective treatment of hypogammaglobulinemia can now be achieved by the injection of purified gammaglobulin obtained from normal donors. Since the half-life of the globulin is approximately 1 month, injections are given in that frequency. Although this treatment is expensive, it is effective, and these individuals can lead relatively normal lives. Recently there have been several successful bone marrow transplants to patients with hereditary hypogammaglobulinemia, and the transplanted cells have produced effective immunoglobulins.

Antibodies do not exist in the normal individual until there has been exposure to the appropriate antigen. When an individual is exposed to an initial dose of antigen, a small amount of antibody is produced in a few days, which then gradually disappears. If a second or booster dose of antigen is now administered, the antibody response is multiplied manyfold, and the decline in blood level is much slower (Fig. 8-4). The optimal

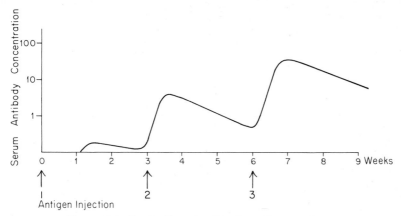

Figure 8-4   Production of antibodies. Repeated exposure to an antigen reduces the time required to produce antibodies and results in a higher and more sustained serum titer.

interval for readministration of the antigen appears to be about 1 month. Since a first exposure to an infection or other antigen source produces a slow and moderate response, other mechanisms of body defense are required until the immunological mechanisms become active. These mechanisms obviously lack the authority of specific immunity. On reexposure, however, the immunologic reactions are prompt and effective. This accelerated response is the rationale for protective immunization. The hyperresponsiveness of antibody production to a specific antigen generally persists throughout life, although the magnitude of response will decrease with time unless reinforced by "booster" immunizations.

Theories of Antibody Production

The actual mechanism of antibody production is intriguing and has given rise to two major theories. The first of these, the *clonal selection hypothesis* of Burnet, postulates that the mechanism for producing all potential antibodies is carried in the genetic information. This is also known as the *selective theory.* All the cells of a particular individual carry the same genes. The total sum of genetic information must be repressed by specialized cells, so that only the information necessary for the ,tructure and function of the specific cell type is manifested. Thus, nerve cells are prevented from secreting digestive enzymes and bone cells from performing rhythmic contractions. During the developmental period, cells which are destined to become immunologically competent develop mechanisms for suppression of the exhibition of immunity to antigenic chemicals native to that individual. Subsequently, exposure to antigens not so coded results in the uncovering of the specific antigenic capacity. These cells then multiply and are subsequently capable of enhanced antibody production in response to the specific antigen. The opposing theory has been termed the *instructional* or *directive hypothesis.* This theory proposes that each antigen specifically instructs the immunologically competent cell to produce an appropriate antibody.

Neither theory is entirely compatible with the available data. The selective theory presupposes that there is genetic information for each potential antigen. However, the potential number of antigens far exceeds the reasonably predicted cellular capacity for storing genetic information. On the other hand, the directive theory proposes that the cell produce antibody proteins for which there is no genetic instruction. Since one of the main tenets of modern genetics is that protein production must be previously encoded in the gene, the mechanism for this instruction is not clearly visualized. It should be noted that both theories visualize that each immunologically competent cell can produce only one specific antibody. At present the selective theory is favored by most immunologists.

Complement

An important component of some antigen-antibody reactions is a complex substance termed *complement.* This material is nonspecific. Recently it has been determined that complement consists of at least nine components which must react in proper sequence. A characteristic of complement is that it can be destroyed by heating serum to $56°$ C. This makes it possible to remove complement without altering antigens or antibodies. The major reactions which involve complement include lysis, activation of opsonin systems, and virus neutralization. Originally it was thought that complement might be necessary for antigen-antibody linkage. It has now been demonstrated that complement acts at the next step. Lysis and other complement-assisted reactions do not occur until complement attaches to both components of the antigen-antibody complex.

ANTIGEN-ANTIBODY REACTIONS

The fundamental assumption of immunology is that the antigen stimulates its host to the production of antibodies, which then react to form antigen-antibody complexes. These complexes either directly inactivate the antigen or make it possible for other body mechanisms to do so. The antibodies are present in the serum and thus have given rise to the science of *serology.* A number of characteristics of the antigen-antibody reaction are well defined, and some are implicit in the previous discussion:

1. The reaction is specific, although some cross-reactions do occur.

2. The fundamental mechanism of antibody action is essentially the same regardless of the ultimate manifestations of the antigen-antibody complex. (Exception may be made in the case of some presumably univalent antibodies.) Antibodies have been characterized as *precipitins* which cause precipitation of soluble antigens, *agglutinins* which cause clumping of bacteria and cells, *lysins* (bacteriolysins and hemolysins) which dissolve antigenic cells, *opsonins* which alter the surface components of bacteria to facilitate phagocytosis, and *antitoxins* which neutralize bacterial and other poisons.

3. The reaction is a chemical one involving entire antigen-antibody molecules without alteration of either.

4. The union is firm but reversible.

5. The antigen and antibody can combine in varying proportions. This is due to the fact that the antibody is bivalent and the antigen, especially if cellular, is multivalent.

6. The reaction is extremely rapid and is almost complete within a few minutes.

The recognition of the presence of antigens and antibodies, as well as of antigen-antibody complexes, requires some overt reaction which can be measured. Fortunately, the antigen-antibody reaction does result in a number of manifestations which can be interpreted by direct and indirect means and which extend the usefulness of serology far beyond the ability to measure immunity to specific disease processes.

Types of Antigen-Antibody Reactions

One of the simplest, earliest, and most widely used reactions is the *precipitin reaction.* In this reaction a visible precipitate forms when proper amounts of serum containing an appropriate antibody are mixed with a solution of antigen. The simplest explanation for precipitate formation would be the production of extremely long molecules of alternate antigen and antibody. However, careful study shows that the optimum ratio for precipitate formation occurs when the number of antibody molecules is slightly greater than two times the number of antigen molecules, although this may vary considerably with the antigen size. This has given rise to the *lattice hypothesis* and is compatible with the concept of antigen multivalency. It is obvious that antibody insufficiency would result in incomplete precipitation of antigen. It is less clear why antibody excess would interfere with complete antigen precipitation. The current belief is that when too many antibody molecules are attached to a single antigen molecule, the extra antibodies block the formation of the lattice structure (Fig. 8-5).

The *agglutination reaction* is of great physiological importance. In this reaction the antibody combines with antigens on the cell wall, resulting in clumping and immobilization. This phenomenon is most frequently observed with bacteria, although the same reaction is seen when red blood cells mismatched for a transfusion result in hemagglutination. Since the bacterial and cellular particles are so much larger than simple antigenic molecules, the agglutination reaction is often easily visible by eye and can be even more acutely observed under the microscope. For this reason much smaller amounts of antibody can be detected by this method than in a precipitation method. Advantage has been taken of this phenomenon to improve the sensitivity of detection of soluble antigens. Specially treated red cells or fine particles of bentonite or latex can be coated with extremely small amounts of antigen. The presence of comparably small amounts of antibody then results in visible agglutination of the coated particles.

Lysis, or the dissolution of cells, requires not only the antigen and the antibody but the presence of complement as well. If serum containing the antibody is allowed to stand a number of days or is heated to $56°\,C$ and then mixed with the appropriate antigenic cells, there will be no visible reaction. If then a nonspecific serum which contains complement but not the appropriate antibody is added to the system, lysis will occur. In

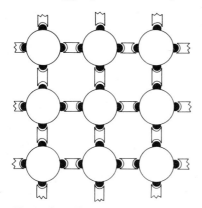

Figure 8-5 The lattice hypothesis. The bivalent characteristics of the antibody make it possible for the antibody to link two antigens together. The presence of multiple antigenic sites on the antigen, in turn, makes multiple linkages possible and gives rise to the lattice hypothesis to explain the optimum relationship between the quantities of antigen and antibody necessary for maximum effect as well as the aggregation of complexes seen in precipitin and agglutinin reactions.

the case of hemolysis, it is believed that there are many small sites on the red blood cell wall where the antibody and complement can fix.   This reaction then injures the wall at that point, allowing the hemoglobin to leak out of the cell and external solution to enter the cell.   When hemolysis is complete, the entire solution takes on the reddish color of the hemoglobin and the destruction of the cell results in clearing of the turbidity previously caused by the cellular particles (Fig. 8-6).

The presence of antitoxins can be detected by *neutralization* techniques.   One of the first uses of this procedure was in the standardization of diphtheria antitoxin.   The usual procedure is to determine the minimum lethal dose (MLD) of diphtheria toxin, which is the minimum amount of toxin which will kill a guinea pig weighing 250 grams within 4 days of subcutaneous inoculation.   The antitoxin can then be standardized by determining how much must be mixed with the standard amount of toxin to prevent a toxic reaction.   In practice, the procedure is more complex because while the antitoxin is stable, the toxin is not.   Therefore, it is customary to establish the potency of the toxin against a known standard of antitoxin prior to using the toxin for standardization of the new batch of antitoxin. Neutralization tests are also used to detect the presence of antibodies to specific viruses.

The type of immunity associated with the production of circulating antibodies is termed *humoral immunity* because it is contained in the fluid, or humoral, portion of the blood and tissues.   It is to be distinguished from *cellular immunity,* which will be discussed later.

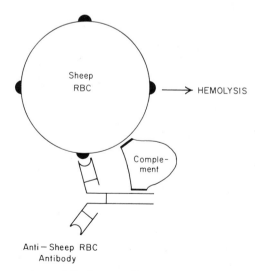

Figure 8-6   The complement-fixation reaction.

Types of Immunity

The most obvious biological purpose for the production of antibodies which results in the antigen-antibody reaction is to provide immunity against infection. From the preceding discussion, it is apparent that there are a number of mechanisms by which immunity can provide protection: the neutralization of toxins, the facilitation of phagocytosis, the immobilization of organisms, and the direct destruction of bacteria and other cells. *Innate immunity* is that component of immunity contributed by the inherited structure and function of the tissues and is unrelated to the presence of antibodies. It is obvious that all antibodies produced by the body must be acquired by exposure to an antigen subsequent to the period of indoctrination as to self and nonself. *Acquired immunity* may be passive or active. *Passive* immunity refers to that immunity conferred by the introduction of externally produced antibodies. This is achieved naturally by the congenital transfer of maternally produced antibodies and can be achieved artificially later in life by the introduction of antibodies from other sources. The most common clinical use has been the injection of diphtheria and tetanus antitoxins. These antitoxins are produced in the horse and are immediately available for administration to patients with diphtheria or individuals who have been exposed to the possibility of tetanus infection. These antitoxins suffer two major disadvantages: (1) Their duration of effectiveness is limited, and (2) the use of horse or other serum as a vehicle exposes the patient to the risk of a reaction to horse serum if readministration is necessary (see immediate hypersensitivity). Another form of passive protection is the administration of purified human gammaglobulin, especially to patients with hypogammaglobulinemia. Occasionally, gammaglobulin is obtained from patients who have just recovered from a disease and therefore can provide specific protection against it.

Active immunity results from direct exposure to the antigen with the subsequent development of antibodies produced within the body. Active immunity may be said to be natural when it results from a natural exposure to antigen as by active infection. Artificially acquired active immunity is produced by the administration of appropriately modified antigens which will cause the recipient to develop antibodies without overt infection or toxic manifestations. The preparation of biological materials which produce artificial, active, acquired immunity has made great strides in the past century. The result of these successes has been that many of the acute infectious diseases, which at one time caused many complications and frequent death, have now become so rare that they are almost medical curiosities. These include such diseases as smallpox, diphtheria, tetanus, pertussis (whooping cough), poliomyelitis, typhoid, measles, German measles (rubella), and yellow fever. (See Table 8-1.)

Table 8-1   Available Active Immunizations

Routine	Special situations (exposure, travel in endemic areas, etc.)
Diphtheria	Cholera
Measles	Influenza
Pertussis	Mumps
Poliomyelitis	Plague
Rubella (routine for children)	Rabies
Smallpox	Tuberculosis
Tetanus	Typhoid–parathyphoid
	Typhus
	Yellow fever

DIAGNOSTIC USES OF SEROLOGICAL TECHNIQUES

If a patient has a disease which is suspected of being caused by an invading organism and which has been present for at least several days, it may be possible to make the exact diagnosis by serological methods. Bacterial suspensions are made from stock cultures of the suspected organisms. To these cultures are added various dilutions of the patient's serum. If very small amounts of serum are capable of agglutinating the bacteria, there is strongly suggestive evidence that the patient's serum contains agglutinins and reflects a response to infection by that organism. A stronger presumption can be made if, during the course of the illness, the concentration of the antibody in the serum appears to increase. This change suggests that the agglutinins are not merely residual from a previous infection or immunization.

Conversely, serum antibodies can be used to identify bacteria. An animal which has a strong antibody-producing response, such as a rabbit or a guinea pig, is generally used. These animals are immunized against a variety of known bacteria and the antibody-containing sera are collected. These sera can then be used to identify the unknown bacteria. The unknown bacteria are mixed with the various sera and the serum which agglutinates the organisms makes the identification. This technique is especially valuable when there are a number of strains of bacteria which otherwise appear to be identical. For example, 70 different strains of pneumococci have been identified on the basis of the antigen found in the capsule. Immunity to one strain does not confer immunity to any of the others. Identification of the exact type of *Pneumococcus* was once of practical importance when the only means of treating pneumococcal pneumonia was the administration of a type-specific antiserum. Another example is the relationship of *Streptococcus* to late complications from streptococcal infection. It has been found that only five of the many strains of *Streptococcus* will produce acute glomerulonephritis (an important and common generalized disease of the kidneys, also known as Bright's disease). This information will, it is hoped, lead to a better understanding of the nature of glomerulonephritis. At present it appears that a *Streptococcus* strain initiates glomerulonephritis but is not necessary for its perpetuation.

Macromolecules have been extremely difficult to identify, not only because of their many components but also because the arrangement of these components is complex and variable. By taking the serum of an animal immunized to a specific antigenic macromolecule and using precipitation and agglutination techniques, it is possible to identify the presence of extremely small amounts of the same macromolecule in solutions made from tissues where the molecule is thought to exist.

The *complement-fixation reaction* was one of the first reactions utilized to demonstrate certain antigen-antibody reactions which produce no visible phenomena. The complement-fixation reaction has already been described: When red blood cells are added to an appropriate hemolytic antibody in the presence of complement, hemolysis results. However, not all complement-fixing reactions produce visible manifestations. If the presence of a complement-fixing antibody is suspected, the serum is inactivated by heating to $56°$ C in order to destroy the complement but not the antibody. The antigen and a measured amount of complement are then added to the serum to be tested, and time is allowed for the complement to become fixed. At this time sheep red blood cells and antisheep cell antibody are added. If the complement has been fixed by the serum antibody and the added antigen, it is no longer available to cause lysis of the sheep cells. On the other hand, if in the original system either antigen or antibody was not present, the added complement is free to unite with the sheep cell–antisheep cell antigen-antibody complex and produce hemolysis. (See Fig. 8-7.) One of the first applications of the complement-fixation reaction was introduced by Wasserman in 1905 for the detection of syphilis. At present, the complement-fixation reaction is widely used for the identification of antiviral antibodies.

The *fluorescent antibody* techniques developed by Coons have extended the range of immunology into fundamental areas, some of which were not anticipated by the original investigators. Coons demonstrated that it was possible to produce antibodies and then attach fluorescent indicators as integral parts of the molecule. The localization of the antibody can then be determined under the microscope by using fluorescent illumination, which causes the fluorescent tag to light up in the characteristic yellow-green color. A typical technique is to obtain a section of

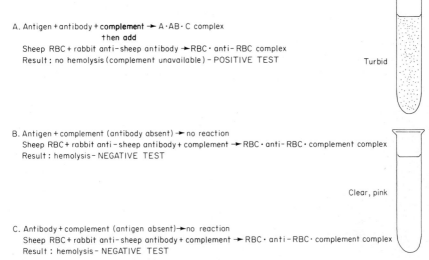

A. Antigen + antibody + **complement** → A·AB·C complex
     then add
   Sheep RBC + rabbit anti-sheep antibody → RBC·anti-RBC complex
   Result : no hemolysis (complement unavailable) – POSITIVE TEST   Turbid

B. Antigen + complement (antibody absent) → no reaction
   Sheep RBC + rabbit anti-sheep antibody + complement → RBC·anti-RBC·complement complex
   Result : hemolysis – NEGATIVE TEST

                                                                         Clear, pink

C. Antibody + complement (antigen absent) → no reaction
   Sheep RBC + rabbit anti-sheep antibody + complement → RBC·anti-RBC·complement complex
   Result : hemolysis – NEGATIVE TEST

Figure 8-7   The complement-fixation test.

fresh tissue, flood it with the fluorescent antibody, and allow the antibody to unite with the appropriate antigen. The excess antibody is then washed off the tissue, and the tissue is then examined, using appropriate equipment. Since antibodies can be made to any antigen and even to antibodies themselves, the possibilities for this technique seem unlimited (Fig. 8-8). For example, the use of fluorescent antibodies made it possible to deter-

●   Specific antigen

⌐⌐   Specific antibody

▬   Anti-human gammaglobulin antibody

٬٬٬٬ Fluorescence

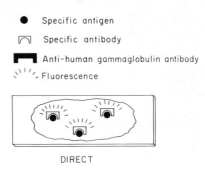

DIRECT

Figure 8-8 Immunofluorescence techniques. In the direct technique, the fluorescent tag is attached directly to the specific antibody. In the indirect technique, it is attached to an antihuman gammaglobulin antibody. This makes it possible to identify where actual antigen-antibody complexes have formed or localized in the tissues.

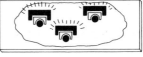

INDIRECT

mine which cells made antibodies and helped in the localization of the various intracellular functions described in Chap. 2. This technique has also been useful in studying a number of diseases thought to be due to immunological abnormalities (Fig. 8-9). Some of these diseases will be discussed in a subsequent portion of this chapter.

The *Coombs test* is a useful method for determining the presence of presumably incomplete or univalent antibodies, particularly those associated with some pathological forms of hemolysis. These antibodies attach to the red blood cell, but because they are effectively univalent they cannot produce agglutination, although they may produce hemolysis. The *direct Coombs test* determines the presence of antibodies already fixed to red blood cells. The patient's blood is drawn and the red cells are separated from the plasma and washed with normal salt solution. They are resuspended in a solution containing rabbit antibodies to human gammaglobu-

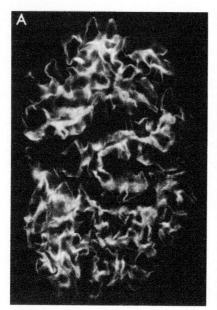 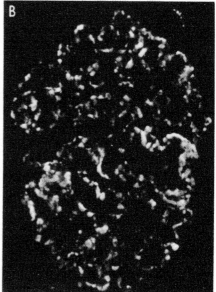

Figure 8-9 Fluorescent antibody reactions. *A:* Fluorescent micrograph of a glomerulus showing linear fluorescence. This suggests that the antibodies have reacted with the basement membranes of the glomeruli. *B:* Granular fluorescence in a glomerulus. This iş associated with the deposition of circulating antigen-antibody complexes which have been trapped on the glomerular basement membrane. Kidney disease can be produced by both mechanisms. [*From F. J. Dixon, C. B. Wilson, and H. Marquardt in J. Hamburger, J. Crosnier and M. H. Maxwell (eds.), Advances in Nephrology, vol. 1., Year Book, New York, 1971, p. 2. By permission of the publishers.*]

lin.   This is an antibody to human antibodies, and if globulin is present on the red cells after washing, the red cells will be agglutinated.   The *indirect test* is used to identify Rh antibodies.   These antibodies to Rh-positive cells are produced by Rh-negative mothers and cross the placenta to hemolyze the fetus's Rh-positive cells.   The antibodies have no effect on the Rh-negative red cells of the mother and cannot be detected by the usual tests.   Fetal blood is not easily available.   Yet it is important to determine if these antibodies are present.   Therefore the maternal serum is added to known Rh-positive cells, the cells are washed, and the rabbit antihuman gammaglobulin serum is added as for the direct test.   Agglutination indicates that anti-Rh-positive antibodies are present.   The test is performed in such a manner that the concentration, or "titer," of antibodies can be estimated, making it possible to evaluate the risk of the fetus (Fig. 8-10).

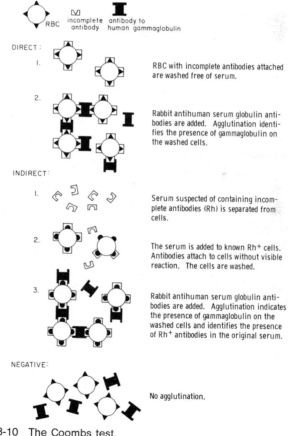

Figure 8-10   The Coombs test.

HYPERSENSITIVITY

Allergy is a term which was introduced by von Pirquet in 1906 to imply an altered capacity to react. However, this could mean increased, decreased, or absent reactivity. The usual connotation is the first of these, and at present immunologists prefer to use the term *hypersensitivity* for this condition. Occasionally, generally following overwhelming disease, the capacity for immunological reaction is completely lost, a condition termed *anergy*. Two general types of hypersensitivity exist. The first can be demonstrated to be due to antibodies circulating in the serum and is termed *immediate hypersensitivity*. The reaction occurs within minutes after the appearance of both antigen and antibody. The second type fails to demonstrate serum components but appears to be mediated by cells. Despite this, the reaction has the characteristics of immunity. The involved cells are lymphocytes, plasma cells, and macrophages. The reaction is specific and manifests acceleration on reexposure comparable to the serum-mediated mechanism. The response usually takes 24 to 36 hours and subsides in 3 or 4 days in the absence of new antigen. This type is generally called *delayed hypersensitivity,* despite the fact that it may appear sooner after antigen exposure than some types of immediate hypersensitivity, such as serum sickness. However, in serum sickness there is a delay only until the antibody appears; the prompt subsequent development of the reaction follows the immediate pattern.

Immediate Hypersensitivity

The most severe type of immediate hypersensitivity is *anaphylaxis.* Anaphylaxis requires previous sensitization at least 10 days earlier. The reaction is initiated by injection of the antigen and is characterized by almost immediate itching of the scalp and tongue, flushing of the skin, difficulty in breathing due to bronchial spasm, and acute hypotension (fall in blood pressure) leading to unconsciousness and often to death. In the past, anaphylaxis has most frequently followed the administration of horse serum antitoxin for the treatment of diphtheria or tetanus. Currently, the most common cause is probably sensitization to some of the breakdown products of penicillin (Table 8-2). The prompt administration of adrenalin followed by adrenal corticosteroids and antihistamines will prevent death. The same mechanism acting more locally on the respiratory mucous membranes (by inhalation) produces the allergic manifestations of *hay fever* and *asthma*. Anaphylaxis in animals varies depending upon the organ most severely affected. The guinea pig responds with intensive spasm of the bronchial muscles. Air gets into the lungs but cannot be expelled, and at death the lungs are greatly overexpanded. The air cannot

Table 8-2   Agents Which Have Produced Anaphylaxis in Man

Proteins	Drugs	Diagnostic reagents
Horse antiserum	Penicillins	Sulfobromophthalein (BSP)
Insulin	Salicylates	Sodium dehydrocholate (Decholin)
Corticotrophin	Para-aminosalicylic acid	Iodinated organic contrast reagents
Allergen extracts	(PAS)	(for x-ray)
Dextran	Local anesthetics	
Liver extract	Procaine amide	
Chymotrypsin	Aminopyrene	
Trypsin	Mercurial diuretics	
Penicillinase	Colchicine	
	Probenecid	
	Indandiones	
	Meprobamate	

SOURCE: Norman in Modell, *Drugs of Choice*, Mosby, St. Louis, 1970.

be forced out even by direct mechanical pressure. The rabbit responds by similarly intense constriction of the pulmonary arteries, resulting in total obstruction to pulmonary blood flow.

Originally it was not possible to demonstrate the presence of circulating antibodies in individuals subject to anaphylaxislike reactions. However, the mechanism was greatly clarified by an ingenious experiment performed by Prausnitz and Küstner and reported in 1921. Küstner was extremely sensitive to the proteins of cooked fish. It was found that extracts of this material would produce a typical wheal with swelling, redness, and itching when injected into Küstner's skin but not when injected into the skin of Prausnitz or of other normal individuals. However, when serum from Küstner was injected into the skin of Prausnitz and followed 24 hours later by the injection of cooked fish protein extract into the same area, a typical wheal and flare developed in the treated area but not in the adjacent normal areas. This experiment demonstrated two important points: (1) that there was a sensitizing component in the serum, and (2) that this component fixed itself in the tissues. It was soon found that the manifestations of localized and systemic anaphylaxis could be duplicated by the administration of histamine, and that excess amounts of histamine could be found in the tissues during experimental anaphylactic reactions. Other studies have shown that at least three other compounds are present which may contribute to the reaction: serotonin, "slow-reacting substance," and bradykinin.

The mechanism and sequence of the reaction can be approximately reconstructed as follows: After appropriate sensitization, a type of antibody is produced which becomes fixed to the *mast cells* in the connective tissue which contain large amounts of histamine. When there is exposure to the specific antigen, a complex forms in the tissue which injures the cells and causes the release of histamine and the other substances enumerated. The major effects of histamine are to cause local smooth-muscle spasm and injury to small vessel walls, resulting in seepage of plasma which results in the local edema.

It is not understood exactly why or under what circumstances these unusual antibodies known as *reagins* are produced. Recently reagin has been identified as a type of antibody which has been designated immunoglobulin IgE. It is present in only minute amounts in the serum of normal individuals but in much larger amounts in patients with hypersensitivity of this type. Patients with clinical allergy tend to have a strong family history of allergic manifestations. The abnormal response to antigens has been termed *atopy* (Fig. 8-11).

Management of patients with allergy consists of removing the allergen when possible; since this is not usually totally effective, symptomatic therapy may be necessary. Antihistamines may be effective and adrenalin and cortisone derivatives are useful in severe and intractable situations. Desensitization is an immunological procedure which has had variable success. The antigen is given in gradually increasing amounts in order to produce antibodies, so that inert antigen-antibody complexes are formed before the antigen reaches the sensitized cell. These have been appropriately called blocking antibodies. Apparently they are not permanent, since it is necessary to desensitize before each allergic season. It should be pointed out that the Prausnitz-Küstner test could be extremely useful both in diagnosis and in research. Unfortunately, at present the possibility of transmitting serum hepatitis is too great to permit its widespread use.

Another type of antibody-mediated hypersensitivity is characterized by the *serum sickness syndrome*. This reaction was initially recognized as a complication of the use of therapeutic antiserum. Symptoms begin 7 to 10 days after exposure and consist of malaise, fever, enlargement of the lymph nodes and spleen, the appearance of an urticarial rash (hives), and usually pain, tenderness, and swelling of the joints. Symptoms and signs may persist for as long as 10 days. If the concentration of the antigen in the serum is followed, it will be found to have a relatively slow but steady decrease for approximately a week. During the next few days the decrease in antigen is much more rapid. Circulating antibodies cannot be detected until the antigen totally disappears. The symptoms and signs of serum sickness coincide with the period of rapid decrease in antigen concentration (Fig. 8-12). It is currently believed that during this period there is antigen-antibody complexing under conditions of antigen excess, and that the antigen excess can account for the acute inflammatory lesions. The

SENSITIZATION

ATOPIC SENSITIZATION

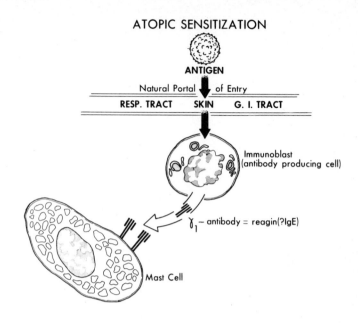

ATOPIC REACTION

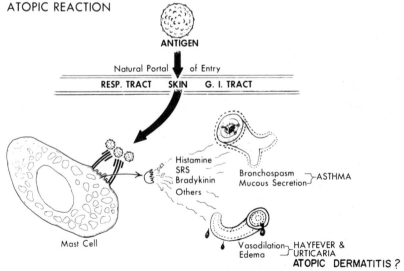

Figure 8-11 Atopy. Recent evidence indicates that IgE is the reagin and that the cell to which it is attached is the mast cell. The mast cell contains histamine granules; injury to this cell releases histamine and accounts for the allergic manifestations. [*From O. L. Frick in T. B. Fitzpatrick (ed.), Dermatology in General Medicine, McGraw-Hill, New York, 1971, pp. 686–687. By permission of the publishers.*]

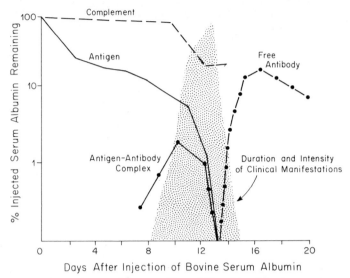

Figure 8-12   Serum sickness. The relationship of the concentrations of antigen, antigen-antibody complexes, and free antibody to the clinical manifestations of serum sickness. Symptoms do not occur until the antibody is developed and begins to react with the antigen. Symptoms subside when all circulating antigen and antigen-antibody complexes are eliminated from the serum. *(Modified from F. J. Dixon, et al., Arch. Pathol. 65:20, 1958. By permission of the publishers.)*

mechanism by which the tissue injuries are produced is not understood. These inflammatory lesions are rather characteristic and generally occur in and around the small blood vessels. The skin manifestations appear to be due to histamine release. At the present time reactions of this type are most commonly due to the administration of sulfonamides and penicillin.

A third group of reactions due to immediate hypersensitivity might be classified as essentially normal antigen-antibody reactions at the wrong time or in the wrong place. Since these reactions appear to account for a number of clinical conditions and diseases, they may profitably be discussed at this point. These reactions are all cytolytic or cytotoxic and usually require complement. In this category are included transfusion reactions, hemolytic disease of the newborn, and some forms of drug hypersensitivity, such as hemolytic anemia and the generalized purpura due to Sedormid, which is a sedative drug. There is also the possibility that some types of acute nephritis are due to the formation of antigen-antibody complexes by bacterial products and the antibodies formed against them, and that these complexes are toxic. Some of the autoallergic phenomena to be discussed later in this chapter may also fall into this category.

Cellular Immunity (Delayed Hypersensitivity)

This type of reaction was first described by Koch in relation to tuberculosis and was originally called *delayed hypersensitivity*. It can perhaps be best illustrated by a description of the Koch phenomenon. If a guinea pig is inoculated with tubercle bacilli, no immediate lesion is produced; but after 10 to 14 days a firm nodule appears, which then ulcerates. At the same time there is gross involvement of the regional lymph nodes. A second injection given 4 to 6 weeks later produces no immediate response, but in the next 18 to 48 hours the area becomes indurated (hardened by infiltrate) and assumes a dark color. This is the delayed reaction. The skin becomes necrotic and sloughs, leaving an ulcer which heals quickly and permanently. The regional lymph nodes are uninvolved by the second injection. This effect can be produced not only by living bacilli but by dead bacilli as well. Koch's recognition of this phenomenon led to the development of the tuberculin test, which has been widely used for the determination of previous exposure to tuberculosis.

Examination of the lesion which follows the second exposure indicates that it is composed almost entirely of mononuclear cells, chiefly lymphocytes and macrophages. The central area of the lesion is usually necrotic tissue, which in tuberculosis is called caseation. The reaction is specific. The time required after first exposure before the delayed reaction is comparable to the time required for the production of serum antibodies, but such antibodies have never been demonstrated either by direct techniques or by the passive transfer of the Prausnitz-Küstner (P-K) type, However, a positive reaction of the P-K type can be obtained if living cells are transferred from a sensitized donor to the test subject. The evidence suggests that during the first exposure to the antigen, large numbers of lymphocytes and possibly macrophages are sensitized to the antigen. These cells then circulate for prolonged periods and are available for local infiltration upon repeated antigenic challenge. At the local site, where they make up the round cell infiltrate of the local granuloma, they are capable of multiplication. Because the mechanism is dependent upon sensitized cells, delayed hypersensitivity is now termed *cellular immunity*. It is of interest that patients with hypogammaglobulinemia are capable of developing cellular immunity.

The role of this reaction in tuberculosis has been extremely difficult to assess and is the subject of much controversy. It has been clearly demonstrated that patients with a positive tuberculin reaction are much less likely to develop disseminated (miliary) tuberculosis on exposure to tubercle bacilli than are individuals with a negative reaction. This protection is far from complete. The production of a necrotic mass containing living tubercle bacilli undoubtedly often facilitates dissemination. For example, in the lung tissue, destruction and caseation produce a semifluid mass which can easily spread bacilli to adjacent areas. For many years a special attenuated (nonpathogenic) strain of tubercle bacilli known as BCG has been given to individuals with negative tuberculin reactions to produce immunity, and there is no question that this offers protection against the development of clinical tuberculosis by localizing the infection and enhancing antibacterial action.

Cellular immunity requires sufficiently prolonged exposure to the antigen and therefore is probably not produced by acute, self-limited infections. Some degree of delayed hypersensitivity has been demonstrated with many prolonged and chronic infections, particularly those in which phagocytosis seems ineffective or in which the organism requires an intracellular habitat. This characteristic has been utilized for the diagnosis of a number of diseases in addition to tuberculosis. These include the bacterial infections of leprosy and brucellosis; the fungus infections of coccidioidomycosis and histoplasmosis; the virus infections of mumps, psittacosis, and lymphogranuloma venereum; the protozoal disease leishmaniasis; and echinococcus disease caused by the dog tapeworm. Delayed hypersensitivity also appears to play a role in some types of contact dermatitis. This type of allergy seems more related to repeated exposure than to hereditary influences, and in certain types of industrial exposures a high percentage of workers can become sensitized. Reactions of this type include those to poison oak and poison ivy, formalin, hair dyes, and metals to name but a few. The skin need not be broken to initiate the action, although open areas may accelerate and aggravate the process.

From the data presented, it can be seen that instead of being an abnormal reaction, delayed hypersensitivity represents a distinct form of immunity which in most instances protects against foreign proteins not defended against by the inflammatory reaction or by immunoglobulin antibodies. Current evidence suggests that the lymphocytes which produce cellular immunity are derived from or are under the control of the thymus, while the lymphocytes which initiate humoral immunity are similarly related to lymphatic tissue in the intestinal tract. The mechanisms of sensitization and reactivation are probably similar. Obviously, the appearance of significant numbers of lymphocytes on the scene will be considerably delayed over the arrival of preformed antibody in the initial inflammatory exudate. Yet accumulating evidence suggests that cellular immunity is probably a more primitive defense mechanism than is humoral immunity (Fig. 8-13).

AUTOIMMUNE DISEASES

A number of disease processes resulting from normal and abnormal immune mechanisms have already been discussed. In almost all cases they have represented the introduction of foreign antigens which have either triggered a normal immune response with disruptive consequences (e.g., transfusion reaction) or have produced one of the hypersensitivity reactions. In the past few years there has been great interest in the possibility that a number of otherwise unexplained diseases may be the result of inappropriate immune responses to body components. At least two classes of antigens can be considered: (1) normal tissues or tissue products which have not previously been identified as self may gain access to the immunologically competent cells and stimulate antibody formation; and (2) normal components may be altered by disease, drug treatment, or some other mechanism and as a result act as antigens. In addition, immunologically competent cells may become altered and not recognize permitted components. Phenomena observed in some diseases of the blood-forming organs and reticuloendothelial system, particularly lymphatic leukemia and multiple myeloma, could be explained in this manner. Under these conditions a constant reservoir of antigen could result in a persistent

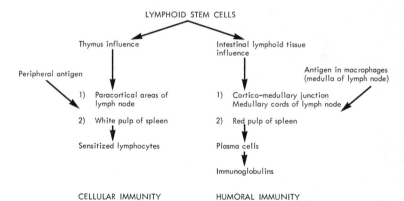

Figure 8-13   The relationship of the development of cellular and humoral immunity. In both instances the antigen stimulates lymphocytes, but cellular immunity results from stimulation of cells of thymus origin while humoral immunity results from stimulation of cells of intestinal origin. *(Modified from Truk, Immunology in Clinical Medicine, Appleton-Century-Crofts, New York, 1969, p. 5. By permission of the publishers.)*

antigen-antibody reaction. Diseases of this type are said to be due to autoimmunity; the antibodies produced are called autoantibodies.

Examples of possible sensitization to normal tissue are as follows:

1. For many years it has been known that injury to one eye may lead to clouding and blindness in the other, a condition termed sympathetic ophthalmia. For this reason it has often been considered wise to remove an extremely damaged eye immediately. There are portions of the eye to which the circulation is extremely limited, and it is possible that these components of the eye have never been identified as "self." The present evidence suggests that the trauma allows unidentified antigens from the eye to stimulate the production of autoantibodies, which then react with the components of the normal eye.

2. One form of chronic thyroiditis is almost invariably associated with antibodies to thyroglobulin. Since thyroglobulin is the storage form of thyroid hormone, it does not normally circulate. It is presumed that, due to some unknown type of injury, thyroglobulin escapes and acts to stimulate antibody production.

3. Mature sperm are not present until after puberty and therefore are not present during the identification of permitted body components. It is possible that some forms of male sterility are due to the formation of antibodies to the sperm. It is also suggested that there may be a relationship between the development of this type of antibody and the fact that the orchitis (testicular inflammation) of mumps rarely occurs until after puberty.

4. The central nervous system is also ordinarily separated from the immune mechanism. It has been known for some time that the intramuscular injection of emulsified brain tissue leads to encephalomyelitis in experimental animals. Evidence has been accumulating to indicate that the mechanism is a delayed type of hypersensitivity reaction. The experimental model very much resembles a number of degenerative neurological diseases for which the etiology had not been established. The response also resembles a type of encephalomyelitis which occasionally follows virus diseases such as measles, mumps, chicken pox, and small pox. In particular, it resembles the disease which may be a complication of the administration of rabies vaccine. This was especially true when the vaccine was made from virus grown in nervous tissue, since it was probable that some of the nerve tissue was present in the material injected. It has been less frequent since the culture medium for virus growth has been changed to duck embryos.

A series of disorders known as the *collagen diseases* has been intensively investigated for a possible autoimmunological etiology. These diseases include lupus erythematosus, rheumatoid arthritis, rheumatic fever, scleroderma, and a number of other apparently related entities. Although these diseases are grouped because of similarities of clinical and pathological patterns, it is probable that disease of connective tissue in general rather than collagen is the factor which causes their similarity. Most of these diseases have abnormal immunological components. An antinuclear antibody to DNA itself has been identified in patients with lupus erythematosus, and a rheumatoid factor has been identified in the serum of many patients with rheumatoid arthritis. A long list of other diseases can be presented in which the etiology is uncertain but in which there is evidence strongly suggestive of immunological abnormality.

TRANSPLANTATION

The obvious potential utility of tissue transplantation has prompted extensive investigation. Transplantations are, in general, of two types. The first is of material which is used primarily as a scaffolding or is immunologically isolated. Included here are blood vessel and bone grafts, which only span defects and are eventually replaced by appropriate body tissues, and corneal grafts, which are protected by the absence of direct blood access. Immunological complications are of little importance to this group. The second type of grafts consist of tissues whose intact function.is required. Grafts of this type include skin, kidney, liver, heart, lung, and endocrine glands. Knowledge of immunology makes it predictable that immune mechanisms would be directed against these grafts. The only exceptions to be expected are *autografts,* which are grafts taken from the same individual, and *isografts,* which are derived from genetically identical twins. *Homografts* and *heterografts*—taken respectively from other members of the same species and from members of another species—would be expected to fail. In general, the predictions are valid. An initial homograft will appear satisfactory for a week or more. However, during the second week there is evidence of disruption and generally by the end of the week the graft has become necrotic. If another graft is then attempted from the same donor, the rejection reaction is greatly accelerated and is usually complete in about 4 days. This is known as the *second-set reaction.* Microscopic examination of the usual rejection reaction reveals intensive infiltration of the graft with mononuclear cells. This finding, in association with the usual inability to demonstrate circulating antibodies, leads to the conclusion that the rejection reaction is a manifestation of cellular immunity. Recent investigations have shown that, under some circumstances, humoral antibodies may be present and are capable of producing a microscopically distinct reaction. Great effort is now being made to protect the grafts by suppressing the immunological response, preferably just to the specific tissue grafted. Unfortunately this is not yet possible, and generalized immunosuppression reduces the defenses against infection and increases the vulnerability of the transplant recipient.

THE IMMUNOLOGICAL ASPECTS OF AGING

One of the most intriguing theories of aging combines the possibilities of somatic mutation and autoimmunity. It is well established that an increasing number of chromosomes show gross changes with age. It seems probable that comparable changes also occur in the genes. Two possibilities exist for autoimmunity to act as a mechanism of aging. First, somatic cells are altered and produce foreign proteins, which in turn stimulate an antibody response. Second, mutations in some of the immunologically competent cells may alter their ability to recognize which compounds are permitted. Either or both of these changes could result in the development of low-grade tissue incompatibility or autoimmune reactions. Although there is no conclusive evidence for this mechanism, there are sufficient suggestive data to warrant further exploration.

BIBLIOGRAPHY

ALEXANDER, J. W., and R. A. GOOD: *Immunobiology for Surgeons,* Philadelphia: W. B. Saunders Company, 1970.

BOYD, W. C.: *Fundamentals of Immunology,* 4th ed., New York: Interscience Publishers, Inc., 1966.

BURNET, M.: "How Antibodies Are Made," *Scientific American,* November, 1954.
——: "The Mechanism of Immunity," *Scientific American,* January, 1961.

GELL, P. T. H., and R. R. A. COOMBS (eds.): *Clinical Aspects of Immunology,* 2d ed., Oxford: Blackwell Scientific Publications, Ltd., 1968.

GOOD, R. A. and D. A. FISHER (eds.): *Immunology,* Stamford, Conn.: Sinauer Associates, Inc., 1971.

HUMPHREY, J. H., and R. G. WHITE: *Immunology for Students of Medicine,* 3d ed., Philadelphia: F. A. Davis Company, 1970.

JAWETZ, E., J. L. MELNICK, and E. A. ADELBERG: *Review of Medical Microbiology,* 9th ed., Los Altos, Calif.: Lange Medical Publications, 1970.

NOSSAL, G. J. V.: "How Cells Make Antibodies," *Scientific American,* December, 1964.

SAMTER, M., and H. L. ALEXANDER (eds.): *Immunological Diseases,* Boston: Little, Brown and Company, 1965.

SPIERS, R. S.: "How Cells Attack Antigens," *Scientific American,* February, 1964.

TURK, J. L.: *Immunology in Clinical Medicine,* London: William Heinemann, Ltd., 1969.

Infection

Pathogenic infections represent the commonest diseases of man. In the past, they have been the most frequent causes of disability and death. The conquest of infectious diseases has undoubtedly been the greatest factor in the extension of life expectancy. This has been accomplished through sanitation and public health measures, the development of immunization methods, antibiotics and chemotherapeutic agents, the control of arthropod vectors, improved nutrition, and by many other factors as well. Nevertheless, infections continue to be a significant source of disability and death. Their control depends upon the continued application of appropriate measures. The structure of our society renders many of these mechanisms relatively invisible. It should never be forgotten that a breakdown in any of these mechanisms would result in the renewed importance of these diseases.

PARASITE FACTORS IN DISEASE

All living material is interdependent. With the exception of that plant life which can convert inorganic to organic material, all other living forms must meet their metabolic requirements by obtaining organic foodstuffs. Thus, herbivorous animals eat plants; carnivorous animals, in general, prey on the herbivores; and the organic material which is left after the death of any of these is eventually decomposed by microorganisms to form nutrient material for plant life. *Parasitism* is a specialized relationship in which one organism takes advantage of another *living* organism in order to survive. This gives rise to the host-parasite relationship, in which the host not only must provide for his own biological needs but also for at least some of the needs of his parasite. It should be appreciated that it is in the interest of the parasite to maintain the well-being of its host, since the death of the host threatens the parasite unless another host can be found. In many instances there is a *commensal* relationship between the host and the parasite, indicating that the parasite produces no apparent effects upon its host. Many bacteria of the skin, mucous membranes, and especially of the intestinal tract may be in this category. A *symbiotic* relationship indicates that both the host and the parasite benefit each other. For example, the bacteria in the rumen* of the ruminant and the protozoa in the stomach of the termite are essential to the lives of their hosts, since without them cellulose could not be broken down into digestible sugars.

Some parasites are capable of independent living and, in fact, may not usually function as parasites. These opportunistic organisms are known as *facultative* parasites. Common examples are the *saprophytic bacteria* which ordinarily live on dead organic material and are responsible for the processes of decomposition. These bacteria become parasites when living in the lower portion of the intestinal tract. Other organisms cannot survive in the absence of a host and are called *obligate* parasites.

Disease is produced only when the parasite causes a detrimental change in its host. It must be understood that these relationships are not always fixed. For example, a saprophyte, which may be a facultative parasite in the intestinal tract and ordinarily has a commensal relationship with its host, may become a pathogen capable of producing disease if it is spilled into the peritoneal cavity as a result of an intestinal perforation.

Infection is the invasion of a host by a parasite. To the extent that parasitism is not synonymous with disease, the same can be said for infection. The *pathogenicity* of an organism is its ability to initiate a disease process. *Virulence* has a slightly different meaning; it refers to the relatively greater ability to produce disease of one strain or sub-species of an organism when compared to another strain of the same species.

---

* The first stomach, where the cud is stored, of cattle and related species.

An *epidemic* disease is one in which a large number of people are involved in a relatively short period of time. An *epizootic* disease is the equivalent situation involving animals. A disease which is present within a community in moderate numbers but at all times is termed *endemic;* one which occurs only occasionally is called *sporadic.* An epidemic which becomes unusually widespread, literally involving all communities, is a *pandemic.*

Infection may be localized in one part of the body or in one organ, or it may be *generalized* if the infection is widespread. A *secondary* or *intercurrent* infection is produced by a second microorganism as a result of the reduced resistance produced by a primary infection. A *mixed* infection is due to more than one organism. Often an individual is debilitated by a chronic disease which paves the way for a *terminal* infection, which is the last, but not necessarily the most important, event leading to death. Infections may be *inapparent* if the entire course evolves without clinical symptoms; inapparent infections often account for immunity in individuals not aware of previous exposure. A *latent* infection is one in which there are no manifestations, either because defense mechanisms hold it in check or because it is in a site where it causes no pathogenic changes.

The presence of bacteria in the circulating blood is termed *bacteremia* and that of viruses, *viremia.* Bacteremia and viremia may not be associated with actual disease. *Septicemia* represents a further evolution of bacteremia and implies serious disease. Septicemia is usually associated with pyogenic organisms and is equivalent to the lay term *blood poisoning.* Septicemia may result in the widespread formation of pyogenic abscesses called *pyemia;* the term literally means "pus in the blood." *Toxemia* is due to the release of toxins into the bloodstream; these are often, but not invariably, of parasite origin.

An infectious disease is generally manifested by a characteristic pattern. After infection there is a period of *incubation,* during which those organisms capable of maintaining infection multiply. This is followed by the *prodrome,* in which mild and usually nonspecific symptoms are manifested. Next is the period of *disease,* during which the manifestations of the disease become overt and clinically specific. If the patient survives, there is a period of *recovery* and finally a period of *convalescence* during which anatomical and physiological integrity are restored. Recovery may take place in a few hours by *crisis* or more gradually over several days by *lysis.* Diseases which run a natural course (excluding complications) are said to be *self-limited;* their duration is usually determined by the length of time required to develop active immune mechanisms or, in the case of some virus diseases, to produce interferon (see page 301).

The Transmission of Infection

The cycle of infection is made up of four components: (1) entrance into the host, (2) establishment and multiplication, (3) exit from the host, and (4) a mode of transportation to the new host. This cycle must be complete if parasitism is to form a repetitive pattern rather than to be a unique episode.

Generalizations can be made which limit the number of portals of entry for purposes of classification and epidemiology.

1. The respiratory tract. Infection via the respiratory tract requires that the infecting organism be carried in relatively small particles which can be inhaled and thus spread through both the upper and lower respiratory system. The commonest mode of spread is via fine, liquid droplets which usually result from the cough or sneeze of an infected individual and which contain pathogenic organisms. Droplet formation associated with quiet respiration and with speech probably contributes to infection. Dust can also be a source of infection, especially by those organisms which can withstand drying.

2. The alimentary canal. Infections of the alimentary canal are usually due to the presence of potential parasites in food and fluid. However, the placement of contaminated objects in the mouth, particularly by young children who mouth their toys, will also complete the cycle.

3. The skin. Only a few organisms can penetrate the intact skin, and therefore the skin is ordinarily an effective barrier. However, the skin is often disrupted and wounds are subject to infection. Generally, infection is by direct contact with a contaminating source, but dust and droplets can contribute. Infections via the mucous membrane of the genitourinary tract, particularly venereal diseases, can also be classified in this category.

4. Arthropod bites. An agent which transmits infecting microorganisms is called a *vector,* and the term is most frequently applied to arthropods. This category could be considered a specialized subclass of (3). However, there are many reasons for maintaining it as a separate entity. The most important of these is the fact that specific organisms are carried by specific arthropods, and the bite of these arthropods will produce the disease in a suitable host. The organisms so transmitted are almost invariably pathogenic. This sequence is so relatively specific as opposed to most other infections that it enables the epidemiologists to attack the chain of infection both through the host and through the insect vector. Insects such as flies, which may spread infection by transferring intestinal pathogens to food and drink, are called mechanical vectors. However, in this instance they are only incidental vectors, and such diseases are not included in the arthropod-borne category.

Factors concerned with the establishment and multiplication of the parasites will be discussed in subsequent sections. The portal of exit is an important component of the cycle and especially relevant to further spread. Respiratory infections are airborne and therefore in most instances localization of the infection in the respiratory tract allows the infected individual to contaminate the atmosphere for future hosts without the necessity of any more complex mode of transmission to the new host.

Transmission of gastrointestinal organisms is usually the result of a simple short circuit from the anal to the oral orifices. Much can be done to break this chain by simple sanitary measures. Modern methods which provide pure water supplies and effective disposal of sewage have undoubtedly been the greatest cause of the reduction in the number of cases of these diseases. However, it is still necessary to train all individuals to wash their hands adequately before handling foods, to eliminate the use of improperly sterilized fertilizers, and to protect against insects which can carry organisms from excreta to food by mechanical means. Not all gastrointestinal infections follow a simple anal to oral pattern. For example, the parasitic flukes have an incredibly complex life cycle. Eggs that are deposited in the stool hatch upon exposure to water. The larvae enter snails, where they multiply and develop further. After they leave the snail, they enter fish or freshwater crustacea. Man then becomes infected by eating the uncooked fish, crayfish, or crab. In this example there are a number of points at which this chain or infection can be broken. Some of the intestinal parasites avoid the anal-oral route entirely. The hookworm and schistosome ova may be lost in the stool, but the larvae enter the body by penetrating the skin.

Many common infections are transmitted by direct contact with a lesion on the surface of the skin. In the case of impetigo, a superficial skin infection due to staphylococci, a local lesion is transmitted from the donor to the recipient. In the case of syphilis, an infectious superficial lesion is the source for the transmission of a systemic infection to the recipient, although a local lesion, the chancre, may mark the point of entry. Contact infections may be transmitted indirectly by contaminated clothing, blankets, and other materials which were in contact with a source of organisms. These infected materials are known as *fomites,* although the term is rarely used. Fortunately, many infectious agents do not survive drying and poor nutrition, and therefore this mechanism is of limited importance.

Arthropods are responsible for the transmission of an extremely large number of diseases, many of which have been of extreme importance because of the number of people infected. Examples include yellow fever, a viral disease, which is transmitted by the aedes mosquito; typhus, a rickettsial disease, which is transmitted by the body louse; plague, a bacterial disease, which is transmitted by the rat flea; malaria and sleeping sickness, protozoan diseases, which are transmitted by the anopheles mosquito and the tsetse fly, respectively; and filariasis, a roundworm disease, which is transmitted by the culex mosquito. These diseases have all been of great historic importance. At one time yellow fever made the American tropics almost uninhabitable. Typhus epidemics have killed millions in central Europe and Asia. It is estimated that the plague killed between one-fourth and one-half of all Europeans during the Middle Ages. Malaria was probably the commonest cause of death in the world until the post-World War II period. Sleeping sickness made much of Africa unproductive; and filariasis, although less important numerically than the others, has produced much disability in the Asiatic and Pacific tropics. Efforts directed at arthropod control have done much to reduce the incidence of all of these diseases.

The previous paragraphs have shown that the following patterns of infection and disease can be demonstrated:

1. Common commensal organisms may become pathogens when some defect in the host defense provides a favorable opportunity.
2. Infections may be passed directly from man to man.
3. Infections may pass from man to man but require an obligate intermediate host or hosts for the complete cycle.
4. Man may be an accidental host in a cycle which ordinarily involves only animals. For example, jungle yellow fever is a disease of monkeys, transmitted in South America by *Haemagogus* mosquitoes. Accidental infection of a jungle worker or transportation of a sick monkey into the city sets up the urban yellow fever cycle of man-to-man transmission by the aedes mosquito.
5. Man may be the accidental host and there may be no way for the organisms to reenter the natural cycle.

An understanding of these patterns is essential for epidemiology and is of particular importance in the management of patients in order to avoid further dissemination of the disease on the ward, in the home, or in the community.

In subsequent sections of this chapter an attempt will be made to catalog the most important organisms infecting man. Obviously, the list will be brief and incomplete. Bacteria, viruses, pathogenic fungi, and protozoa are all termed microorganisms because complete individuals are microscopic or submicroscopic in size. Helminthes, or worms, and arthropods complete the list of parasites. Arthropods will not be discussed in detail. However, their greatest importance lies in the smaller parasites

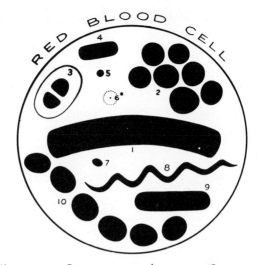

MORPHOLOGIC RELATIONSHIPS of INFECTIOUS ORGANISMS
1. *B. anthracis,* 3-8μ x 1-1.2μ.
2. *S. aureus,* 0.7μ -0.9μ
3. *D. pneumoniae,* .8-1.25μ x 1.5-2.5μ.
4. *H. influenzae,* 1-1.5 x 0.3-0.4μ.
5. *Vaccinia virus,* 0.15μ.
6. *Yellow fever virus,* 0.018μ.
7. *Rickettsia prowazekii,* 0.3μ x 0.3-0.5μ.
8. *Tr. pallidum,* 0.2μ x 4-14μ.
9. *E. Coli,* 2-3μ x 1-1.2μ.
10. *S. pyogenes,* 0.6μ -1.5μ.

* APPROXIMATELY THREE TIMES LARGER THAN
A MOLECULE OF SERUM GLOBULIN

Figure 9-1 This diagram shows the relative size and shape of a number of important microorganisms. The symbol μ represents 1/1,000,000 of a meter. [*From H. C. Hopps in W. A. D. Anderson (ed.), Pathology, 6th ed., Mosby, St. Louis, 1971, p. 274. By permission of the publishers.*]

that they transport, and this relationship will be presented. Figure 9-1 shows the size and shape of a variety of bacteria in relation to a red blood cell and two viruses as a point of reference for the subsequent discussion.

BACTERIA

Antony van Leeuwenhoek first reported the observation of "animalcules" in 1683, based on his work with a simple, homemade microscope. However, it was not until nearly two hundred years later, in 1876, that Pasteur and Koch both demonstrated independently that injections into animals of small amounts of a culture of *Bacillus anthracis* would produce anthrax in the inoculated animals. These experiments unequivocally established that bacteria could produce disease. However, concepts of contagion had existed for at least several centuries, and in the fifty years preceding their work a number of experiments had been conducted which inevitably led to the final demonstrations by Koch and Pasteur. In 1865, Joseph Lister, impressed by some of Pasteur's earlier work, had initiated techniques using phenol to reduce the risks of infection in surgery. Dubos has stated that the era opened by Pasteur, Lister, and Koch probably represents the greatest single contribution so far made to the theory and practice of medicine.

Identification

Bacteria are complete cells, with nuclei, cytoplasm, and cell walls. They range in size from 0.3 to 15.0 micrometers in length; a red blood cell is approximately 7.5 micrometers in diameter (see Fig. 9-1). Rod-shaped bacteria are called *bacilli,* spherical bacteria are called *cocci,* and spiral bacteria are called *spirilla* if rigid and *spirochetes* if flexible. Organisms which have variable shapes, depending upon growth conditions, are said to be *pleomorphic.* In general, the spiral forms are motile, as are some bacilli that are equipped with whiplike flagella.

Further visual differentiation can be achieved with light microscopy by various staining techniques which show a number of relatively gross differences. An important technique for the differentiation of many bacteria is the use of the *Gram stain.* In this procedure the organisms are stained first with crystal violet, a basic dye. A solution of iodine is then applied and rinsed off, and the bacteria are treated with acid alcohol. The gram-positive cells remain stained a dark blue color, but the gram-negative bacteria are washed free of the dye. A counterstain is then applied, usually one which gives a red color to contrast with the blue of the gram-positive stain. The slide is then examined under the microscope. Recent evidence indicates that the crystal violet-iodine complex attaches to bacterial cytoplasm within the cell wall, and that the alcohol is unable to penetrate the wall to wash out the complex. The Gram stain not only serves to aid in bacterial identification but also indicates a significant difference in the structure of the cell wall itself.

The use of the electron microscope has added an important new dimension to the evaluation of bacterial structure; however, this technique is too complex at the present time to be useful in clinical differentiation. Other important procedures for bacterial identification include observations of the nature of cell growth on various culture media, the demonstration of specific biochemical characteristics, and serological typing as described in Chap. 8.

Mechanisms of Bacterial Pathogenesis

Since pathogenic bacteria produce disease, it is of great importance to understand the mechanisms by which they affect structure and function. There are two general groups of factors which are considered to affect pathogenicity. The first of these is the ability to enter tissues, survive, multiply, and spread, a quality known as *invasiveness*. The second is the ability to produce toxic or poisonous substances and is termed *toxigenicity*.

Many pathogenic bacteria possess a capsule outside the cell wall. This capsule is generally somewhat gelatinous and literally makes the organism so slippery that phagocytosis is relatively unsuccessful. Under certain conditions many of these organisms can be grown without the capsule, and these modified bacteria tend to be nonpathogenic. This is one example of the mechanisms by which virulence can vary within a single species of organisms. Other bacteria, not equipped with a capsule, have substances within the cell wall proper which are deterrents to phagocytosis. These capsules and cell walls have varying antigenic properties. However, when antibodies are formed, they usually are of the opsonin type, and phagocytosis destroys their pathogenic properties. Ordinarily, it requires a week to produce antibodies after a primary exposure, and the spread of virulent organisms may be sufficient within that time to produce severe complications or death.

Other bacteria induce anticapsular antibodies but are not destroyed by this mechanism, although antibodies to other components may be effective in host defense. Some organisms, notably the streptococci, contain hyaluronic acid, a substance which is also antiphagocytic. Hyaluronic acid is a normal component of tissues and is, therefore, nonantigenic. As a result, protective antibodies cannot be developed against this substance. There are other instances in which lack of antigenicity enhances the pathogenic capacity of specific microorganisms. A number of other organisms produce hyaluronidase, an enzyme which destroys hyaluronic acid. Hyaluronic acid is an important component of connective tissues; its dissolution enhances the ability of these bacteria to spread through the tissues. The enzyme streptokinase, which is produced by some of the most pathogenic streptococci, has a similar action. This enzyme digests fibrin and probably also accounts for the fact that the pus from streptococcal infection is thin and watery by comparison to that of staphylococcal infection, which tends to enhance fibrin formation. A number of other enzymes which disrupt and dissolve tissues have also been recognized. Finally, some organisms are able to survive within the cell, despite phagocytosis. An important example is the tubercle bacillus. This organism contains a large amount of fat in the capsule which apparently renders it relatively resistant to intracellular digestion.   Other organisms, such as the rickettsiae, are actually incapable of multiplying unless they are within cells.

There are three groups of bacterial toxins: (1) exotoxins, (2) endotoxins, and (3) enzymes.   These are distinguished by the mechanisms whereby their toxic manifestations are produced.   *Exotoxins* are produced by living cells and diffuse into the tissues.   Four important exotoxins are those of botulism, tetanus, diphtheria, and gas gangrene.   The toxin of *Clostridium botulinum* is one of the most potent known; a little more than one trillionth of an ounce is sufficient to kill a mouse.   This exotoxin is produced by bacteria growing in improperly preserved foodstuffs and is absorbed from the gastrointestinal tract without the necessity of living organisms being present.   It is a neurotoxin and kills by its action on the central nervous system. Tetanus toxin is also a neurotoxin and is present after the contamination of wounds by the spores of *Clostridium tetani.*   Invasiveness is not necessary, since the presence of a few growing organisms will produce sufficient toxin. The toxin produces neuromuscular hyperirritability with resultant spasm, which causes the characteristic manifestation of "lockjaw."   The etiological agent of diptheria, *Corynebacterium diphtheriae,* is also noninvasive and usually remains in the upper respiratory tract.   One of the most important effects of the diptheria toxin is to damage heart muscle cells.   The only exotoxin associated with invasiveness is that of gas gangrene, produced by *Clostridium perfringens* and other related clostridia.   This exotoxin injures and kills tissue cells, resulting in enhanced growth and spread of the invading bacteria.   Gas gangrene is usually associated with extensive wounds, and the mortality is extremely high.

Endotoxins are released only with the death and disruption of certain types of bacteria, chiefly the bacilli, both commensal and pathogenic, most commonly associated with intestinal infections.   The endotoxins do not appear to be metabolic products but are actually components of the cell wall.   The most notable effects of endotoxins include fever; circulatory changes, of which the most important is shock; a transient decrease in the number of circulating leukocytes (leukopenia); and possibly the subsequent increase in circulating leukocytes (leukocytosis).   These manifestations will be discussed further in the section on host responses.   *Enzymes* produced by bacteria or released in their destruction can produce a variety of manifestations comparable to those already examined in relation to invasiveness.

The accumulative effects of the infectious process may produce manifestations which are in a sense distinct from the individual processes themselves.   Thus, the formation of an abscess may interfere with the function of an organ or even totally destroy it.   The mechanical presence of a large, inflammatory exudate in the pericardial space may compress the heart, and large inflammatory exudates in the pleural spaces may compromise respiration. Inflammation of the urethra by *Gonococcus* may result in scarring and obstruction to urine flow. These and other similar manifestations will depend upon the characteristics of the specific organism and the location of the infection. Finally, the effects of the microorganisms may be due not to their inherent pathogenic capacity but to the induction of a delayed hypersensitivity response, of which tuberculosis may be the classical example. These responses—gross tissue destruction,

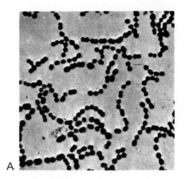

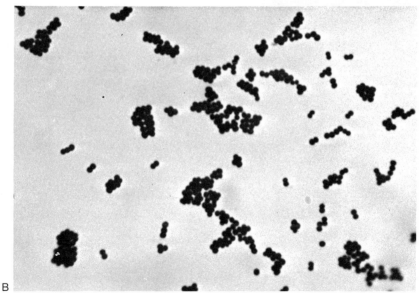

Figure 9-2 *A: Streptococcus pyogenes* (×1900). *B: Staphylococcus aureus* (×1300). *(From M. J. Pelczar, Jr., and R. D. Reid, Microbiology, 3d ed., McGraw-Hill, New York, 1970, pp. 571 and 630. By permission of the publishers.)*

mechanical interference with function, and delayed hypersensitivity reactions—all represent not just the pathogenicity of the organisms but host response factors as well.

Because the number of pathogenic bacteria is quite large, it would be impossible to discuss them all in detail. However, the major groups and their characteristics will be presented. The major criteria for detailed discussion include the frequency or importance of the disease produced and the demonstration of important principles.

The Cocci

The pathogenic cocci include the gram-positive streptococci, staphylococci, and pneumococci and the gram-negative neisseriae. The *streptococci* are characterized by long chains of organisms when examined on a stained slide, although paired organisms are frequent (Fig. 9-2). A very large number of antigenic types have been recognized. An important characteristic of most pathogenic streptococci is the production of a hemolytic exotoxin which helps to identify this group of cocci. This can be easily demonstrated by culturing the cocci on media containing blood. Around each colony of organisms will be found a clear area in which the hemoglobin has been destroyed. Interestingly, this exotoxin appears to have relatively little relationship to the pathogenicity in humans.

The hemolytic streptocci have been divided into serological groups A to O. Group A is the one which has most frequently been associated with human disease, and more than fifty serologic subtypes have been identified. In addition to carbohydrate substances in the cell wall which have antigenic capacities on which classification is based, at least twenty antigenic extracellular products are produced by group A. Several of these, including streptokinase and hyaluronidase, as already discussed, are important in enhancing invasiveness. Streptodornase is a deoxyribonuclease which breaks down DNA, thus increasing the fluidity of the exudate. The erythrogenic toxin is responsible for the rash of scarlet fever. There is recent evidence which indicates that this toxin is produced only by streptococci which are themselves parasitized by a virus called bacteriophage.

Streptococci are widespread and are frequently found in the respiratory tract. One group of streptococci, the enterococci, are normal intestinal residents. The enterococci belong to group D, rather than the more commonly pathogenic group A. Disease depends upon the presence of virulent strains or a decrease in local resistance. Common diseases produced by streptococci include sore throat, scarlet fever, erysipelas (a spreading subcutaneous infection), wound infections, puerperal (childbirth) fever, bacterial endocarditis, and occasional urinary tract infections (particularly by enterococci). Acute glomerulonephritis (Bright's disease of the kidney) and rheumatic fever generally develop 1 to 4 weeks after a streptococcal infection; the present evidence indicates that these diseases are not due to the presence of streptococci but result from an immunological response to products produced by the infection.

Streptococcal infections may be transmitted through the air, by direct contact, or occasionally through food. Milk is a good culture medium and was a frequent source of infection prior to the general acceptance of pasteurization. Control is difficult because of the widespread distribution and prevalence of carriers. However, patients with virulent disease should be isolated, and aseptic, protective measures should be carried out to prevent wound infections and puerperal sepsis in other patients. The multiplicity of strains makes immunization procedures impractical. Fortunately almost all strains are sensitive to antibiotic treatment.

The *staphylococci* are characterized by irregular grapelike clusters when examined on stained smears (Fig. 9-2). Serological typing has not been particularly successful. However, by other techniques over twenty strains have been identified. The staphylococci produce several toxins and enzymes. One of these, a coagulase, has been linked with pathogenicity and initiates the deposition of fibrin. Only the coagulase-positive staphylococci are pathogenic. The role of fibrin has been under much debate (see section on inflammation), with evidence that it both enhances and interferes with phagocytosis of the bacteria. The coagulase may play a role in the rather characteristic "walling off" of staphylococcal infections. Several antigens are produced which are capable of killing white blood cells in the test tube, but only one appears effective against human leukocytes. An increasing number of strains of staphylococci are capable of elaborating penicillinase, an enzyme which breaks down penicillin and renders it ineffective. Some strains of staphylococci produce an enterotoxin when grown in carbohydrate food. This toxin, even in the absence of the organism, produces vomiting and diarrhea in 1 to 6 hours and is responsible for one type of acute food poisoning.

Cultures of normal adults show that 30 to 50 percent have staphylococci on the skin, 10 to 20 percent in the anterior nares, and 20 to 30 percent in the intestinal tract. Almost all individuals carry staphylococci at one time or another. The characteristic pathogenic effect is the production of superficial abscesses (Fig. 9-3). Common initial sites are in traumatized sebaceous glands and hair follicles (pimples). More extensive infections may result in abscess formation (boils) or carbuncles, an infection which becomes loculated or compartmented due to the presence of strong bands of connective tissue. Dissemination of organisms may result in abscess formation wherever the organisms succeed in implantation.

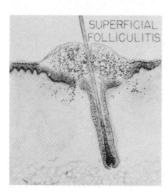 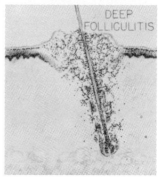

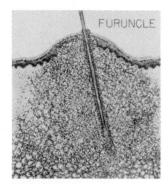 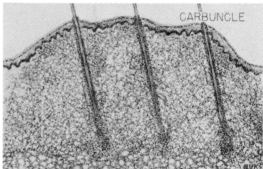

Figure 9-3   Infections of the hair follicle.   These are perhaps the most common of all infections and are usually caused by staphylococci.   The "pimple" is a folliculitis.   A "boil" caused by infection introduced through the hair follicle is a furuncle, and a number of confluent furuncles become a carbuncle. *(From D. M. Pillsbury et al., Dermatology, Saunders, Philadelphia, 1956, p. 461.   By permission of the publishers.)*

Staphylococcal infections are generally transmitted by direct contact, and appropriate precautions must be taken to avoid wound contamination. Airborne infection may also be important.   The production of immunity to staphylococci has not been successful.   The evolution of strains that are resistant to antibiotics, such as the penicillinase-producing, penicillin-resistant strains, poses difficult problems of control.

The *pneumococci* generally appear paired on smear and are called *diplococci*.   Each organism has roughly the shape of an isosceles triangle, with the two short sides of the triangle back to back (Fig. 9-4).   Virulent strains have a very marked capsule which is antigenic and characterizes more than seventy-five different types.   Between 40 and 70 percent of humans harbor virulent pneumococci at some time.   However, they become pathogenic only when there is a reduction in the resistance of

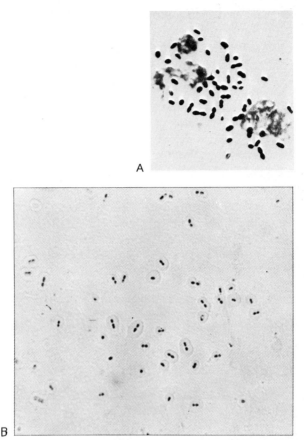

Figure 9-4   *A:* Pneumococci in pus (×1500).   *B:* Pneumococcal capsule (the capsules have been enlarged by the presence of specific antiserum). *(From M. J. Pelczar, Jr., and R. D. Reid, Microbiology, 3d ed., McGraw-Hill, New York, 1970, pp. 579 and 556. By permission of the publishers.)*

the lower respiratory tract.   The most common cause for this reduced resistance is a viral respiratory infection.   The pneumococci have no demonstrated toxins; their multiplication in the respiratory epithelium results in an inflammatory reaction with leukocyte and serum exudation. The capsule prevents phagocytosis, the exudate fills the alveoli, and the characteristic manifestations result.   The pneumococci are susceptible to most antibiotics and to specific capsular antisera.   The multiplicity of strains, the relative infrequency of disease due to a specific strain, and antibiotic sensitivity render immunization ordinarily impractical.

The *neisseriae* are gram-negative diplocci.   They are kidney-shaped, with the concave sides of the pair facing each other (Fig. 9-5). The non-pathogenic variety are extracellular and are not infrequently found in the respiratory tract. The two human pathogens, *Meningococcus* and *Gonococcus,* are intracellular organisms. Normally, a significant number of individuals carry the *meningococci* in the respiratory passages without evidence of disease. However, during epidemics the carrier rate may go up to 70 or 80 percent. In actual cases of meningitis the organisms enter the bloodstream and eventually localize in the meninges, where an acute purulent reaction ensues. Until recently the meningococci were sensitive to sulfonamides, but resistant strains have recently appeared which, fortunately, respond to penicillin. Since transmission usually is not from case to case but by carriers, effective interruption of an epidemic can be achieved only by administering small doses of sulfonamides or oral penicillin to the entire population. In the past this was successful in closed groups, such as military training camps, but the emergence of sulfonamide-resistant strains may modify the outlook.

Gonorrhea is a strictly human disease which produces a purulent

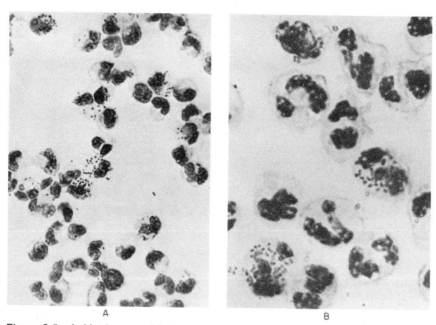

A   B

Figure 9-5 *A:* Meningococci in pus cells; spinal fluid ($\times$1350). *B:* Gonococci in urethral pus ($\times$2250). *(From M. J. Lynch, S. S. Raphael, L. D. Mellor, P. D. Spare, and M. J. H. Inwood, Medical Laboratory Technology and Clinical Pathology, 2d ed., Saunders, Philadelphia, 1969, pp. 836–837. By permission of the publishers.)*

inflammatory reaction in the mucosa of the urethra and genital organs. Immunity does not develop and infection can become chronic. The usual mode of transmission is by venereal contact. An exception is *ophthalmia neonotorum,* an eye infection of the newborn which is transmitted during passage through the genital canal. Since this type of conjunctivitis can produce blindness, state laws generally require the instillation of silver nitrate into the eyes of all children at the time of birth. Unlike the meningococci, the gonococci developed resistance within only 5 years of the introduction of the sulfonamide drugs. These organisms are still sensitive to penicillin, although increasingly large doses are necessary.

The Gram-positive Bacilli

Bacillus anthracis and the *clostridia* are all large rods which are capable of forming spores. They are independent of moisture and able to survive for long periods of time in the soil, where they are commonly found. *Bacillus anthracis* causes anthrax, which is usually a disease of animals. It was as a result of his study of sheep anthrax that Pasteur first established the pathogenicity of bacteria and developed his first techniques for immunization. In man, the disease is produced by entry through injured skin or mucous membranes, although it may occasionally be the result of inhalation of spore-laden dust. The organisms multiply rapidly, are resistant to phagocytosis, and appear to cause death by allowing the plasma fluid to leak into the tissues. Active immunization is effective.

The *clostridia* include three groups of organims producing botulism, tetanus, and gas gangrene (Fig. 9-6). As previously noted, all produce extremely potent exotoxins. The relationship of invasiveness to pathogenicity shows a remarkable range. *Clostridium botulinum* need not be present to produce disease if the toxin is present in the food. Tetanus and gas gangrene follow the introduction of organisms into injured tissue. Invasiveness is not important in tetanus, although the organisms must be in the tissues to produce the toxin. The exotoxins of gas gangrene serve specifically to enhance bacterial invasion. Both active and passive immunizations are possible, although they are only of questionable value in gas gangrene. All of the clostridia are anaerobic; that is, they grow preferentially in the absence of oxygen. The recent use of hyperbaric chambers, rooms in which oxygen can be administered at several times atmospheric pressure, has greatly improved the treatment of gas gangrene by preventing toxin production.

The *corynebacteria* are small, slender, nonspore forming gram-positive rods which may have club-shaped ends. Various strains of corynebacteria are common inhabitants of the upper respiratory mucous mem-

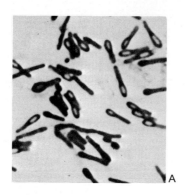

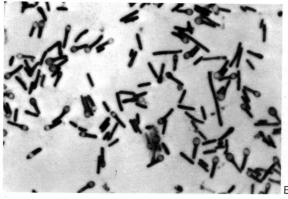

Figure 9-6 A: Clostridium botulinum (×1500). *B: Clostridium tetani.* Both figures show clostridial bacilli changing to spore forms with characteristic drumstick appearance. *(From M. J. Pelczar, Jr., and R. D. Reid, Microbiology, 3d ed., McGraw-Hill, New York, 1970, pp. 616 and 636. By permission of the publishers.)*

branes, of the conjunctiva of the eye, and occasionally of the genito-urinary tract. The important organism of this group is *Corynebacterium diphtheriae,* the etiological agent for diphtheria. This bacterium is relatively noninvasive but destroys the mucous membrane, causing a dirty gray "pseudomembrane" composed of fibrin and leukocytes to form over the denuded area. The organisms grow in the pseudomembrane and damaged tissue, which also serves as an area for toxin absorption. As with the erythrogenic strains of streptococci, viral parasitism of the diphtheria bacillus is necessary to produce the exotoxin. Diphtheria is more frequently transmitted by carriers than cases. The best means of control is by widespread immunization. Occasionally *C. diphtheriae* may infect wounds. This is most frequent in the tropics. Since this localization is not anticipated, it is often overlooked and the mortality is high.

The Enteric Gram-negative Bacilli

This is a large and diverse group of organisms which normally either inhabit the gastrointestinal tract or produce disease as a result of gastrointestinal invasion.   Many organisms in these groups have flagella and are, therefore, motile when examined alive in a wet preparation.   Many also produce endotoxins upon disruption of the cell wall.   The *coliform group* includes *Escherichia coli, Aerobacter aerogenes, Klebsiella pneumoniae,* and the paracolon bacilli.   These organisms are normally found in the gastrointestinal tract, where they are essentially nonpathogenic.

The almost invariable organism of the gastrointestinal tract is *E. coli* (Fig. 9-7).   It is so commonly present that it is generally used as a marker to identify fecal contamination of water sources; the presence of *E. coli* on

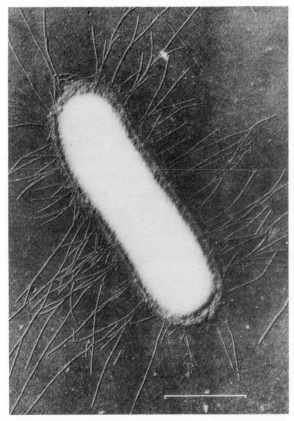

Figure 9-7   Electron micrograph of *Escherichia coli* (×33,000).
(From R. Y. Stanier, M. Doudoroff and E. A. Adelberg, The Microbial World, 2d ed., Prentice-Hall, Englewood Cliffs, N.J., 1970, p. 370. By permission of the publishers.)

culture of drinking water indicates that sewage has had access to the water. Although these organisms are commensal in the intestinal tract, they can become extremely pathogenic elsewhere in the body. Rupture of the lower intestinal tract, such as occurs with acute appendicitis, bowel injury, and occasionally intestinal obstruction, will produce severe peritonitis which is often fatal. *E. coli* is also the commonest cause of urinary tract infection. There is evidence that the coliform bacteria produce thiamine and niacin and reduce the dietary need for these vitamins. Drugs which reduce the normal bacterial flora often allow overgrowth by other organisms, particularly by monilia, a form of yeast.

Although a member of the coliform group, *Klebsiella pneumoniae* is a frequent resident of the respiratory tract and is occasionally pathogenic, producing a characteristic and frequently suppurative pneumonia. The proteus group and *Pseudomonas aeruginosa* resemble the coliform group in that they are gram-negative motile rods, commonly found in the soil and in the intestinal tract where they are not pathogenic. They are, however, occasionally found as pathogens in other parts of the body (Fig. 9-8). In particular, *Pseudomonas* produces a resistant urinary tract infection. Until recently this infection responded only to the polymyxin antibiotics, which are difficult to administer and not always effective. Several new antibiotics have been introduced which seem to be more effective.

The *salmonellae* are a large group of organisms which often produce disease in man (Fig. 9-8). They are not normally found in the gastrointestinal tract and are generally transmitted by anal-oral contamination. Carriers are probably the common source of sporadic infection, but contaminated water supplies are of greater importance in producing epidemics. The clinical manifestations are divided into three types: enteric fevers, gastroenteritis, and septicemia. The enteric fevers are caused by *Salmonella typhosa, S. paratyphi, S. schottmulleri,* and *S. hirschfeldii. S. typhosa* and *S. paratyphi* are strictly human parasites. Man is an alternate host for the other salmonellae. Manifestations of the disease are due to local intestinal lesions, body invasion via the intestinal lymphatics, and the presence of endotoxins. The most important is *S. typhosa,* which produces typhoid fever. Gastroenteritis (one of the forms of "food poisoning") is usually due to *S. typhimurium, S. enteritidis,* or *S. derby.* As opposed to staphylococcal food poisoning, which occurs in 1 to 6 hours, salmonella gastroenteritis has an incubation period of 8 to 48 hours. In other respects it resembles staphylococcal food poisoning except that there is a fever and the toxic manifestations are more persistent. Septicemia is most frequently due to *S. choleraesuis.* Intestinal involvement is usually absent. Localized infections may involve the gall bladder, kidney, endocardium, meninges, bones, perineal and pelvic regions, and the lungs.

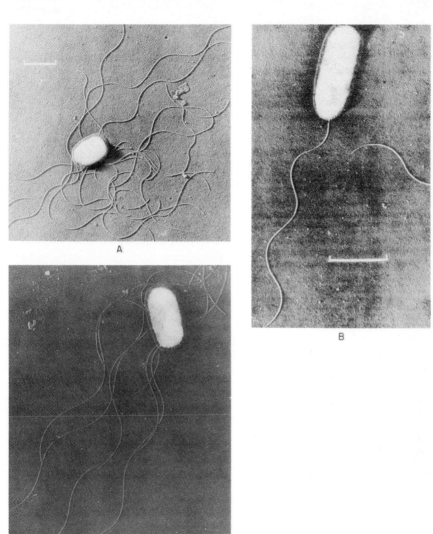

Figure 9-8 Electron micrographs. The measuring bar indicates
one micrometer. *A: Proteus vulgaris. B: Pseudomonas aeruginosa. C: Salmonella typhosa.* Motile bacilli showing flagella.
*(From M. F. Wheeler and W. A. Volk, Basic Microbiology, 2d ed.,
Lippincott, Philadelphia, 1969, pp. 17, 251. By permission of the
publishers.)*

Active immunization is effective in controlling the typhoid and paraty-phoid enteric fevers; however, the large number of strains limits the useful-ness of immunization to other organisms. Sanitation, carrier control, and antibiotic treatment have greatly reduced the frequency of these diseases.

The *shigellae* differ from the foregoing in that they are nonmotile. They are found only in the gastrointestinal tracts of primates, and in man they cause bacillary dysentery. The endotoxins chemically resemble those of salmonella and coliform organisms. These bacteria produce inflam-mation in the large bowel and occasionally the terminal ileum, followed by ragged ulcerations. The symptoms are probably produced by endotoxins and are dominated by abdominal pain, profuse watery diarrhea, and fever. Since the organisms do not enter the body, immune mechanisms play a limited role.

Cholera, the most dramatic of the dysenteric diseases, is caused by *Vibrio cholerae.* This organism is a comma-shaped rod and is, therefore, often designated *V. comma.* It possesses a single flagellum at one end and is motile. Cholera bacilli appear to be pathogenic only for man. They are not invasive; all clinical manifestations are the result of endotoxin release. The toxin damages the gastrointestinal epithelium, resulting in an outpouring of a copious amount of electrolyte-rich fluid. There is no fever or abdominal pain. All clinical and pathological changes can be attributed to the depletion of fluid and electrolytes.

The *Bacteroides* group make up the greatest number of organisms in the human stool. Yet information regarding them is surprisingly sparse. The two most important strains are *Bacteroides fragilis* and *B. funduliform-is.* They are strictly anaerobic, pleomorphic, and of variable size. In additon to the gastrointestinal tract, they have been found in the upper respiratory and genitourinary tracts. Despite their ubiquitousness and great numbers, these organisms rarely initiate disease. However, once tissue injury has occurred, they may perpetuate a serious infection.

Small Gram-negative Bacilli

The *brucellae* are small coccobacilli which are obligate parasites of animals and man, usually residing within cells. These organisms usually infect animals, the reservoirs including goats, cattle, and pigs. However, in man they cause undulant fever. The clinical manifestations are proba-bly due to the release of endotoxin. The pathologic lesion is that of small granulomas, and it is thought that endotoxin release may stimulate a delayed hypersensitivity response resulting in further bacterial destruction of tissue and clinical cycling. Transmission to man is usually through contaminated milk and less commonly by direct contact with infected animals.

Pasteurella pestis is the organism which causes plague.   It is a short gram-negative rod with rounded ends that stain at both poles during the parasitic stage (Fig. 9-9).   Plague is primarily a disease of wild rodents which is transmitted by the rat flea.   Man enters the cycle only accidentally, usually as the result of an epizootic among susceptible urban rats. When this occurs, large numbers of rats die, and the fleas may find man in their search for a new host.   In the absence of epidemiological intervention, the epizootic continues until the community is repopulated with resistant rats.   In the usual case there is the rapid development of bacteremia with toxemia, and the death rate is 60 to 90 percent.   The lymph nodes draining the inoculation site become swollen and are called buboes, hence bubonic plague.   Man-to-man respiratory transmission can occur as a result of fulminant pneumonic plague.   The persistent reservoir of infected wild animals poses a constant threat of urban epidemics.

Tularemia is a disease which very much resembles plague.   It was first recognized in Tulare, California, but is now known to be worldwide in distribution.   It is naturally a disease of wild rodents and the commonest human source is contact with wild jackrabbits.   The causative organism was previously called *Pasteurella tularensis* but has been reclassified as *Francisella tularensis.*

The *Hemophilus* group contains a number of organisms which produce rather diverse diseases.   The most important is *Hemophilus influenzae,* so named because it was frequently found in patients dying during the influenza epidemic after World War I and was once thought to be the etiological factor in that disease.   It is a frequent invader in respiratory

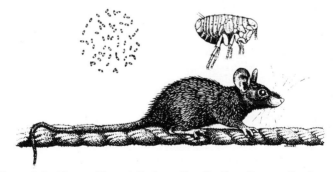

Figure 9-9   Plague: The rat, *Rattus rattus;* the flea, *Xenopsylla cheopis;* and the bacillus, *Pasteurella pestis.   (From W. H. Hargreaves, and R. J. G. Morrison, The Practice of Tropical Medicine, Staples Press, London, 1965, p. 101.   By permission of the publishers.)*

tissue already damaged by the influenza virus. The organism is quite pleomorphic, varying in shape from coccobacilli to long rods. The non-encapsulated form is frequently found in the normal respiratory tract. The pathogenic encapsulated form produces pneumonia comparable to pneumococcus pneumonia, but the endotoxin may contribute to its pathogenicity. However, antibodies to this toxin do not appear related to recovery. In infants under the age of 2 years, *H. influenzae* is a frequent cause of severe meningitis. In older children and less frequently in adults it may produce a sudden severe inflammation with swelling of the epiglottis which often produces death by asphyxia unless an immediate tracheotomy is performed. *H. ducreyi* produces a relatively mild venereal disease called chancroid or soft chancre. *H. aegyptius* (Koch-Weeks bacillus) and the Morax-Axenfeld bacillus produce forms of conjunctivitis.

The *Bordetella* organisms resemble the *Hemophilus* group structurally but are antigenically different. The most important is *Bordetella pertussis,* which causes whooping cough. The organisms grow in mucous membranes and the endotoxins cause cell necrosis, respiratory symptoms with the characteristic cough, and marked lymphocytosis. Secondary infection is common and the cause of often serious complications. Very little maternal immunity is passed on to the infant, and the most serious infections usually occur in very young children. The natural mortality is relatively high and almost half the deaths occur in the first year of life. Immunization is effective but should be started early. All the organisms of the *Hemophilus* and *Bordetella* groups are pathogenic only for man; case-to-case transmission is usual, and carrier infection is rare.

The Mycobacteria

The mycobacteria are slender rods which stain poorly and are not characterized by Gram techniques. When stained by basic dyes using special methods, the dye cannot be washed out by 3 percent acid and alcohol and the organisms are said to be "acid-fast." Many of the characteristics of mycobacterial infections appear to be the result of the large fat content of the cell. No known toxins are produced. *Mycobacterium tuberculosis* is the etiological agent of tuberculosis, and two strains, the human and the bovine, are pathogenic for man. Bovine tuberculosis is usually transmitted through infected milk and entry is through the gastrointestinal mucous membranes. Clinical infection most frequently involves the cervical lymph nodes (scrofula), the abdominal lymph nodes, and bone. Human tuberculosis is generally transmitted by droplet infection with primary involvement of the lungs (Fig. 9-10). Subsequent dissemination is generally from that tissue. Initial infection results in an exudative inflammatory

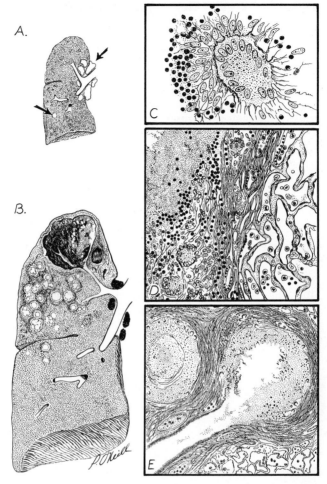

Figure 9-10 Pulmonary tuberculosis. *A:* The primary lesion. The arrows indicate the Ghon tubercle and the large caseous regional lymph nodes. *B:* Secondary tuberculosis with cavitation, bronchogenic spread, and tubercle formation. The bronchus opens into the cavity. The regional lymph nodes are uninvolved in the active process. *C:* Hard tubercle. There is an outer layer of mononuclear cells, an inner layer of epithelioid cells, and a central giant cell. *D:* A caseous tubercle. Caseous necrotic material is visible on the upper left. There are peripheral mononuclear cells, epithelioid cells, and giant cells. Normal lung tissue is seen to the lower right. *E:* A well-encapsulated tubercle is seen on the left and a similar tubercle opening into a small bronchus and discharging caseous material is seen on the right. *(From B. D. Fallis, Textbook of Pathology, McGraw-Hill, New York, 1964, pp. 224–225. By permission of the publishers.)*

reaction with mononuclear phagocytosis of organisms and extension to the regional lymph nodes (Ghon complex). Multiplication of bacteria is chiefly intracellular. The fatty cell wall resists lysis. Cellular immunity develops in an average of 40 days. As a result, the following four phenomena can be demonstrated:

1. The exudative response is replaced by a productive granulomatous inflammatory response.
2. Mononuclear phagocytosis is enhanced with increased destruction of bacilli and inhibited multiplication of the remaining viable organisms.
3. The lesions remain localized and lymphatic spread is inhibited.
4. Caseous necrosis becomes apparent.

The first three of these responses are protective to the host; however, the fourth facilitates dissemination since the necrotic material containing living bacilli infects adjacent tissue during drainage and may enter the bloodstream through eroded vessels. Recently it has been recognized that other mycobacteria can produce similar lesions, although they are not as clinically severe or frequent as tuberculosis. The development of antituberculous drugs, such as streptomycin, para-amino salicylate (PAS), and isoniazid (INH), has completely altered the outlook for tuberculous patients.

Mycobacterium leprae was isolated by Hansen 4 years before Koch isolated the tubercle bacillus. Since the organisms cannot be cultured or transmitted to animals, their role as the etiological agent in leprosy is uncertain, despite the presence of many organisms in the lesions. The exact mode of transmission is still unknown. The incubation period is at least several years. The lesions are granulomatous but no caseation is evident. A number of chemical compounds of a group called sulfones are effective in curing this infection.

The Spirochaetaceae

These organisms are extremely slender, motile spirals. They are best observed in wet preparations using dark-field illumination. This is an indirect illumination which acts in much the same way as a beam of light that makes dust particles in the air visible when seen from the side. They stain poorly with the usual dyes; however, they reduce silver nitrate to metallic silver, which renders them visible. Culture in artificial media is generally difficult and susceptible animals have been more widely used. *Treponema pallidum* is the etiological agent for syphilis (Fig. 9-11). It is a fine spiral organism measuring 5 to 20 millimeters in length, having from 4

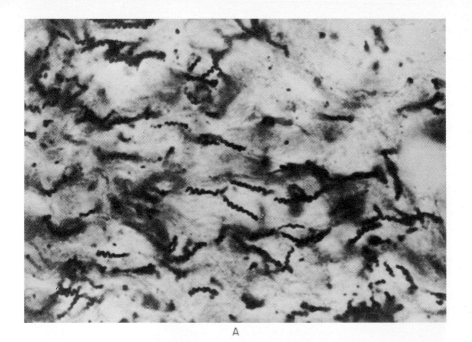

A

B

Figure 9-11 *Treponema pallidum. A:* Silver nitrate stain of *T. pallidum* in tissues *(From Smith and Gault, Essentials of Pathology, McGraw-Hill, 1948, p. 151. By permission of the publishers.)* *B: T. pallidum* by dark-field microscopy (×3400). *(From M. J. Pelczar, Jr., and R. D. Reid, Microbiology, 3d ed., McGraw-Hill, New York, 1970, p. 624. By permission of the publishers.)*

to 14 spirals, and moving with a rotating and somewhat undulating motion. *T. pallidum* is transmitted by direct, usually venereal contact, probably entering through a break in the epithelium, although the ability to penetrate intact skin and mucous membranes has been postulated. Very little is known of the relation between the nature of the organism and the type of pathological changes which it induces (Figs. 9-12 and 9-13). A number of

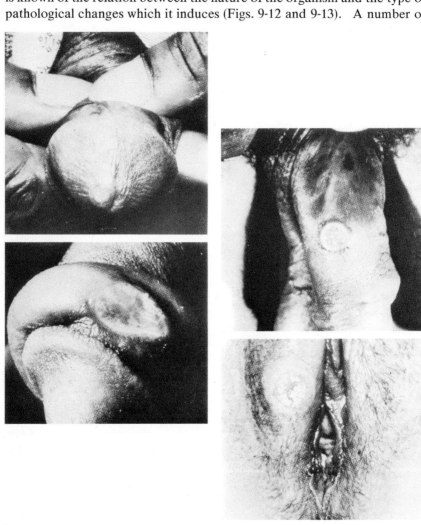

Figure 9-12 The primary lesions of syphilis, chancres. These are firm, painless ulcers. In the woman they are usually internal on the cervix, and thus not visible. [*From T. B. Fitzpatrick (ed.), Dermatology in General Medicine, McGraw-Hill, New York, 1971, p. 1957. By permission of the publishers.*]

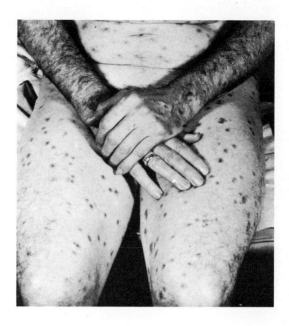

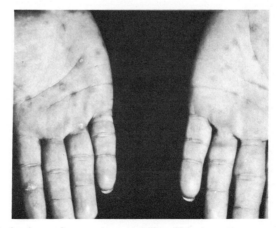

Figure 9-13   Lesions of secondary syphilis.   This is a common
form in which the lesions are of copper color, symmetrical, do not
itch, and, unlike most rashes, also appear on the palms and soles.
[*From T. B. Fitzpatrick (ed.), Dermatology in General Medicine,
McGraw-Hill, New York, 1971, pp. 1961.   By permission of the
publishers.*]

nonvenereal diseases are caused by treponemes which appear identical with *T. pallidum*. These include bejel in Arabia, yaws in many tropical areas of high annual rainfall, and pinta, which is prevalent from Mexico south to Colombia. All treponemataceae are extremely susceptible to penicillin.

The *leptospirae* are of approximately the same size as the treponemes but are more tightly coiled and move with a nonundulating, rotational movement. A large number of species have been serologically identified. They are normally animal parasites and transmission is via the urine and feces. Human infection is most frequently due to skin exposure to leptospira-infected water and less frequently to ingestion. The best known is *Leptospira icterohaemorrhagiae*. This infection causes a form of hepatitis, often with jaundice; less frequently a nephritis with acute uremia; and occasionally a mild meningitis. Although this *Leptospira* causes the most serious disease, at least a dozen others have been shown to produce similar patterns although with different levels of organ involvement.

The *Borrelia* spirochetes are longer than the treponemataceae and leptospirae. The spirals are proportionately larger and less numerous and the movement is more flexible. These organisms produce relapsing fever. The mortality of this disease is normally low, but it may approach 50 percent in some epidemics. The natural reservoir hosts are not known but are assumed to be wild rodents, and transmission is by tick bite. Louse-borne infections are probably most common in man-to-man epidemics. *Spirillum minus* is a parasite of rats which is transmitted to man by the bite of that animal. The disease produced is appropriately called rat-bite fever. A number of spirochetes are found normally in the human mouth. It is suspected that the combined effects of spirochetes and fusiform bacilli, a type of *Bacteroides,* produces Vincent's angina (trench mouth). At present this association is less certain than previously believed.

The Rickettsiae

The rickettsiae are very small obligate intracellular parasites existing either as short rods or as cocci. These organisms can be cultured in the yolk sac of embryonated eggs. The living organisms produce a toxin, which is therefore probably an exotoxin, which may cause direct injury to host cells. One of the manifestations is injury to capillary endothelium with leakage of plasma into the tissues and a progressive loss of blood volume. A hemolysin is also present, but this seems to play little role in human infection. The rickettsiae multiply inside the endothelial cell lining of small blood vessels. The cells swell and proliferate. Thrombosis may result. In addition, polymorphonuclear leukocytes, macrophages, and lymphoid cells surround the blood vessel and increase the inflammatory mass. These vascular lesions lead to small microinfarcts. Thrombosis of large vessels is relatively rare. Sulfonamides potentiate rickettsial growth whereas para-aminobenzoic acid inhibits it; the reverse of what is found in many other bacterial species. Rickettsiae are transmitted to man by a large variety of arthropods whose principal hosts are normally rodents (Fig. 9-14). However, it appears that at least some of the arthropods can perpetuate their infection by direct transmission to their ova.

The rickettsial diseases are divided into five major groups: typhus, spotted fever, scrub typhus, Q fever, and trench fever. With exceptions to be noted, all are characterized by fever and hemorrhagic skin lesions due to the vascular response previously described. In the typhus group the rash starts centrally and spreads peripherally. Epidemic typhus is louse-borne, is due to *Rickettsia prowazeki,* and has a high mortality. Murine typhus is sporadic, transmitted to man by the rat flea, caused by *R. mooseri,* and much less lethal. Rocky Mountain spotted fever is due to *R. rickettsii* and is transmitted by ticks. It is characterized by a rash which starts on the extremities. The untreated mortality is approximately 20 percent. A number of less severe tick-borne spotted fevers are found in the Eastern Hemisphere. Scrub typhus is found in western Asia and

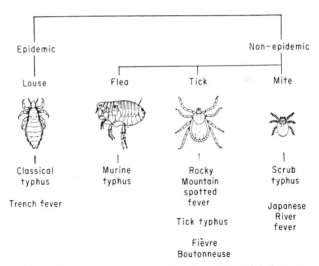

Figure 9-14   The arthropod vectors of various rickettsial diseases. *(From W. H. Hargreaves, and R. J. G. Morrison, The Practice of Tropical Medicine, Staples Press, London, 1965, p. 138. By permission of the publishers.)*

adjacent islands. It is caused by *R. tsutsugamushi* and is transmitted by a mite. The disease is also known as tsutsugamushi fever. Mortality is comparable to epidemic typhus and Rocky Mountain spotted fever. Trench fever is due to *R. quintana,* which is capable of extracellular growth in culture. It is transmitted by the body louse. During World War I over a million cases were observed. The disease was severely incapacitating but not fatal. Rickettsialpox is a member of the spotted fever group but produces a rash which resembles smallpox. It is caused by *R. akari* and is transmitted by mites normally parasitic on mice. The disease is mild and no fatalities have been reported. Q fever is an animal disease, now well established in cattle and maintained by animal-to-animal transmission. The etiologic agent is *Coxiella burneti.* Q fever resembles an atypical pneumonia more than it does the other rickettsial diseases. Transmission is through infected milk or by respiratory contamination from infected animals.

Psittacosis-Lymphogranuloma Organisms

These organisms are extremely small and are at the limit of visibility by light microscopy. Originally, they were classified as large viruses because of their size and their intracellular habitat. However, further study has demonstrated that they contain both DNA and RNA, have a cell wall, possess enzymes, and can perform metabolic functions. For these reasons they are now often classed with the rickettsiae, despite the fact that none has an arthropod host. Little is known about their specific pathogenetic mechanisms. Human diseases produced by these organisms include psittacosis, ornithosis, lymphogranuloma venereum, trachoma, and inclusion conjunctivitis. Psittacosis and ornithosis are normally relatively nonpathogenic infections of birds, which when transmitted to man produce a severe but rarely fatal pneumonia. Lymphogranuloma venereum is transmitted by venereal contact and produces a local lesion, followed by a regional lymphatic inflammatory reaction and severe late scarring. The organisms producing trachoma and inclusion conjunctivitis are classed together as TRIC agents. They are transmitted by direct contact and, particularly in the case of trachoma, produce a chronic purulent infection which causes scarring and resultant blindness.

Mycoplasmataceae

The mycoplasmas are extremely small organisms which cannot be seen by light microscopy but which can be cultured on suitable extracellular media, where they demonstrate a characteristic growth pattern. They lack the characteristic rigid bacterial cell wall, but they do have a cell membrane. *Mycoplasma pneumoniae* produces a wide spectrum of respiratory manifestations, including a characteristic, clinically severe, but rarely fatal pneumonia in young adults. During World War II the incidence among military personnel was ten times that of bacterial pneumonia. Interestingly, the organism often stimulates the production of a cold agglutinin to type O erythrocytes and an agglutinin for a strain of *Streptococcus* called *Streptococcus MG;* this characteristic aids in clinical diagnosis. *M. hominis* type 1 produces an acute febrile respiratory illness with sore throat and tonsillar exudate. Over 50 percent of normal adults have specific antibodies to this organism. Other mycoplasmas cause disease in animals.

VIRUSES

When it was realized that disease could be produced by bacteria, an intensive search was instituted to find the etiologic organisms for all diseases that showed evidence suggesting an infectious origin. It soon became apparent that a large number of apparently infectious diseases failed to yield to efforts to demonstrate appropriate bacteria. About the turn of the century it was shown that filters with ultramicroscopic pores so small that all microscopically visible particulate material was removed would allow the passage of infectious material from tissues obtained from patients and animals dying from some of these diseases. At that time the word *virus* was equivalent to *germ,* and the infectious agent was termed a *filterable virus.* It is only recently that the simpler term *virus* has been used in its present connotation. Early studies on viral diseases were hampered by the fact that they would grow only on living tissue and that this, coupled with their small size, made it impossible to handle them directly, as could be done with bacterial cultures. Nevertheless, steady progress was made. Serological responses were characterized; culture techniques, particularly those using tissue cultures, were developed; and viruses were finally directly visualized by electron microscopy. One of the most unexpected aids to the development of knowledge concerning the viruses was the elucidation of the structure and function of DNA and RNA.

It is presently known that all viruses contain either a DNA or an RNA core, which is called the *viral genome.* Surrounding the nucleoprotein core is a protein shell or *capsid.* The capsid is made up of a variable number of protein subunits known as *capsomeres,* although this number is fixed for each specific virus strain. Animal viruses have two basic configurations. In one the nucleoprotein is wound in a helix (spiral) which is enclosed by individual capsomeres. In the other configuration the nucleoprotein is enclosed by a cubical capsid. This cube is an icosa-hedron, which is a 20-sided figure each side of which is made up of an equilateral triangle. In addition to the capsid, some virus particles have an outer envelope which has no characteristic configuration. The complete virus is termed a *virion* (Figs. 9-15 and 9-16).

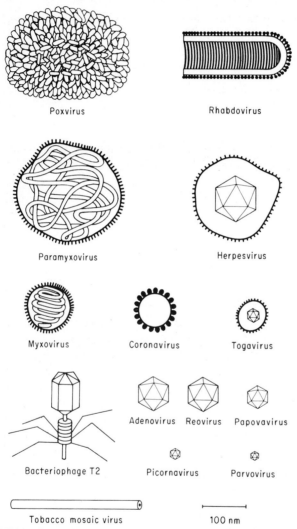

Figure 9-15   Diagramatic configuration of important viruses. The coronaviruses are a newly described group which cause respira-tory diseases in man. The togaviruses comprise the majority of the arboviruses. *(From F. Fenner and D. O. White, Medical Virol-ogy, Academic Press, New York, 1970, p. 16. By permission of the publishers.)*

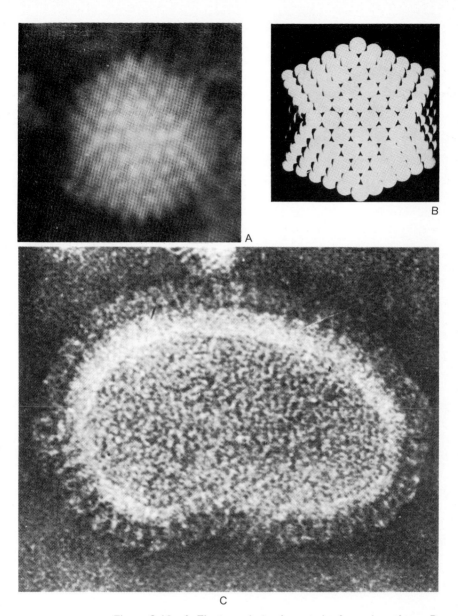

Figure 9-16   *A:* Electron photomicrograph of an adenovirus.   *B:*
Model of adenovirus particle showing icosahedral structure and
configuration of 252 capsomeres.   [*From C. H. Kempe and V. A.
Fulginite in R. E. Cooke (ed.), The Biologic Basis of Pediatric
Practice, McGraw-Hill, New York, 1968, p. 600.   By permission of
the publishers.*]   *C:* Electron photomicrograph of influenza virus.
*(From A. Cohen, Textbook of Medical Virology, Blackwell, Oxford
and Edinburgh, 1969, p. 70.   By permission of the publishers.)*

One of the major problems in virus study has been the fact that viruses will not live outside living cells and that in many instances the cell must be specific. Stanley showed in 1935 that the tobacco mosaic virus could be crystallized and kept indefinitely, but that when it was applied to the tobacco leaf it would again become active and reproduce itself as it damaged the leaf. Similar crystallization has been achieved for polio virus (Fig. 9-17).

Mechanisms of Viral Pathogenesis

Present evidence indicates that the contact between the virus and the susceptible cell to be parasitized is entirely random and undirected. The protein capsid is essential only for the extracellular portion of the virus existence. It aids in the fixation of the virus on its host's cell and in the penetration of the virus through the cell wall. The plant virus capsid remains outside the cell, and the animal virus capsid is immediately disassembled as soon as it enters the cell. The DNA virus then immediate-

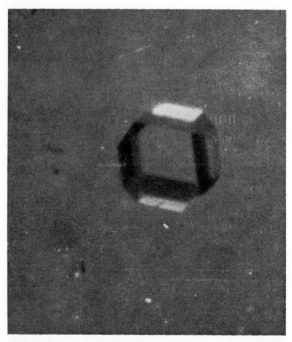

Figure 9-17 Light micrograph of poliovirus crystals (×320). [*From R. E. Cooke (ed.), The Biologic Basis of Pediatric Practice, McGraw-Hill, New York, 1968, p. 601. By permission of the publishers.*]

ly insinuates itself into the cellular genome, and the RNA virus immediately attaches to ribosomes. Viral reproduction must involve the replication of the genome, and the genome must carry information which enables the production of the capsid components and those enzymes necessary to provide for the structural components and their assembly. In the process of viral replication, the cell is cannibalized for necessary components. Even relatively active cells have a limited reserve of nucleotides, and therefore cellular DNA and RNA are broken down for this purpose. One of the interesting problems is how the viral nucleotide is protected while all other nucleotides are being destroyed. If the virus capsule has a lipoprotein component, the cell can discharge the virus as soon as it is assembled and virus release is continuous. Other viruses are retained until the cell is disrupted and they are all released at once.

Viral reproduction with cell destruction is not the only outcome of viral infection of cells. At least two other possibilities are well established. There may be complete or incomplete reproduction of virus which fails to destroy the cell and results in a relatively stable relationship. Manifestations of the infection may become apparent when this relationship is disturbed. The classic example is herpes simplex (fever blister), which is due to such an infection early in life. The effects of the viral infection become apparent when the individual develops certain febrile illnesses, particularly pneumonia and other respiratory infections. When inapparent infection exists, it can be transmitted to each of the daughter cells of the initially infected cell. Thus, the complete virion need not be reconstituted in order for it to be transmitted from cell to cell.

A second type of response is the induction of proliferation. This can be induced by either DNA or RNA viruses and is believed to be due to incorporation of the viral nucleotides into the cellular genetic mechanisms. Once this occurs the viral effect can be transferred from cell to cell. Although no virus-induced cancer has been demonstrated for man, a large number have been clearly demonstrated for other animals. These observations underlie the resurgent interest in the possibility that at least some human cancers may be of viral origin. Gross chromosomal abnormalities have been noted in a number of cancers, and it seems possible that they may be the visible result of this process.

Most viral infections produce their clinical effects in the epithelial cells in which they make first contact. Typical examples are the respiratory and gastrointestinal infections. These diseases have a relatively short incubation period and produce relatively little specific immunity. Other infections may be associated with viremia, and infection generally produces a solid immunity. In these the incubation period is usually several weeks. The protein capsid and envelope are antigenic and antibodies are obviously effective only against the extracellular virus, since the antigenic proteins are destroyed when the virus enters the cells.

Viremia is associated with two general types of infection. The first is that transmitted by arthropods, since viremia provides the mechanism by which the infectious cycle can be completed (Fig. 9–18). The second group consists of those infections in which the first generation of viruses reproduce in the epithelial cells and the second generation enters the circulation to infect more deep-lying susceptible cells. Poliomyelitis is a typical member of this group; the first generation of virus reproduces in the epithelial cells of the gastrointestinal tract and the second generation is then disseminated through the circulation to infect neural cells. The effectiveness of immunization procedures depends upon the ability of the antibodies to neutralize the virus during the period of transportation. Once within the cell, the virus is most vulnerable between the time the capsid is disassembled and either the DNA incorporates with the nuclear DNA or the RNA attaches to the ribosome.

Viral infection often causes characteristic cellular changes resulting in cellular degeneration and necrosis. Vacuole formation, swelling, the fusion of several cells, hypertrophy, and hyperplasia have been noted. There may be changes in the nucleus and the nucleolus may be displaced. At one time *inclusion bodies* were important for specific diagnosis. The Negri bodies of rabies, which were found in certain brain cells, were often used to determine whether an animal which had inflicted a bite was rabid. Inclusion bodies when present are often quite characteristic. They are found either in the nucleus or cytoplasm, depending upon the virus.

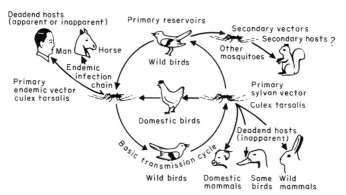

Figure 9-18   The normal cycle and accidental hosts of the parasite of Western equine encephalitis. *(From A. D. Hess and P. Holden, Annals of the New York Academy of Science, 70:294, 1958. By permission of the publishers.)*

Initially, they were thought to represent the virus; however, it is now believed that they represent the site at which the virus is assembled. More reliable methods are now used for diagnosis. The inflammatory reaction appears to be a response to the cellular injury and possibly not to the virus itself. There is usually considerable edema, and the cellular infiltrate is largely mononuclear and lymphocytic, with relatively little polymorphonuclear involvement except in the presence of secondary bacterial infection.

Classification of Viruses

The initial classification of viruses was hampered by the fact that the characteristics of the viruses themselves could not be determined. As a result viruses were classified by their effects, and those which produced primarily neural or dermal manifestations were grouped together. This classification was patently unsatisfactory, since the same virus occasionally produced primary manifestations in different organ systems and often affected different organ systems in different species. The development of new techniques has now made it possible to classify viruses on inherent virus properties. In 1963 an international committee on virus nomenclature adopted a system of classification based on these criteria. The major division separates those viruses with a DNA genome from those with an RNA genome. Further separation is based on whether the capsid is helical or icosahedral, the presence of an envelope, particle size, and sensitivity to ether. Other bases for classification include the number of capsomeres and immunologic properties. (See Table 9-1.)

The *DNA viruses* include the papovavirus, adenovirus, herpesvirus, and poxvirus groups. These groups have been listed in increasing order of size. The *papovaviruses* include a number which cause papillomas in animals and man, the polyoma of mice, which under a variety of conditions has produced 20 distinct types of tumors, and the simian vacuolating virus. The name derives from the lesions produced by these viruses and includes the first two letters of papilloma, polyoma, and vacuolation. At present, about 11 species have been identified. The only one pathogenic for man is the human papilloma virus, which produces simple warts. *Adenoviruses* were first isolated from the adenoids of children with respiratory infections. Thirty distinct types have been identified in humans and others have been isolated from primates, cattle, dogs, mice, and birds. These viruses apparently can persist for a long time in lymphoid tissue. In addition to respiratory infections, one type can produce conjunctivitis. The *herpesvirus* group includes the viruses of

Table 9-1 Classification of Animal Viruses

Group	Capsid	Envelope	Size, mμm	Multiplication site	Ether sensitivity	Common diseases
DNA viruses						
Papovavirus	Icosahedral	—	40–55	Nucleus	—	Warts
Adenovirus	Icosahedral	—	70–80	Nucleus	—	Mild respiratory disease
Herpesvirus	Icosahedral	+	120–180	Nucleus	+	Herpes simplex, herpes zoster, chickenpox, cytomegalic virus
Poxvirus	Helical	+	150–300	Cytoplasm	±	Smallpox, vaccinia (cowpox), molluscum contagiosum
RNA viruses						
Picornavirus	Icosahedral	—	18–30	Cytoplasm	—	Enteroviruses: Over 60 identified including polio-, coxsackie- and echoviruses Rhinoviruses: Over 60 identified; common cause of colds
Reovirus	Icosahedral	—	70–75	Cytoplasm	—	Mild respiratory and enteric infections
Arbovirus	Icosahedral	+?	40–50	Cytoplasm	+	Over 200 identified, including yellow fever, dengue, and encephalitis
Myxovirus						
I	Helical	+	80–200	Nucleus and cytoplasm	+	Influenza
II	Helical	+	100–300	Nucleus	+	Measles, mumps, parainfluenza, distemper

herpes simplex, chickenpox (the same virus also produces herpes zoster), and the cytomegalovirus. The *poxvirus* group produces characteristic cutaneous lesions in many species. Diseases infecting man include smallpox, vaccinia, cowpox, and molluscum contagiosum. Note that chickenpox does not belong to this group but is a member of the herpes-virus group.

The RNA viruses include the picornavirus, reovirus, arbovirus, and myxovirus groups. The *picornaviruses* are extremely small, and the name derives from *pico* (small) and RNA. This group is subdivided again into rhinovirus (respiratory) and enterovirus (gastrointestinal tract) groups. Over 60 serotypes of human rhinoviruses have been identified. Most of these produce respiratory infection. The enteroviruses also number over 60 serotypes and include the polioviruses; the Coxsackie viruses, which cause herpangina, minor summer illnesses, pleurodynia, meningitis, carditis, and mild respiratory infections; and the ECHO (*e*nteric *c*yto-pathogenic, *h*uman, *o*rphan) viruses, which produce meningitis, fevers and colds. The picornaviruses of lower animals include, among others, the virus of foot and mouth disease.

The *reovirus* group was initally classed with the ECHO viruses; however, their RNA was found to be double-stranded, a unique feature, and therefore they contain more RNA than other RNA viruses. The name derives from *r*espiratory, *e*nteric, *o*rphan viruses. Three types are recognized which produce respiratory and enteric diseases. The name *arbovirus* derives from *ar*thropod-*bo*rne viruses. This is an extremely large and clinically varied group, representing over 160 recognized agents. Commonly known diseases produced by arboviruses include yellow fever; dengue; equine, St. Louis, and Japanese encephalitis; sandfly fever; and vesicular stomatitis. The *myxovirus* group is so named because of an affinity for mucoproteins, which appears to be part of the mechanism for cell entry. This group is further divided into subgroups 1 and 2, also called orthomyxoviruses and paramyxoviruses. The viral genome of the latter is exactly twice the diameter of the former. Subgroup 1 includes the influenzas and subgroup 2 includes mumps, measles, respiratory syncytial virus, and parainfluenza, as well as the virus of animal distemper.

A number of viruses are unclassified. Melnick has recently proposed a rhabdovirus group, which would include the virus of rabies. These viruses have a characteristic morphology; they contain an RNA core and a helical capsid resembling a bullet, flat on one end and rounded on the other. Other important human viruses which have not yet been classified are those of rubella (German measles), infectious and serum hepatitis, infectious mononucleosis, and lymphocytic choriomeningitis.

THE MYCOSES

The mycoses are diseases due to fungi. The pathogenic fungi represent only about fifty of the thousands of known species. *Actinomyces, Nocardia,* and *Streptomyces* belong to the order Actinomycetales, which falls between the true bacteria and the true fungi. They exhibit a nonbacterial branching and produce spores; however they break into bacteria-sized particles. *Actinomyces* are sensitive to penicillin and *Nocardia* are sensitive to sulfonamides, while the higher fungi are resistant to these drugs. Almost all the remaining mycoses belong to the Deuteromycetes or Fungi Imperfecti. The true fungi are characterized by long branching filaments called *hyphae.* The hypha may divide and become a chain of cells. The intertwined growth of hyphae produces a dense mat called a *mycelium.* Fungi reproduce by spores, which have characteristic modes of formation and configuration that aid in their classification. The Fungi Imperfecti reproduce by asexual spores, in the formation of which no fusion of nuclei occurs.

The true fungi are generally differentiated by their spores. They all grow well on Sabouraud's medium, and material for microscopic identification is readily available from this source. In diseased individuals various immunologic reactions are often produced which may be used to facilitate the identification of the infecting fungus. These reactions include skin tests utilizing delayed hypersensitivity as well as serological tests for precipitins and complement-fixation reactions. The fungi are widely present in the air and soil, and many potential pathogens are normally resident on the skin and mucous membranes. Man-to-man and animal-to-man transmission is extremely unusual except in the case of the dermatophytes (skin fungi).

Superficial Mycoses

Fungus infections are generally divided into two groups: superficial and deep. *Superficial mycoses* include tinea pedis (athlete's foot), tinea corporus (ringworm), tinea capitis (ringworm of the scalp), tinea versicolor (a skin infection with brownish-red scaling on the trunk, neck, and arms), piedra (black or white nodules attached to the hair), and erythrasma (an infection of the axillary or pubic skin). As a group these diseases are called the *dermatophytoses.* These diseases are caused by fungi from three genera: *Trichophyton, Microsporum,* and *Epidermophyton.* The organisms live in keratin and do not invade the living cells. However, they may produce a local inflammatory reaction, either as a result of altering the defensive properties of the keratin or as the result of sensitization (Fig. 9-19).

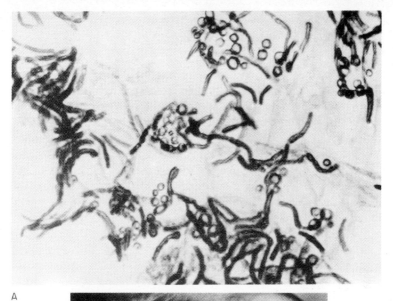

A

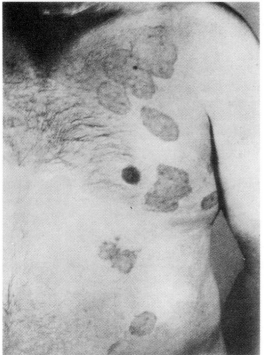

B

Figure 9-19 *A:* Hyphae and budding cells of *Malassezia furfur,*
the agent causing tinea versicolor. *B:* Tinea corporis, or ringworm.
*(From N. F. Conant, D. S. Martin, D. T. Smith, R. D. Baker and J. L.
Calloway, Manual of Clinical Mycology, Saunders, Philadelphia,
1944, pp. 224, 275. By permission of the publishers.)*

Deep Mycoses

The *deep mycoses* represent more complex and potentially dangerous infections. The fungi produce no toxins and the response to the organisms is a direct inflammatory one. These spores tend to be extremely resistant to phagocytic and immunological destruction, and some may, in fact, survive within phagocytes. The persistence of infection leads to granuloma formation and to delayed hypersensitivity. As in tuberculosis, but probably to a lesser extent, the role of delayed hypersensitivity in the perpetuation of the infection is not entirely established. However, the preparation of an appropriate antigen may be utilized in some fungal diseases in the same manner as tuberculin to help establish the diagnosis. The deep mycoses are often progressive, and death may occur as the result either of the expansion of the primary lesion or of generalized dissemination.

The frequency with which deep mycoses are being diagnosed has increased as a result of a number of factors other than improved recognition. The administration of adrenal corticosteroids for the treatment of a number of diseases impairs the inflammatory response and encourages the resident fungi to proliferate and often to produce disease. A similar effect is induced by the use of various immunosuppressive drugs in the treatment of autoimmune diseases and in organ transplantation. The most common cause, however, is the widespread use of antibiotics. Suppression of normal bacterial flora, especially in the mouth, gastrointestinal tract, and vagina, results in the overgrowth of a number of fungi of which *Candida (Monilia)* is the most prominent.

Actinomycosis is caused by *Actinomyces israelii,* which is a common inhabitant of the mouth. About half the cases of actinomycosis start as chronic abscesses of the face and neck which break down to yield chronic draining sinuses. Other lesions involve the lung or the abdomen. The pus contains characteristic "sulphur granules" which are mycelial fragments (Figs. 9-20 and 9-21). *Blastomycosis braziliensis* also causes extensive chronic granulomas of the mucous membranes of the mouth, skin, and associated lymph nodes or of the intestines, abdominal lymph nodes, and other abdominal viscera.

Coccidioides immitis is a common pathogen in the arid regions of California, Arizona, and West Texas. It produces a mild respiratory disease known as San Joaquin Valley fever which usually subsides without complications. In an occasional individual, particularly in non-Caucasians, the disease may disseminate and be eventually fatal. The primary lesion is generally in the respiratory tract or lungs, but dissemination may involve lymph nodes, bones, and often the meninges. Precipitin and

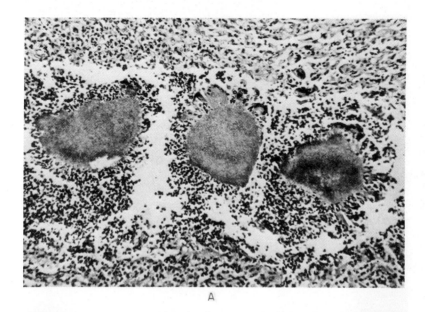

A

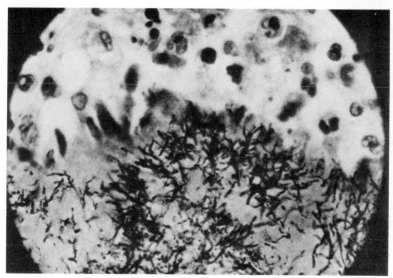

B

Figure 9-20   A: "Sulfur granules" of actinomycosis.   These are characteristic mycelia which occur in the tissues.   B: Higher power showing the hyphae which make up the mycelium.   (From N. F. Conant, D. S. Martin, D. T. Smith, R. D. Baker, and J. L. Calloway, Manual of Clinical Mycology, Saunders, Philadelphia, 1944, pp. 17 and 20.   By permission of the publishers.)

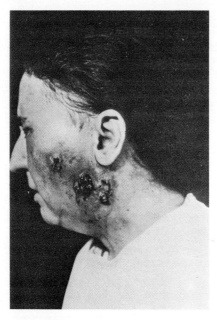

Figure 9-21 Actinomycosis. Characteristic lesions at the angle of the jaw with
multiple, persistent sinuses. *(From N. F.
Conant, D. S. Martin, D. T. Smith, R. D.
Baker and J. L. Calloway, Manual of Clinical Mycology, Saunders, Philadelphia,
1944, p. 2. By permission of the publishers.)*

complement-fixing antibodies can be demonstrated; a rising titer of the
latter is of ominous significance. Hypersensitivity can be demonstrated
by the coccidioidin skin test. The tissues and exudates contain endo-
spores filled with spherules which are noninfectious but which, when cultured, produce extremely infectious arthrospores. These spores must be
present in infectious dust, but the life cycle has not been established.

   Histoplasmosis is produced by *Histoplasma capsulatum.* This disease
resembles that caused by *Coccidioides* in that it is dustborne and usually
associated with only a mild respiratory infection. However, progressive
and disseminated infections may be fatal. In the United States this disease
is prevalent in the drainage area of the Mississippi River. In contrast to
the disease caused by *Coccidioides,* histoplasmosis is more severe in
Caucasians than non-Caucasians. The general pattern of primary respiratory infection followed by disseminated granulomatous abscesses and
occasional meningitis is also seen in *cryptococcosis, North American
blastomycosis, nocardiosis,* and *aspergillosis.* In all these diseases differentiation depends upon identification of the organism.

   Another pattern of mycotic infection involves initial subcutaneous
inoculation. This may occur in a *North American blastomycosis, sporotri-
chosis, maduromycosis,* and *chromoblastomycosis.* The skin and regional
lymphatic systems are involved with chronic granulomatous draining
lesions; however, dissemination is rare. A severe clinical manifestation is

the *mycetoma,* or *madura foot.*   In this lesion there is destruction of bone and muscle and a marked deformity of the foot, which takes on a clubbed appearance.

PROTOZOA

The protozoa are single-celled organisms variously classified as animals or as higher protists by those who prefer to avoid the distinction between plant and animal forms at this level of development.   Four classes are recognized: (1) the Mastigophora or flagellates, (2) the Sarcodina, (3) the Sporozoa, and (4) the Ciliophora or Ciliata.   All four classes have representatives pathogenic for man.   A number of nonpathogenic protozoan parasites have been identified but will not be discussed in this section.

Mastigophora

The *trypanosomes* cause sleeping sickness and Chagas disease in man. When in the free form in the blood they are elongated organisms made motile by a lateral undulating membrane terminating in a single anterior flagellum.   They multiply in the tissues, where they form compact bodies not recognizable as protozoa.   The trypanosome of *sleeping sickness* is transmitted by the bite of the tsetse fly in tropical Africa.   Man is the only known host for the trypanosome of Gambian sleeping sickness, although an animal reservoir is suspected.   The parasites multiply in the tissues and enter the blood via the lymphatics in about 3 weeks.   Severe fever and general debility result, and intercurrent infections often cause death. About 2 years after onset the parasites enter the central nervous system and the classic picture of sleeping sickness develops.   The untreated mortality is 25 to 50 percent.   Rhodesian sleeping sickness is more severe and usually causes death within 1 year.   Antelopes are known reservoirs (Fig. 9-22).

Chagas' disease or American trypanosomiasis occurs from Southern Mexico to South America.   The vector is the reduviid bug (often called "kissing bugs" because they frequently bite the lip); the parasites are most frequently found in macrophages, skeletal and heart muscle, and the central nervous system.   The predeliction of the parasites for the heart muscle is extremely important since acute and chronic heart failure are frequent complications and often cause death.

Leishmaniasis consists of three distinct diseases: kala-azar, Oriental sore, and American mucocutaneous leishmaniasis.   The etiologic agents are *Leishmania donovanni, L. tropica,* and *L. braziliensia* respectively.   All three are transmitted by the bite of sand flies.   Kala-azar is found through-

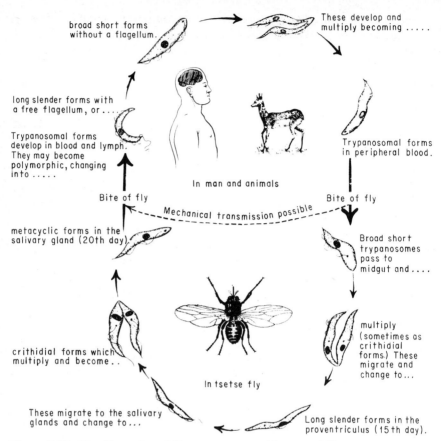

broad short forms without a flagellum.

These develop and multiply becoming .....

long slender forms with a free flagellum, or ....

Trypanosomal forms develop in blood and lymph. They may become polymorphic, changing into .....

Trypanosomal forms in peripheral blood.

In man and animals

Bite of fly

Mechanical transmission possible

Bite of fly

metacyclic forms in the salivary gland (20th day).

Broad short trypanosomes pass to midgut and ....

crithidial forms which multiply and become ..

multiply (sometimes as crithidial forms.) These migrate and change to...

In tsetse fly

These migrate to the salivary glands and change to...

Long slender forms in the proventriculus (15th day).

Figure 9-22 The life cycles of *Trypanosoma gambiense* and *T. rhodesiense* (sleeping sickness). *(From Medical Protozoology and Helminthology, U.S. Naval Medical School, Bethesda, Md., 1962, p. 108. By permission of the publishers.)*

out Asia and the Mediterranean and in a few areas of Central and South America. In some areas animal reservoirs, including dogs, have been demonstrated, but in others none have been found. The organisms proliferate in the reticuloendothelial system, where small rounded forms can be found packing the cells. These are known as Leishman-Donovan bodies and are diagnostic when they are seen on microscopic examination. Many of the manifestations of the disease may be due to the tremendous number of organisms in the cells. The free form of these flagellates is not usually found in man but occurs in the sand fly. However, they can be produced from Donovan bodies in media containing blood. The cutaneous and mucocutaneous forms are generally less severe and may heal spontaneously.

Trichomonas vaginalis is a mildly pathogenic flagellate found in the urethra and vagina. It produces a mild urethritis; however, in women it also causes a persistent vaginitis characterized by itching, burning, and a profuse vaginal discharge. *Giardia lamblia* is another mildly pathogenic flagellate which inhabits the intestinal tract and may produce diarrhea, particularly in children. Both *Trichomonas* and *Giardia* are quite common, although infrequently the cause of symptoms.

Sarcodina

The sarcodina are represented by a number of nonpathogenic species and by one significant pathogen, *Entamoeba histolytica. E. histolytica* exists as a motile trophozoite and as a cyst. The trophozoites (active forms) are fragile and rarely transmitted; the cysts survive for relatively long periods and therefore are the form in which the infection is usually transmitted. After ingestion, the cysts pass through the stomach and are activated in the small intestine. Parasitism is generally of the large intestine, although the terminal ileum may be involved. The amoebae produce characteristic intestinal ulcerations with ragged overhanging edges and sometimes enter the portal veins and infect the liver, where they can produce abscesses. It has been proposed that the amoebae produce a histolytic enzyme, but this has not been established. Interestingly, the pathogenicity may depend upon the number and variety of bacteria in the normal intestinal flora. In most individuals the infection will be asymptomatic; however, all grades of chronic and acute colitis are possible.

Sporozoa

The most important sporozoan parasite is the *malarial plasmodium.* The three important species in man are *Plasmodium vivax, P. malariae,* and *P. falciparum.* The sexual cycle of the parasite occurs in the female anopheles mosquito (Fig. 9-23). The mature parasites, called sporozoites, migrate to the salivary glands and are injected into man when the mosquito bites. Initially the organisms undergo asexual multiplication in the liver and then infect the red cells. When sufficient red cells have been parasitized, a cycle ensues in which the parasites multiply and eventually rupture the cells. This is associated with a chill lasting from 15 to 60 minutes. Subsequently there is a sudden high fever, during which the parasites infect new cells. The fever subsides as the patient has a profuse sweat, and in a short time the patient feels relatively well until the next turn of the cycle.

P. vivax causes tertian malaria in which the cycle is 48 hours. *P. malariae* produces quartan malaria in which the cycle is 72 hours. *P. falciparum* causes malignant tertian malaria with an irregular cycle of 36 to 48 hours. Tertian and quartan malaria rarely cause death directly, but

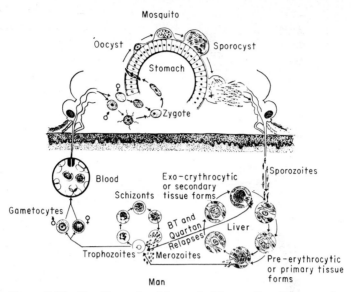

Figure 9-23   The life cycle of the malarial parasite.   The sexual phase of the malarial parasite occurs in the intestinal wall of the female aedes mosquito.   There are two asexual cycles in the human.   The first cycle is in the liver and may be entirely asymptomatic.   The second cycle is in the bloodstream and gives rise to the characteristic clinical manifestations.   *(From W. H. Hargreaves, and R. J. G. Morrison, The Practice of Tropical Medicine, Staples Press, London, 1965, p. 3.   By permission of the publishers.)*

debility increases susceptibility to other diseases.   Malignant tertian malaria is more severe and may cause death.   Extremely heavy parasitism may cause obstruction of small blood vessels, which results in a variety of clinical manifestations.   In the absence of superinfection or malignant complications, *P. falciparum* malaria will generally terminate spontaneously.   However, *P. vivax* and *P. malariae* persist in the liver cycle, and recurrence of active disease is possible after many years.   As recently as 1945, malaria was probably the most important disease in the world, with 10 percent of the population having active symptoms at any one time.   Intensive programs aimed at destroying mosquitoes and decreasing the human reservoirs have achieved marked success, with almost total elimination of the disease in many areas.

Toxoplasma gondii produces an infection whose importance has only recently been recognized.   Serological surveys indicate that toxoplasmosis is widespread; one-third of subjects tested in a number of American cities have shown significant levels of antibody in the serum.   Except for transmission from the mother to the fetus, which produces overt manifestations in the infant, the mode of transmission is unknown. The organism grows in and destroys macrophages and parenchymal cells. Infected infants may be stillborn, show signs of neonatal infection, or later develop hydrocephaly, convulsions, eye defects, and psychomotor retardation.

Ciliata

Balantidium coli is an unusually large protozoan organism which inhabits the large intestine. It is transmitted by ingestion of cyst forms. The range of manifestations is comparable to those of *Entamoeba histolytica,* but there are no liver complications and the colitis is not usually as severe.

HELMINTHS

Helminth, or worm, infestations are of worldwide distribution; their greatest importance is limited to the tropical areas where infection is widespread and the consequences are measured not only in clinical disease but in extensive economic and social loss as well. Three classes of worms produce disease in man. These include the Cestoda (tapeworms) and Trematoda (flukes) of the phylum Platyhelminthes (flatworms) and the nematode roundworms of the phylum Nemathelminthes.

Cestoda

The mature *tapeworm* consists of a *scolex* (head), which is especially adapted for adhesion to intestinal mucosa, and reproductive organs called *proglottids* (Fig. 9-24). The scolex produces the proglottids at the distal end opposite the point of attachment. As the proglottids mature and enlarge, they are separated from the scolex by the formation of new, less mature proglottids. Thus the scolex is at the upper end of a long chain of proglottids of gradually increasing size. The mature proglottids at the end of the chain detach and release their ova, which are then passed in the feces. When the ova are ingested by the intermediate host, digestion releases the larvae, which penetrate the intestinal wall, enter the circulation, and are deposited in various tissues, where they encyst. The most common site of cyst formation is in striated muscle, although, depending upon the species, almost any organ may be involved. Ingestion of the larvae by man, most commonly as a result of eating undercooked beef, pork, or fish, releases the larvae, which then become scolices and renew the cycle.

The tapeworms of importance in man are *Taenia saginata,* the beef

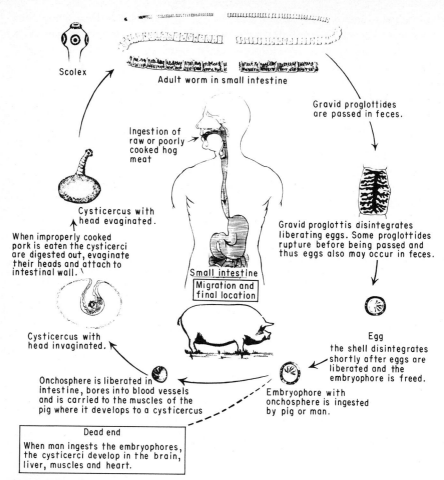

Figure 9-24   The life cycle of the pork tapeworm, *Taenia solium.*
(From Medical Protozoology and Helminthology, U.S. Naval Medical School, Bethesda, Md., 1962, p. 155.   By permission of the publishers.)

tapeworm; *T. solium,* the pork tapeworm; *Diphyllobothrium latum,* the fish tapeworm; and *Hymenolepis nana,* the dwarf tapeworm.   The beef and pork tapeworms generally produce only minor symptoms in man. The fish tapeworm may produce anemia resembling pernicious anemia. This worm competes with the body for the vitamin B_{12} in the diet.   Since vitamin B_{12} is essential for the production of red blood cells, anemia results.   The dwarf tapeworm undergoes a complete cycle in the same host, and self-reinfection is possible.   When present in large numbers, this tapeworm can produce symptoms of intestinal irritation and obstruction.

Occasionally man can be the intermediate host in various tapeworm cycles, in which case serious complications can ensue. Regurgitation of a pork tapeworm into the stomach can result in activation of larvae and the formation of *cysticerci* (larval cysts) in various parts of the body, of which the most important are the eye and brain. *Echinococcus* is particularly common where dogs are used for sheepherding. These dogs are infected by the tapeworm *Echinococcus granulosus,* which they get by eating the sheep offal. The accidental ingestion of the ova by man results in cyst formation, primarily in the liver and lungs. Dangerous tissue destruction can result.

Trematoda

The *schistosome trematoda* are widespread, with important endemic foci in the Nile Valley, the Philippines, Japan and China, and the Caribbean, including Puerto Rico. The adult schistosome worms reside in the veins draining the intestines and the pelvic organs. The female worm lays the eggs within a venule, where they produce an inflammatory response with tubercle formation. In the case of *Schistosoma mansoni* and *S. japonicum,* some of the ova eventually work through the intestinal mucosa and into the feces. However, a number of ova are trapped in the tissues by the inflammatory response or fail to penetrate the blood vessel wall and are carried by the portal circulation to the liver. In addition to some intestinal penetration, many of the ova of *S. hematobium,* which are deposited in the pelvic venous plexus, erode through the bladder wall and are excreted in the urine. If the eggs reach water, free-swimming miracidia are hatched. The miracidia in turn enter snails of specific species which serve as the intermediate hosts. The miracidia multiply and numerous cercariae emerge from the snails. When man works, bathes, or swims in fresh water contaminated with cercariae, they penetrate the skin or mucous membranes, enter the lymphatics, progress to the circulation, and then mature in the branches of the portal vein in the liver. The mature worms then travel against the bloodstream to the veins draining the intestines and bladder. The disease manifestations are probably due primarily to inflammation and scar formation, although sensitization may be important. The ultimate complication of *S. mansoni* and *S. japonicum* is severe liver fibrosis with all the characteristics of fulminant cirrhosis. *S. hematobium* produces scarring and contracture of the bladder with urinary obstruction, infection, and frequent bladder carcinoma.

Other trematodes, including the *lung and liver flukes,* have an even more complicated life cycle (Fig. 9-25). The ova hatch and produce

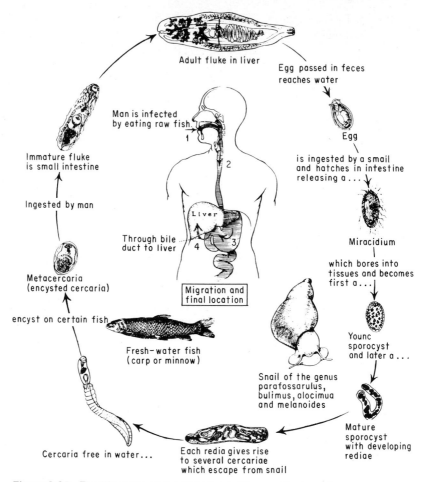

Figure 9-25   The life cycle of the liver fluke, *Clonorchis sinensis*.
(From Medical Protozoology and Helminthology, U.S. Naval Medical School, Bethesda, Md., 1962, p. 135.   By permission of the publishers.)

miracidia, which penetrate snails, where metamorphosis and multiplication occur.   The cercariae leave the snails and enter crayfish, crabs, or fish, where they encyst.   Man is infected by eating these intermediate hosts either raw or inadequately cooked.   The metacercariae are released in the duodenum and migrate to the liver or lungs, where the mature worm develops.   Unless extremely heavy infestation results, the symptoms and pathological changes are relatively mild and nonspecific.

Nematoda

A large number of nematodes are pathogenic for man. However, their epidemiology can be reduced to a smaller number of patterns. *Ascaris lumbricoides* inhabit the small intestine, where they are usually asymptomatic, despite their size. They are 15 to 30 centimeters in length and 0.2 to 0.6 centimeters in diameter. Occasionally they may obstruct the bile ducts, intestines, or appendix. Eggs are passed with the feces and infection is initiated by ingestion. The larvae are released from the eggs

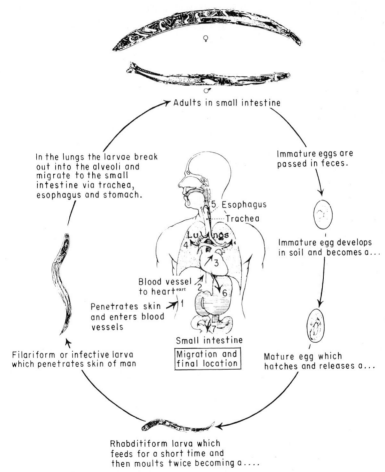

Figure 9-26   The life cycles of hookworms. *(From Medical Proto-zoology and Helminthology, U.S. Naval Medical School, Bethesda, Md., 1961, p. 175. By permission of the publishers.)*

in the small intestine, where they penetrate the wall and reach the lungs by way of venules of lymphatics. Here they pass into the alveoli, ascend the respiratory passages, and are then reswallowed and grow into adult form in the small intestine. *Enterobius vermicularis,* the pinworm or threadworm, deposits its eggs in the anal and perianal regions. Local pruritis causes scratching and oral recontamination. The ova mature in the intestine; both the male and female die after producing fertile eggs, and persistence depends upon reinfection.

The *hookworms (Ancylostoma duodenale* and *Necator americanus)* and *Strongyloides stercoralis* have similar life cycles (Fig. 9-26). The adult worms reside in the intestinal tract. Ova are passed with the feces and the larvae are hatched in the soil. The larvae penetrate the skin, enter the venules, and are carried to the lungs. In the lungs they penetrate the alveolar epithelium, ascend the respiratory passages, are swallowed and reach the small intestine, where they mature. The hookworm infections are significant primarily because they produce a chronic anemia, initiating a cycle of chronic debility and poor productivity. The resultant low economic status in endemic areas interferes with sanitation, the purchase of shoes, and other factors which would interrupt the cycle. Strongyloides can also produce a hyperinfection of the colon with pathologic changes and local symptoms.

Trichinosis is caused by *Trichinella spiralis,* a nematode which infects a large variety of mammals (Fig. 9-27). In animals the disease is transmitted by raw meat, and a common cycle is pig-rat-pig, and so on. The disease is initiated in man after ingestion of inadequately cooked meat, most frequently pork. Larvae are liberated from the cysts and enter the intestinal mucosa, where they mature. The female then discharges living larvae, which enter the circulation, are distributed throughout the body, and encyst. Most of the manifestations are due to larval migration and include intestinal and muscular inflammation, fever, a rash and skin hemorrhages, and occasionally central nervous system manifestations. Since a large percent of the population can be demonstrated to have cysts (15 to 20 percent), most infections must be asymptomatic or nonspecific in their manifestations. However, symptoms occur in heavy infestation, and deaths have been reported.

Filariasis includes a group of nematode diseases in which the filarial larva is transmitted by the bite of an arthropod. Manifestations of these diseases are rather diverse, and only one will be discussed. The term *filariasis* is often used specifically to indicate the disease produced by *Wuchereria bancrofti,* the agent which produces elephantiasis. This disease has a wide distribution, and American experience was increased by the presence of filariasis in some Pacific islands during World War II.

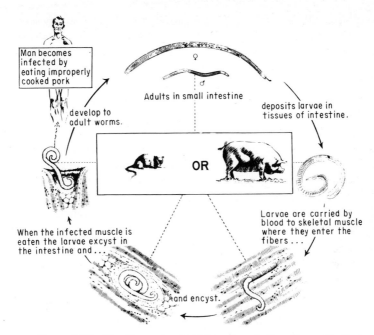

Figure 9-27   The life cycle of *Trichinella spiralis. (From Medical Protozoology and Helminthology, U.S. Naval Medical School, Bethesda, Md., 1962, p. 188.   By permission of the publishers.)*

The mature worms may survive in human lymphatics for 5 to 10 years. The microfilarial larvae are released into the blood only between 9 P.M. and 2 A.M., a fact which delayed early elucidation of the life cycle.   Patients bitten during this period will transfer the microfilariae to the appropriate mosquito vector, where further development occurs.   Full maturation results on inoculation into a new host.   Acute filariasis may represent a hypersensitivity as well as an inflammatory reaction.   Chronic filariasis results in scarring of lymphatic channels and lymph nodes.   The granulomatous inflammatory reaction does not occur until death of the worm. Lymphedema and elephantiasis result from this mechanism; however severe forms are noted only in endemic areas where superinfection has occurred.

HOST FACTORS IN DISEASE

Susceptibility and Resistance

Species and tissue resistances are important to the development and nature of disease, yet little is known about these factors.   Why can one species of parasite affect man while another closely related species is unable to do so but will infect another host? In the last section a number of extremely intricate life cycles were described which required highly specific hosts through several stages. Man is susceptible to very few of the many parasitic helminth infections in nature. An illustrative example is "swimmer's itch," which is found in many localized areas of the world. These itches are due to the penetration of the skin by cercariae comparable to those which produce schistomiasis. However, after penetrating the skin and producing local symptoms, the cercariae die and the cycle is not completed. This phenomenon is undoubtedly repeated many times in nature until the appropriate host is found. The opportunity for infection is apparently the same. There must be subtle differences in genetically controlled chemical processes which account for these phenomena. Still, it would seem easier to explain why one group of parasites would be successful with an animal host and another would be successful with man than it is to explain why apparently similar parasites are pathogenic for different species.

An attempt has been made to indicate the mechanisms of localization of many of the infections discussed. Mechanical factors of exposure are obviously the most important. The course of the disease and the biological interaction between the parasite and the host determine the subsequent course, and many of these factors are known. However, many striking examples such as the localization of *Neisseria meningitidis* to the meninges and *N. gonorrhoeae* to the urethra require further study for complete understanding.

It has been demonstrated that strains of animals can be bred which are unusually resistant or unusually susceptible to a particular pathogen. This may explain the unusual resistance of some individuals to a particular infection. Such studies cannot be clear since the entire previous infectious experience of the individual is not known. Genetic studies in humans will undoubtedly be hampered by similar factors. The same problems obscure questions of so-called racial immunity and susceptibility. The exposure of primitive populations to measles often results in severe epidemics with a high mortality. The extent to which this represents failure of natural selection as opposed to lack of appropriate prior exposure cannot always be determined.

Age is one of the most important factors affecting the individual response to infection. Young children and the aged have the highest mortality from infectious diseases. In the case of children, it is readily understood that it takes some time before the immune mechanisms are fully developed. What is not generally appreciated is that the increased susceptibility of the aged is not an isolated phenomenon. When allowances are made for differential risks of exposure, the case fatality rate increases with every increase in age beyond puberty. Some of the factors underlying this phenomenon will be discussed in Chap. 12.

The presence of malnutrition, fatigue, and other disease usually increases the risk and severity of infection. In addition, many diseases predispose to specific infectious complications. Mention has been made of influenza and *Hemophilus influenzae* pneumonia. Silicosis predisposes to tuberculosis, nephrosis to pneumococcal peritonitis, chronic leukemia to herpes zoster, and hypoparathyroidism to candidiasis. Such a list could be greatly extended.

A number of metabolic factors are known to alter host resistance. Two of these are clinically obvious and have been extensively studied: diabetes mellitus and abnormalities in adrenocorticosteroid levels. Diabetes is clinically frequently associated with uncontrolled urinary-tract infections and cutaneous pyogenic infections, usually staphylococcal. It was previously assumed that the high levels of sugar in the extracellular fluids provided favorable nutrients for the bacteria. This concept was not substantiated; it is now believed that, instead of producing normal amounts of lactic acid, the inflammatory cells in the diabetic produce metabolic end products which are less antibacterial than lactic acid.

Adrenal insufficiency, which causes an inadequate output of corticosteroids (adrenal cortical hormone), results in an inadequate response to stress and a failure to mobilize body defenses. On the other hand, excess corticosteroid, now frequently due to the administration of cortisone and prednisone for therapeutic purposes (rather than to pathological oversecretion by the adrenal gland), results in suppression of inflammation. This may be beneficial when disease manifestations are primarily due to the inflammatory response, as in hypersensitivity reactions. However, at the same time the corticosteroids block many of the defense reactions essential to the localization and destruction of infectious organisms.

Host Defenses

Many local factors serve as defenses against infection. The most important is the mechanical barrier of the intact skin and mucous membrane. Relatively few organisms can penetrate the keratin barrier of the epidermis. In addition, the normal secretions of the skin have considerable antibacterial activity. When measured quantities of bacteria are placed on the skin, there is a rapid decrease in the number of living organisms as sequential cultures are taken from the area. The mucous membranes of the respiratory tract are protected by the secretion of mucus, which entraps organisms, and by the constant brushing action of the cilia of cells of the intact mucous membrane, which tend to sweep the mucus and particulate matter out of the respiratory tract. The normal cough mechanism is especially important, as is demonstrated by the increased frequency of pulmonary infection which follows unconscious states such as anesthesia and coma. The gastrointestinal tract destroys many potentially pathogenic organisms as the result of action by the gastric acids and the digestive enzymes. Unfortunately, this barrier is not totally protective, and in some instances, such as following the ingestion of protozoan cysts and helminth ova, it serves to activate the parasite. The tears contain bactericidal lysozyme, a proteolytic enzyme similar to that found in the lysosomes.

General Factors

Most of the important general factors in host resistance have been discussed in previous chapters. These include the inflammatory reaction, phagocytosis, and the immune response. The role of phagocytosis varies, depending upon the mode of infection. Bacteria which gain entrance directly into the circulation are cleared very rapidly by the fixed macrophages, particularly those of the spleen, liver, and bone marrow. Organisms introduced into the tissues are less rapidly phagocytosed, and those which escape from the local lesion are generally taken up in the regional lymph nodes. Organisms in various serous cavities, which for mechanical reasons are less accessible for phagocytosis than the blood or tissues, are more likely to have the opportunity to multiply without disturbance. It is for this reason that the control of infections in the peritoneum is often difficult and that peritonitis is such a grave disease. The same is true of the pleural and pericardial cavities, joint spaces, sinuses, gall bladder, and urinary bladder. The numbers of organisms of a given type necessary to produce a persistent infection is related inversely to the time required for effective phagocytosis. Organisms which can survive within the phagocytes present additional problems of host defense.

Host defense mechanisms to virus infection are less well understood than are those mechanisms which can be examined more directly. Recent techniques indicate that virus particles are phagocytosed. However, the role of phagocytosis is not clear. Patients with virus diseases often recover normally, even during periods of agranulocytosis. Similarly, patients with hypogammaglobulinemia recover normally from virus diseases, despite the fact that the production of antibodies cannot be demonstrated. Cellular immunity and delayed hypersensitivity appears in response to many viruses. A hypersensitive phagocyte may be more effective than one which is not sensitized, as is the case in tuberculosis and other bacterial diseases.

The most promising evidence for a specific antiviral defense has been the recognition of *interferon*. Interferon is a relatively low-molecular-weight protein which is specific for the host but nonspecific for the parasite. It has been demonstrated to increase in host cells following infection with picornaviruses, arboviruses, myxoviruses, papovaviruses, and poxviruses. Less interferon is found after infection with virulent than with avirulent strains of the same virus. Nucleic acids will also stimulate the cells to produce interferon. Experimental mouse infections with influenza virus show that peak amounts of interferon are found at 3 days, coincident with subsidence of infection but considerably before the production of significant antibodies. Other studies have shown that the information for interferon production resides in the cellular DNA. It has been suggested that interferon plays a fundamental role in cellular function and that, in response to the presence of foreign genetic material, a gene is uncovered which interferes with the replication of the foreign material. This defense might be effective against many types of mutation as well as against viruses. It may be that interferon was developed primarily to protect the integrity of the genome from all types of alteration. The presence of one viral infection often blocks infection with another virus, and resistance to any second virus infection persists for some time. This phenomenon is probably due to interferon.

Systemic Responses to Infection

Many of the characteristic responses to infection have been shown in the preceding sections to be determined by the nature of the parasite as well as by specific host reactions. However, a number of host reactions are nonspecific and appear to be related to the general fact of infection. The patient appears ill or "toxic" and he feels general malaise and weakness. Often there is a dissociation between how ill the patient appears and the threat of the situation. A patient can appear quite ill with influenza yet at the same time obviously not be in danger. Symptoms can include weakness, fatigability, loss of appetite, headache, and muscle aching. Relatively little is known of the exact mechanism which produces these symptoms. They often run parallel to the fever, but they may be due to the *pyrogens* (fever-producing substances) causing the fever rather than to the fever itself. Often, sensations of weakness, lassitude, and vasomotor instability persist for several weeks after recovery. These symptoms may be out of proportion to the severity of the initial disease and have been noted especially after upper respiratory infections, infectious mononucleosis, hepatitis, and brucellosis. Occasionally specific lesions are found in muscle, but these are infrequent and inconstant.

Fever

The body temperature depends upon the relationship between heat production and heat loss. This regulation is controlled by a center in the brain except when there are extensive environmental factors beyond the capacity for physiological compensation. The administration of extremely small amounts of endotoxin from gram-negative organisms results in an immediate and transient drop in the number of circulating polymorphonuclear leukocytes, followed by the rapid appearance of fever. The bacterial endotoxin causes destruction of the leukocytes, which in turn release a pyrogen which acts on the heat regulating center to increase heat production and decrease heat loss, thus causing a rise in the body temperature. The endotoxin may act directly as a pyrogen as well, since injection of endotoxin into the brain, where there are no white cells, also produces a temperature rise. Damage to other cells may also release pyrogens. The destruction of white cells by pyogenic processes would therefore be expected to be a consistent cause of fever, and the persistence of fever in patients with well-walled-off abscesses could be explained by the continuing leakage of pyrogen from the purulent material. *Fever is continuous or*

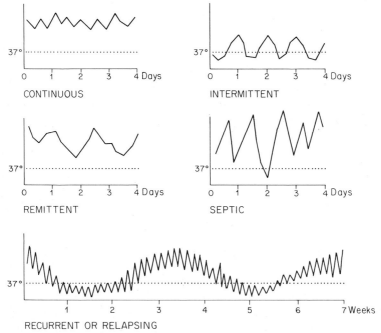

Figure 9-28 The variety of fevers which can be associated with infectious diseases.

sustained when it is present throughout the day (Fig. 9-28). It is *intermittent* if it returns to normal at least once daily, and *remittent* if it shows variations but does not return to normal. *Hectic* or *septic fevers* show very wide swings over short periods of time. *Recurrent* or *relapsing fevers* are fevers lasting for several days with intervals of normal temperature between. There is no substantial evidence that fever is a necessary part of the defense mechanism and, except in unusual circumstances, the patient usually benefits by procedures designed to lower the temperature.

Circulatory Changes

Fever is usually associated with an acceleration in the heart rate on the order of approximately 10 beats per minute per degree Fahrenheit of elevation. Unless the heart itself is involved by the inflammatory process, there is little evidence of cardiac difficulty. However, patients with cardiac disease tolerate fever poorly and may go into acute heart failure. In some diseases, such as typhoid and yellow fever, the increase in the heart rate is not as much as would be anticipated from the level of the fever. Peripheral circulatory failure with a fall in the blood pressure may occur as a result of specific manifestations of disease. There are two types, one due to excessive loss of body fluids and the other due to blood vessel injury with loss of normal tone. Blood volume may be decreased by large losses of fluid either into the tissues, such as with rickettsial diseases, or through the intestinal tract, as with dysentery or cholera. There is generally a fall in the blood pressure following a chill and after the subsidence of a fever. This may produce a sense of lassitude and weakness, but it is not generally of serious significance. An important cause of loss of vascular tone is endotoxin shock produced by the endotoxins from gram-negative bacteria. It is due to septicemia and is almost invariably fatal.

Blood Changes

The changes in the number and distribution of the white blood cells in infection are often characteristic and help in establishing the diagnosis. The most common response is an increase in the number of circulating polymorphonuclear leukocytes (specifically a *granulocytosis,* but usually termed *leukocytosis*), although in overwhelming infections there may occasionally be an actual decrease. In particular, pyogenic infections almost invariably produce a polymorphonuclear leukocytosis. Some bacterial infections, such as typhoid, tularemia, and brucellosis, produce a decrease in the number of leukocytes, or *leukopenia.* Most viral diseases, particularly measles, influenza, smallpox, and dengue also produce a moderate leukopenia. *Eosinophilia,* which is an increase in the number of circulating eosinophils, is common in worm infestations and is also noted in certain extensive skin diseases and some hypersensitivity reactions. A marked *lymphocytosis,* a relative or absolute increase of lymphocytes, is noted in pertussis (whooping cough), and a moderate lymphocytosis is seen in many viral diseases, such as mumps and measles. *Monocytosis,* an increase in monocytes, may be observed in tuberculosis. *Agranulocytosis,* the total absence of polymorphonuclear leukocytes (granulocytes), usually results from nonbacterial toxins, but when it is present it renders the patient extremely vulnerable to bacterial infection.

Infection generally causes the red blood cells to clump together, so that, if blood is placed in a test tube, the red blood cells settle out with unusual rapidity. This reaction has been standardized and has been called the *sedimentation rate.* *Anemia* is rarely seen with acute infections; however, a moderate anemia is quite common in chronic infections. There is a reduction in the rate of red cell production, and the number of red cells in the circulation tends to stabilize at a lower than normal concentration.

THERAPY

It is not appropriate to enter into an extensive discussion of therapy in this text. However, certain principles can be profitably examined on the basis of the foregoing discussion. The role of active and passive immunization techniques was discussed in the last chapter and will not be examined further. Antimicrobial chemotherapy depends upon the concept of selective toxicity, which was first developed by Paul Ehrlich. He believed that each organism had specific chemical characteristics, and that it would be possible to find chemical mechanisms which would take advantage of the specificity to destroy the parasites without affecting the host. The first mechanism recognized was that of competitive inhibition. For example, many bacteria require folic acid, whose synthesis includes para-aminobenzoic acid (PABA) as a component. The sulfonamides are structurally very similar to PABA, and when present compete with PABA for incorporation into the folic acid molecule. However, the sulfonamide-containing folic acidlike molecule is metabolically ineffective and interferes with the bacterial cell function. Second, like plants, bacteria have a rigid outer layer which lends strength to the cytoplasmic membrane, which actually is the limit of the metabolically active cell. Antibiotics related to penicillin interfere with the synthesis of the cell wall, and as a result the bacteria are extremely susceptible to disruption by local physical factors. The members of a third group of antibiotics exert their effects directly upon the cytoplasmic membrane. Examples include the polymyxins, which act on gram-negative bacteria, and the polyenes, which act on fungi. These compounds alter the permeability of the cell membrane, which then allows the outward leakage of nucleotides and proteins and perhaps the inward diffusion of undesirable chemicals as well. A fourth mechanism, demonstrated by chloramphenicol, the tetracyclines, and the streptomycins, is the inhibition of protein synthesis. Chloramphenicol interferes with the attachment of messenger RNA to the ribosomes. Streptomycin seems to interfere with messenger RNA function but not with its attachment. A final group of drugs inhibit nucleic acid synthesis. Actinomycin binds with DNA and blocks messenger RNA formation; it also inhibits DNA virus replication. Mitomycin breaks down DNA. Unfortunately both these compounds, while extremely valuable in experimental studies, also exert their effect on animal cells and are not practical therapeutic agents.

Systematic explorations for antiviral chemical agents have also been initiated. A number of steps in viral reproduction has been defined: absorption of virus into cells, penetration and attachment of the viral genome to the cellular genome or ribosome, the replication of viral DNA or RNA, the synthesis of viral protein, assembly of virus particles, and virus release. These all represent points of vulnerability against which therapeutic drugs can be directed. Several antiviral chemicals have already been demonstrated and their sites of action identified. L-Adamantanamine appears to block the penetration of myxoviruses into cells and has been effective in modifying experimental influenza. Satin betathiosemicarbazone inhibits the synthesis of viral protein or the assembly of virus particles. It has a specific effect upon poxviruses, and field trials against smallpox have been promising. IUDR, 5-iodo-2′-deoxyuridine, blocks DNA synthesis and, although its systemic use is not possible because of toxicity, it has been found effective in treating the eye lesions produced by the cold-sore virus, herpes simplex. IUDR and a number of similar purine and pyrimidine analogs become incorporated into DNA and RNA and prevent normal function. This approach to virus chemotherapy is relatively new, but it is promising because it is rational.

CHANGING PATTERNS IN HUMAN INFECTION

The risk of disease and death as a result of organisms which produce specific diseases, such as diphtheria, typhoid, and poliomyelitis, has been greatly reduced during the past century. Many factors have contributed to these changes. They include improved knowledge and better education, sanitary developments which reduce the risk of exposure to contaminated food and fluid, arthropod control techniques including insecticides, specific immunizations, and the availability of a wide range of chemotherapeutic and antibiotic products.

At the same time there has been a relative and an absolute increase in the risk of infection by some normally resident, usually commensal organisms. This change may result from a number of factors. The widespread use of antibiotics often results in the elimination of many normal commensal bacteria which ordinarily compete effectively with potentially pathogenic species. The use of antibiotics also often results in the development of resistant strains which are more difficult to control. The use of steroids and immunity-suppressing drugs in the treatment of a large number of diseases carries the unfortunate hazard of decreased antimicrobial defense. There may also be an increased carelessness engendered by the apparent security from infectious complications.

We must be grateful for the decrease in specific infections and epidemic diseases, continuing our vigilance with the realization that the changes are not all irreversible, and that epidemics are still possible if there is a social breakdown. This is exemplified by the recrudescence of malaria where mosquito control programs have been abandoned; by the widespread increase in the incidence of venereal diseases; and by the epidemics of typhoid, cholera, and typhus among refugees. Control of infections by ordinarily commensal parasites will require the continued use of proved principles and a search for new solutions.

BIBLIOGRAPHY

BRAUDE, A. I.: "Bacterial Endotoxins," *Scientific American,* March, 1964.

BURNET, M.: "Viruses," *Scientific American,* May, 1951.

CHRISTIE, A. B.: *Infectious Diseases,* London: Livingstone, 1969.

DUBOS, R. J., and J. G. HIRSCH (eds.): *Bacterial and Mycotic Infections of Man,* 4th ed., Philadelphia: J. B. Lippincott Company, 1965.

GORDON, J. E., (ed.): *Control of Communicable Diseases in Men,* 10th ed., New York: The American Public Health Association, 1965.

HORNE, R. W.: "The Structure of Viruses," *Scientific American,* January, 1963.

HORSFALL, F. L., JR., and I. TAMM (eds.): *Viral and Rickettsial Infections of Man,* 4th ed., Philadelphia: J. B. Lippincott Company, 1965.

HUNTER, G. W., W. W. FRYE, and J. C. SWARTZWELDER (eds.): *A Manual of Tropical Medicine,* Philadelphia: W. B. Saunders Company, 1966.

JAWETZ, E., J. L. MELNICK, and E. A. ADELBERG (eds.): *Review of Medical Microbiology,* 9th ed., Los Altos, Calif.: Lange Medical Publications, 1970.

MANSON-BAHR, P.: *Manson's Tropical Diseases,* 16th ed., Baltimore: The Williams & Wilkins Company, 1966.

Medical Protozoology and Helminthology, Bethesda, Md.: U.S. Naval Medical School, 1962.

RHODES, A. J., and C. E. VAN ROOYEN: *Textbook of Virology,* 5th ed., Baltimore: Williams & Wilkins Company, 1968.

TOP, F. H.: *Communicable and Infectious Diseases,* 6th ed., St. Louis: The C. V. Mosby Company, 1968.

Special Circulatory Disorders: Hemorrhage and Shock; Thrombosis, Embolism, and Infarction; Arteriosclerosis

The subjects to be discussed in this chapter could be equally well described in a section on diseases of the blood vessels as part of a review of diseases by organ systems. However, these processes represent mechanisms by which isolated disease can be produced in every organ system. In addition, with the exception of hemorrhage, they are generally unfamiliar to students being introduced to disease concepts. Yet the related processes of thrombosis, embolism, and infarction probably account for over 50 percent of deaths in modern societies. Therefore it seems appropriate to include these disorders in this section.

Before discussing the processes affecting blood vessels, it is necessary to introduce some information regarding the structure of the vascular system (Fig. 10-1). The inner layer of a blood vessel is a thin endothelium called the *intima*. The middle layer, or *media*, is composed of elastic fibers, collagen, and smooth muscle cells. The outer layer, or *adventitia*, is fibrous connective tissue, mostly collagen, and binds the vessel to the surrounding tissues. The media of the arteries near the heart is primarily

307

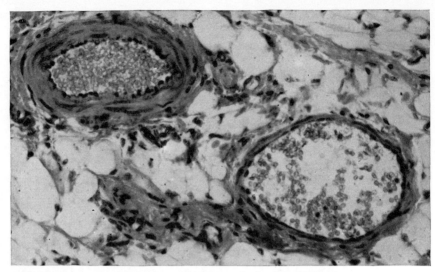

Figure 10-1   Cross section of a small artery and vein. The internal layer, or intima, consists of endothelium, lying directly upon the wavy internal elastic membrane. The media consists of encircling smooth muscle cells. The external adventitia consists of connective tissue. The wall of the vein consists of the same three layers which are considerably thinner and therefore do not maintain the tubular configuration unless filled with blood. [*From R. J. Barrnett in R. O. Greep (ed.), Histology, McGraw-Hill, New York, 1966, p. 276. By permission of the publishers.*]

elastic tissue which cushions the accelerating pressure of the heartbeat. Further away, the smooth muscle becomes the predominant component and, by differential contraction, helps direct blood flow to areas of greatest need. Eventually, the muscular arteries give way to the *arterioles,* small arteries with only one layer of muscle cells which are extremely reactive and even further control distribution of blood flow. Finally, the capillaries consist of the intimal endothelium only, without media or adventitia. This thin layer of squamous epithelium is the minimal barrier to the exchange of metabolic materials and products between the bloodstream and the tissues.

The *venules* and the veins are the counterparts of the arterioles and arteries. At this point, the hemodynamic force of the heart is expended (see Chap. 2), and these vessels have thinner walls. Since the return of the blood to the heart is passive, there are valves in the walls of the veins which direct the blood. Passive filling of the veins and muscular movements of the body and extremities lift the blood stepwise, from valve to valve, through the venous system toward the heart.

HEMORRHAGE

Hemorrhage is the escape of blood from vascular channels. The most commonly recognized form of hemorrhage is the free flow of blood following injury. Arterial hemorrhage is characterized by the spurting flow of bright blood under pressure. Venous bleeding is identified by a slower flow of darker blood. Capillary hemorrhage is the oozing of bright blood. Internal hemorrhage may be due to trauma or to a variety of disease processes, including congenital defects of blood vessel walls, arteriosclerosis (often in combination with high blood pressure), infection, and erosion by tumor. In addition, a large number of diseases affect the integrity of the capillary walls. These diseases may be manifest by small lesions visible under the skin or mucous membranes. If these hemorrhages are quite small, measuring less than 1 to 2 millimeters in diameter, they are known as *petechiae.* They are frequently found in such diseases as scurvy, typhoid fever, bacterial endocarditis, and thrombocytopenia (platelet deficiency). Larger hemorrhages of the same general type but measuring 5 to 10 millimeters or more in diameter are called *purpura.* This type of rash may often be seen with the rickettsial diseases—especially the spotted fever group, after some drug poisons, and rarely in association with an extremely lethal form of meningococcal meningitis. The distinction between petechiae and purpura is not absolute. Many more diseases than those listed will produce one or both of these lesions. Larger, irregular subepithelial hemorrhages are termed *ecchymoses;* they are most commonly seen after injury, the commonest form being the bruise. Senile ecchymoses are often seen on the backs of the hands of older individuals; they do not appear to be of significance. A *hematoma* is blood in the tissues in sufficient quantity to create a demonstrable mass.

The presence of a hemorrhage initiates a number of local and general responses. If the blood leak is quite small, and especially if it involves only capillaries, large numbers of platelets will aggregate at the defect and, by virtue of the adhesiveness of their surfaces, form a plug which seals the breach. If an artery is cut, the natural elasticity of the vessel causes it to retract, and the muscles of the wall at the cut end constrict in such a way as to narrow the orifice. In the case of the veins, the flow of blood is relatively low under little pressure. The chemical factors associated with blood vessel and tissue injury and the deposition of platelets trigger the mechanism for blood clotting.

Blood clotting, or *coagulation,* may be activated by an injury which causes blood to escape from the blood vessels, or it may be activated within the vessels by a variety of factors, some of which will be discussed

later.   In either case, the first step is the activation of thromboplastin
(Fig. 10-2).   Tissue thromboplastin is released by injury.   In the presence
of calcium ions it initiates the activation of a series of factors, VII, X, and
V, which then convert *prothrombin to thrombin.*   Roman numerals have
been given to many of these factors which previously had many names
assigned by scientists who did not at first recognize that they were the
same.   Thrombin activates the conversion of *fibrinogen to fibrin.*   Fibrinogen is a soluble protein of the blood plasma which deposits as long insoluble strands when converted to fibrin, adheres to the blood vessel
walls, and traps red and white blood cells within its network.   The effectiveness of the fibrin clot is enhanced by the presence of platelets, which
cause the fibrin to contract.   This, in turn, brings the vessel walls closer
together, increases the strength of the clot, expresses the serum, and pre-
pares for subsequent organization of the clot by invading fibroblasts.
    Coagulation within intact blood vessels proceeds by a different initial
course, termed the *intrinsic* pathway when compared to the *extrinsic* or

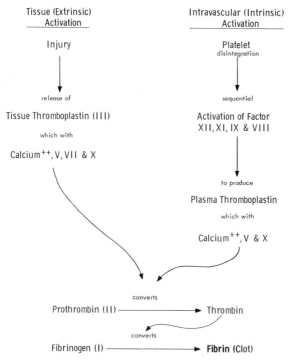

Figure 10-2   The mechanism of blood coagulation. The Roman
numerals represent the standardized nomenclature of the coagulation factors.

tissue pathway described above. This pathway starts with platelet disintegration, which activates in turn factors XII, XI, IX, and VIII. The resultant plasma thromboplastin, in the presence of calcium ion, factor V, and factor X, converts prothrombin to thrombin, followed by the conversion of fibrinogen to fibrin as in the extrinsic system. We have previously observed that fibrin is also precipitated in the tissues during inflammation. The source of tissue fibrin is also the plasma fibrinogen which is carried to the site by the inflammatory exudate.

The mechanisms designed to arrest blood flow are ordinarily effective, although they may fail under a number of circumstances. The clotting mechanism may not act soon enough to prevent death from exsanguination if the vessel is too large or if for some anatomical reason hemostasis is not possible. Arteriosclerosis may make the vessels so rigid that they do not contract to favor clotting, and each pulsation interferes with clot formation. Occasionally failure may be due to a defect in the clotting mechanism itself. It is obvious that this intricate system prevents the coagulation of circulating blood but is prepared to promote coagulation when needed. It is understandable that such a complex system should be subject to potential defects. For example, it is the absence of factor VIII which causes classical hemophilia and of factor IX which causes the clinically indistinguishable hemophilia B. An important class of bleeding disorders is associated with a platelet deficit. Both inherited and acquired defects have been observed in almost all the coagulation factors.

Whenever hemorrhage is severe or persistent, there are compensatory physiological mechanisms which are brought into immediate action to restore effective blood volume. Blood which is normally sequestered in the spleen and other reservoirs is immediately put into the circulation, and fluid from the cells and interstitial spaces is moved into the circulatory system. Because the tissue fluid contains no cells, the hematocrit (red blood cell concentration) decreases. As the blood volume falls, the blood vessels constrict, so that most of the blood circulates through the heart muscle and central nervous system, the two organs which require a high oxygen intake in order to survive. Normally the heart and brain receive 20 to 25 percent of the heart's output of blood; this may increase to as much as 75 to 80 percent after severe hemorrhage.* The remaining tissues naturally receive a proportionately reduced share of the already decreased flow. If hemorrhage continues, or if it stops and less than a critical amount of blood is available, the individual will die. Although remarkably

---

* All of the blood circulates through the heart, but the heart muscle requires its own blood supply which is delivered through the coronary arteries.

small amounts of hemoglobin are necessary if the decrease has been gradual and chronic, the rapid, unreplaced loss of 30 percent of the blood volume is usually fatal.

The diagnosis of hemorrhage is obvious when there is external blood loss, but it may be obscure with internal losses even when these are large. Hemorrhage into vital structures, such as the brain, may produce acute and characteristic symptoms. Losses of blood into the peritoneal cavity and the intestinal tract can be quite large before their presence is suspected. The symptoms of hemorrhage are usually characteristic. The patient, if conscious, is alert and restless. The skin is pale. Thirst may be a prominent symptom. The pulse rate is almost always rapid and weak; as the hemorrhage continues, the blood pressure falls. If the rate of blood loss is very rapid, the patient will lose consciousness and die of simple circulatory inadequacy. Slower bleeding over a period of hours or arrest of bleeding before critical exsanguination will lead to shock if blood replacement is delayed or inadequate. Continuous small losses of blood generally produce anemia.

Brisk hemorrhage, along with cardiac and respiratory arrest, is one of the critical emergencies in medicine. Everyone, professional or not, should be prepared to arrest most forms of external hemorrhage as directed by first aid handbooks.

SHOCK

The medical application of the term *shock* describes a number of conditions in which the amount of blood delivered by the heart is inadequate to meet the mechanical and metabolic needs of the body. In general, the most characteristic manifestation of shock is a fall in the blood pressure below the normal physiological range. The causes of shock may be divided into two major groups: (1) those due to the failure of the heart as a pump, and (2) those due to extracardiac factors which lead to a reduction in the effective blood volume. An extremely common cause of shock is the acute reduction in cardiac output which results from a coronary artery occlusion with myocardial infarction (death of heart muscle). This is the most common form of "heart attack" and will be described more fully later in this chapter. Other acute causes of heart failure are sudden, inefficient, rapid, or irregular heart rhythms and cardiac tamponade. *Tamponade* is due to rapid accumulation of fluid or blood in the pericardial space. Since this cavity is of limited volume, the pressure compresses the heart and interferes with its function. Chronic heart failure is not included as a cause of shock since, like chronic hemorrhage, the slow development allows adaptive mechanisms to become functional.

The types of shock due to a reduction in the effective blood volume result from either an increase in the vascular compartment or a decrease in the total blood volume. There are a number of causes for an increase in the size of the vascular compartment. The usual nonmedical use of the term *shock* is in association with a sudden emotional blow (shock) which may cause immediate fainting or collapse. This has also been called *neurogenic* or *primary shock* and is ordinarily inconsequential. It is due to the relaxation in the blood vessels and a slowing of the heart-beat as a result of vagus nerve stimulation and is often termed vasovagal syncope. This combination of pooling of blood in the dependent portions of the body plus reduced heart output diverts blood from the brain, and weakness or unconsciousness ensues. This is the mechanism which causes fainting after an injection or on the military parade ground. The individual either falls or assumes a recumbent position which restores the blood flow to the central nervous system, and then the symptoms subside. A somewhat similar mechanism seen in aged individuals and after some acute illnesses is termed *orthostatic hypotension.* Normally, when an individual arises, especially from a recumbent position, the size of the blood vessels must be adjusted to prevent the pooling of large amounts of blood in the lower extremities. The rigidity of older vessels and neurologic deficits after acute illness may interfere with a prompt response, resulting in a fall in blood pressure, transient giddiness, and occasional fainting. Many drugs used in the treatment of hypertension (high blood pressure) will also produce orthostatic hypotension.

Anaphylactic shock may operate in a similar manner; however, at least in some animals, the interference with the return of the blood to the heart is due to local vascular spasm with obstruction rather than relaxation with pooling. Some toxic states, especially those associated with bacterial endotoxin, may result in vascular paralysis and pooling of blood in the veins. This, in turn, causes a reduction in the return of the blood to the heart and a decrease in the cardiac output. This type of shock is more resistant to treatment than are most others which are due to increases in the size of the vascular compartment.

The most important cause of shock, usually called *surgical* or *trau-matic shock,* is an actual decrease in the circulating blood volume. Hemorrhage is a cause of shock that has long been known, but an identical clinical pattern of shock can be seen when hemorrhage is not evident. For this reason there was much speculation that other factors must be involved. Improvement in the ability to measure blood volume has demonstrated that in almost all instances inadequacy of blood volume is the critical factor. Two examples are illustrative. Experience with fractures of the femur has shown that shock is an almost invariable component, even when the fracture is closed and there is no evident blood loss. However, careful measurement shows that several liters of blood and fluid can be lost into the thigh with only relatively moderate evidence of swelling. This localized sequestration of blood and fluid is sufficient to initiate shock. In World War II, "crush" injuries due to falling debris from bombing were frequently associated with shock in the absence of overt hemorrhage. It was later proved that in crush injury the blood vessels and lymphatics in the crushed area are so damaged that fluid leaks into the tissues faster than it can be removed by the blood vessels and lymphatics.

Shock is an extremely important component of burns; a copious inflammatory exudate forms, and if the burned surface is large, the loss of plasma can be extensive. In many situations the loss of water by both sensible and insensible sweating can be extremely large. Skin losses of over 10 liters per day have been reported in desert studies. It is this mechanism which produces dehydration and death in the absence of water replacement in hot climates. Similar excessive losses of fluid may occur from the intestinal tract either by copious vomiting or diarrhea. The classic example previously mentioned is cholera. In this disease the diarrheal losses may amount to 500 to 1,000 milliliters per hour. In a recent study, the average total daily replacement requirement was 20 liters of intravenous fluid.

If the reduction of blood volume is due to the loss of whole blood, fluids are mobilized from the cells and tissues and the remaining blood is diluted. Therefore the hemoglobin concentration falls. If, on the other hand, the decrease in blood volume is due to the loss of fluids alone, the red blood cells become more concentrated, and at the same time the hemoglobin concentration must also increase.

The *clinical picture of shock* is generally modified by the symptoms of the underlying disorder. Most commonly the patient is conscious but listless at first and gradually sinks into unconsciousness and coma as the condition progresses. The pulse is usually rapid but thin; the skin is cold and clammy. In addition, the skin often appears gray due to the slow movement of inadequately oxygenated blood. The most characteristic finding is a low blood pressure which, in the absence of treatment, falls inexorably. The early compensatory mechanisms prevent the fall in blood pressure, and shock should be diagnosed at this time. The diagnosis of shock before the fall in blood pressure can be made only if the clinical condition is known to be one which predisposes to shock and the medical attendants are alert to the appropriate signs. Often the knowledge that, if untreated, these various etiologies can lead to shock results in the appropriate corrective therapy and shock does not develop.

For example, standard therapy for burns includes plasma replacement and measures designed to reduce plasma seepage. When possible, venous pressure and blood volume determinations are made to guide therapy. However, these procedures are not always available. If the blood pressure falls despite these measures, the therapy has been inadequate and shock becomes manifest. Therefore the monitoring of the blood pressure is a most important guide to the presence and progress of shock.

The physiological compensations for shock are essentially the same as those for hemorrhage. This should be expected, since hemorrhage is one of the commonest causes of shock. Small amounts of blood can be mobilized from blood pools; the most important is probably the spleen, which can expel 100 milliliters or so by splenic contraction. Fluid is mobilized from uninvolved tissues to compensate for the decreased blood volume; blood is diverted away from the skin and muscles to the vital viscera, in particular the brain and heart muscle. However, after a period of time even the measures designed to restore the normal blood volume may become ineffective. For example, if blood replacement after hemorrhage is delayed beyond a critical time, even though full replacement is achieved and the blood pressure is elevated, the course of shock may not be reversed. There is then a gradual secondary fall in the blood pressure and inevitable death. This has led to the classification of reversible and irreversible shock.

Although it is now generally agreed that the initiating cause of most shock is an inadequate blood volume, the mechanism for irreversible shock has not been specifically established and may be a result of a number of factors. Prolonged anoxia (inadequacy of the oxygen supply), lack of nutrition, and inadequate removal of cellular wastes may result in irreversible damage to tissue cells. This concept seems most attractive. There is also considerable evidence to support the concept that beyond a certain time the veins lose their tone and cause pooling of blood. However, overtransfusion is ineffective, and evidence for pooling is not completely convincing in postmortem examination. There is also evidence to suggest that in some animals prolonged shock results in an inability to handle the normal amount of endotoxins absorbed from dying intestinal bacteria. There is no direct evidence for this mechanism in humans.

The *treatment of shock* depends upon the prompt elimination of its cause and the institution of measures designed to restore and maintain effective blood volume. The ideal replacement fluid matches the fluid lost: blood for hemorrhage, plasma for burns, and various salt solutions appropriate for evaporative and gastrointestinal losses. The management of shock is one of the most critical problems in medicine and nursing.

Treatment must be prompt, correct, and sustained. There must be diligent monitoring of every patient in whom shock may be a complication of the fundamental disorder.

The ultimate outcome of tardy, inadequate, or otherwise unsuccessful treatment of shock is death. However, the successful treatment of shock is generally associated with remarkably few complications. One of the most important, especially since it is potentially reversible, is acute kidney failure. The diversion of blood away from the kidney during shock results in a reduced urine output. If the shock persists for a sufficiently long period of time, the limited blood supply becomes inadequate to sustain the kidney cells. Necrosis occurs and, although all other functions may be restored, the kidneys may fail to produce urine. Proper management of these patients, which often requires the use of the artificial kidney, may allow time for the kidneys to recover. Another fairly frequent complication of shock is the development of thrombi. This is almost entirely confined to older individuals, especially those suffering from cardiovascular diseases. The severity of this complication depends, of course, upon the extent of the vascular occlusion and the resulting ischemia.

THROMBOSIS

Thrombosis is the development of blood clots within the circulatory system during life. A *thrombus* is the special type of clot which is initiated by the deposition of platelets on the endothelium (Fig. 10-3). This is followed by the agglutination of more platelets until a platelet mound develops. Possibly as the result of thromboplastin release due to platelet damage, fibrin forms on the platelet mound and traps white cells, some red cells, and more platelets. The thrombus increases in size and may eventually completely occlude the vessel. The blood, in the direction of flow behind the thrombus, now becomes stagnant and can form into a blood clot. If the blood clot extends to a junction where another vessel feeds blood into the same channel, there may be reestablishment of the process of thrombosis with the deposition of alternate layers of platelets, cells, and fibrin until the tributary vessel is occluded as well.

An important distinction must be made between a thrombus and the usual blood clot. A thrombus develops during life and requires the presence of moving blood. It can be identified by microscopic examination because of the presence of the alternating layers of platelets, cells, and fibrin which are called the lines of Zahn. In addition, the thrombus is attached to the endothelium. Usually the thrombus is relatively pale, since it is made up primarily of fibrin and white blood cells with a relative

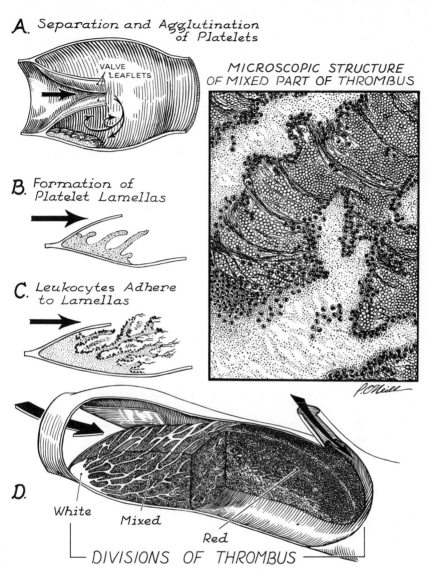

A. Separation and Agglutination of Platelets

VALVE LEAFLETS

MICROSCOPIC STRUCTURE OF MIXED PART OF THROMBUS

B. Formation of Platelet Lamellas

C. Leukocytes Adhere to Lamellas

D.

White

Mixed

Red

DIVISIONS OF THROMBUS

Figure 10-3 The formation of a thrombus. The thrombus forms in the area of slow blood flow behind the valve. There is initial platelet deposition, followed by leukocyte adherence, fibrin formation, entrapment of red blood cells, and the formation of new platelet lamellae. The lines of Zahn can be seen in D and in the microscopic section. *(From B. D. Fallis, Textbook of Pathology, McGraw-Hill, New York, 1964, p. 87. By permission of the publishers.)*

scarcity of red blood cells. On the other hand, a blood clot may develop whenever there is sufficient blood stasis within or without the body, whether the individual is alive or dead. The blood clot is produced by the conversion of soluble fibrinogen into insoluble fibrin. Because the blood is static, red cells are generally incorporated into the clot. When this is the case, it is often called a "currant jelly" clot. If the red cells have settled out so that large portions of the clot are composed only of plasma, it is called a "chicken fat" clot. These descriptions are apt. (Morehead refers to this as "delicatessen nomenclature," a frequent practice in pathology.) The distinction between thrombi and blood clots, especially postmortem clots, is of great clinical importance.

It is obviously necessary that the blood remain fluid while within the circulatory system. It is equally important that there be a mechanism for the prevention of blood loss due to disruption of the vascular system. The normal role of the platelets appears to be the preservation of the integrity of the endothelial lining, which they ordinarily achieve without the concomitant production of thrombosis. Intravascular clotting is generally prevented by the normal integrity of the endothelium, the streamlining of blood flow, the complexity of the intravascular clotting mechanism, and the presence of normal circulating anticoagulants.

The concept of thrombosis was first enunciated a little over a century ago by Rudolph Virchow, who was the father of modern pathology. At that time he described three factors predisposing to thrombosis. These factors, which are still accepted, are (1) changes in the blood vessel wall, (2) slowing of the bloodstream, and (3) changes in the character of the blood. At the time of Virchow's studies infection was common, and his attention was drawn primarily to thromboses which resulted from bacterial injury to endothelium. Since the thrombi were produced in association with infection of the blood vessel wall, the thrombi themselves contained microorganisms and were called *septic thrombi*. Thrombi which did not contain organisms were *bland thrombi*. At the present time most thrombi are not infected, and it is assumed that they are bland unless otherwise stated. Trauma to the venous endothelium is probably the most common cause of thrombi. This trauma may be quite minimal when other factors are favorable for thrombosis. For example, prolonged riding in an automobile or even sitting watching television has produced sufficient trauma to the veins in the legs to initiate the process.

Injury due to intravenous injection of irritating substances and the prolonged administration of intravenous fluids are frequently associated with venous thrombosis. The recent increase in the use of narcotics and other drugs, often impure and unsterile, has led to many serious complications. A common cause of arterial thrombi is roughening of the arterial intima (endothelium) as the result of arteriosclerosis. The slowing of the bloodstream is another important factor and underlies the frequency of thrombosis in older individuals with heart disease. Bed rest may slow venous drainage of the legs and increase thrombosis. Varicose veins may result in pooling of blood and contribute to the slowing of the blood flow. Pregnancy may achieve the same result by pressing on the large veins of the abdomen which drain the blood from the lower extremities. One of the principal changes in the blood is manifested by the number and character of the platelets. Injuries in general, but in particular abdominal surgery, fractures, and childbirth, are associated with an increase in the number and adhesiveness of circulating platelets. Other factors include changes in blood viscosity, variations in blood anticoagulation factors, and a variety of disease states.

From the foregoing discussion it should be obvious that there are certain conditions which predispose to thrombosis and in which it can be anticipated. In general, thrombi are most common in older individuals with arteriosclerosis, who have heart disease, who are undergoing surgery, who have suffered trauma, and who are placed in bed with inadequate attention to drainage of blood from the legs, which generally requires active movement of the leg muscles. The other period of relatively increased vulnerability is in younger women during pregnancy and parturition. At this time there may be changes in concentration of some of the components of the blood clotting system which increase the likelihood of inappropriate thrombosis. In some respects the use of contraceptive medications simulates some of the endocrine aspects of pregnancy and may also cause increased thrombosis. The commonest sites for the development of thrombi are the veins of the lower extremities and lower abdomen, the arteries subject to arteriosclerosis, and certain specific areas in the heart itself (Fig. 10-4).

Once a thrombus is formed, there are several alternatives through which it may evolve, assuming that death has not resulted from obstruction of a vital vessel. A small thrombus may contract and eventually be absorbed. This presupposes that it has not been occlusive. Organization may occur, especially if an arterial wall was involved. Macrophages, endothelial buds, and fibroblasts enter the thrombus as in any healing process. The thrombus is converted into scar tissue, and in a relatively short period of time endothelium may cover any surfaces presenting to the vessel lumen. There may be canalization of the clot, in which new but restricted passages are formed which reopen the continuity of the blood vessel. An important complication of thrombosis may be continued propagation of the clot, which not only increases the obstruction to flow but also increases the possibility of detachment of clot fragments.

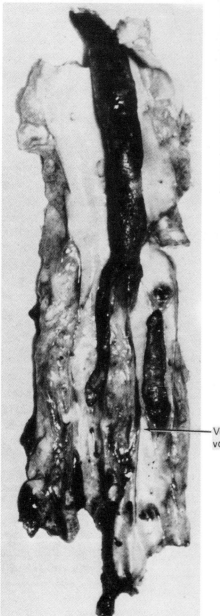

Venous
valve

Figure 10-4 Development of thrombi. The veins have been opened, showing the deep femoral vein on the right joining the superficial femoral vein on the left to form the common femoral vein above. A thrombus has formed on the valve cusps at the junction of the superficial and common femoral veins and a smaller thrombus can be seen propagating in the deep femoral vein. The valve cusp is most easily seen at the lower edge of the smaller thrombus. [*From S. Sevitt in A. A. Sasahara and M. Stein, (eds.), Pulmonary Embolic Disease, Grune & Stratton, New York, 1965, p. 269. By permission of the publishers.*]

EMBOLISM

An *embolus* is a solid particle, liquid droplet, or gaseous bubble floating in the bloodstream which, in the process of *embolism,* impacts in a vascular tributary and causes obstruction. The commonest source of emboli is from a thrombus. However, the thrombus itself is less likely to detach from its original site than is the blood clot, which forms downstream from the thrombus. Venous thrombi are the most common source of emboli. Since venous flow is from smaller to larger veins, they pass freely to the heart and into the pulmonary artery, where they eventually impact when the arterial branches in the lung become too small for further passage (Fig. 10-5). *Arterial emboli* are less common and are most often associated with the diseases of the heart. They are usually relatively small as compared to venous emboli. However, in some instances, especially associated with arteriosclerosis of the aorta, fairly large emboli may develop. One frequent form is the *"saddle embolus"* which straddles the aorta as it divides into the right and left iliac arteries to supply the legs. If the occlusion is sufficiently complete, it causes gangrene of the legs and possible death. A rare form of embolus is the so-called crossed or *paradoxical embolus.* This embolus arises in the veins, bypasses the lungs by traversing a congenital defect in the tissue which separates the right and left sides of the heart, and eventually lodges in a systemic artery. Emboli which arise from thrombi may undergo an evolution indistinguishable from that of the original thrombus. It is often difficult to determine whether the embolus is, in fact, an embolus or whether it is a thrombus. The ultimate proof may depend upon the demonstration of a primary source.

Malignant tumors may invade blood vessels and produce *tumor emboli.* These emboli are generally small and do not survive, but a successful implantation is termed a *metastasis.* Similarly, clumps of microorganisms may embolize and set up inflammation and often abscesses at sites remote from the original infection. These are called *septic emboli.* This pyemic process has been previously noted. Fragments of arteriosclerotic material within the blood vessel wall may erode the intima, detach, and form emboli. Since this process involves the arteries, embolization is via the systemic circulation to all parts of the body. *Gas emboli* arise from two sources: (1) laceration of veins, especially of the lungs, may be associated with negative pressure at the site of injury which sucks air into the vessel; and (2) reduction of external pressure, such as rapid ascent after diving or in an unpressurized airplane, results in the liberation of gases already in the system. As was noted in Chap. 6, gas emboli may not only obstruct flow through blood vessels but may also interfere with cardiac action; a large bubble in the heart may prevent entry of blood and

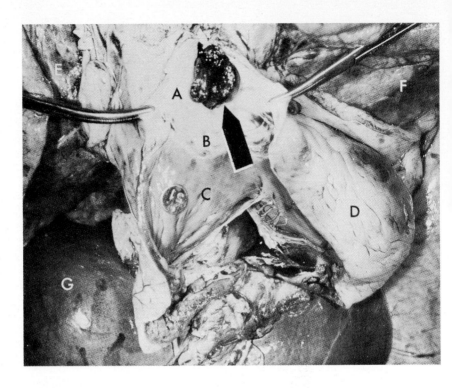

Figure 10-5 Massive pulmonary embolus occluding the entire pulmonary artery *(A)*. Just below the pulmonary artery is the pulmonary valve *(B)* and the opened right ventricle *(C)*. The left ventricle *(D)*, the right lung *(E)*, the left lung *(F)*, and the dome of the liver *(G)* are also visible. *(From B. D. Fallis, Textbook of Pathology, McGraw-Hill, New York, 1964, p. 99. By permission of the publishers.)*

at the same time, by its compressibility, fail to be dislodged by the heart's contraction.

Finally, droplets of fat may enter the circulation and cause *fat embolism*. The commonest cause of fat embolism is severe trauma to the fatty bone marrow, which is usually associated with severe fractures, especially of the lower extremities. Frequent fat embolization is also seen in alcoholics with fatty livers. Two patterns have been noted. In the first, the lungs are heavily embolized and death frequently occurs within 2 days or less. In the second, most manifestations are produced in the brain and may lead to coma and death in 2 to 7 days. In both these conditions large quantities of fat have been observed in the lungs and brain. It has been noted recently that these fatty emboli contain large amounts of cholesterol. Since this could not be derived from the marrow, liver, or fat depots but only from the blood, a new interpretation of the mechanism producing fat emboli may be necessary.

INFARCTION

An infarct is necrosis of tissue due to *ischemia,* which is a relative inadequacy of blood supplied to the involved tissue. Obviously, both thrombosis and embolism can lead to infarction. In fact, infarction is the common-

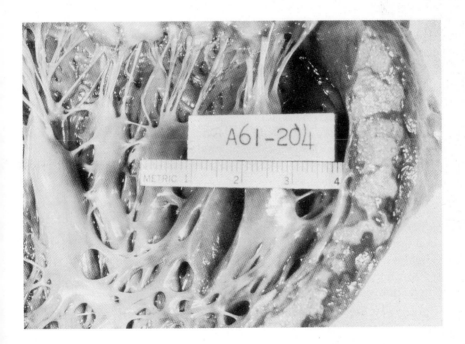

Figure 10-6 Acute myocardial infarct. The chamber of the left ventricle is shown to the left and the cross-section of the heart muscle is on the right. White necrotic tissue can be seen extending almost entirely through the muscle wall. *(From B. D. Fallis, Textbook of Pathology, McGraw-Hill, New York, 1964, p. 406. By permission of the publishers.)*

est and most important complication of thrombosis and embolism. However, infarction is not an inevitable sequel. At one extreme the results of vascular obstruction may be so catastrophic as to produce somatic death before tissue necrosis can develop. Such a situation is frequently observed with coronary occlusion (the so-called heart attack), cerebral-vascular occlusion (stroke), and sudden massive pulmonary occlusion. At the other extreme a vascular occlusion may obstruct only one of several vessels supplying a specific tissue and no demonstrable effect may be observed. Such an alternate blood supply is termed a *collateral blood flow*. The vulnerability of tissues to ischemia is quite variable. Cardiac failure greatly increases the effects of vascular occlusion. In general, parenchymatous tissues show a much greater effect than do the supportive tissues.

The general pattern of infarction is fairly uniform. Infarction usually results from arterial rather than venous obstruction. If the occluded artery is an end artery and is the only source of blood for the affected tissue, the infarcted area will become quite pale and is termed a *white infarct* (Fig. 10-6). If the tissue borders an area in which vascular integrity has not been affected, there will be injury of blood vessels at the junction between the living and dead tissue, red blood cells will escape into the tissue, and the white infarct will be surrounded by a hemorrhagic border. If some collateral vessels to the infarcted tissue exist, there will be tissue damage in the infarcted area and the collateral vessels will spill blood into the infarcted tissues, producing a *red infarct*. Some organs have a double blood supply, and unless both supplies are occluded, the evidences of infarction can be quite minimal. Most infarcts will then undergo a period of necrosis followed by absorption and organization with scar formation (Fig. 10-7). This process is essentially the same as the repair which follows inflammatory tissue destruction (Fig. 10-8). However, the parenchymatous organs do not regenerate functional tissue and the residual defect remains. Most important is the fact that the heart and brain, the organs most likely to be the sites of infarction, both have relatively poor collateral circulation and are unable to repair tissues damaged by ischemia. Isolated venous obstruction, although often symptomatic, rarely produces infarction. Occasionally the twisting of an organ or a tumor on its pedicle (stalk) may produce sufficient pressure to obstruct the venous outflow without blocking the arterial inflow, in which case the manifestations of a hemorrhagic infarct would be evident.

A number of infarcts are of major importance because they destroy or impair vital organs or extremities. Vascular occlusion of the heart, lungs, and brain have already been noted. Other common sites of occlusion include the kidneys, spleen, intestines, liver, and lower extremities.

The results of vascular occlusion due to thrombosis or embolism can be summarized briefly as follows: There may be death, infarction, or an absence of significant manifestations. Infarction may lead to death or there may be recovery, usually with significant tissue deficit and functional disability.

ARTERIOSCLEROSIS AND ATHEROSCLEROSIS

Arteriosclerosis, literally hardening *(skleros)* of the arteries, is almost universal in older individuals. Several types of arteriosclerosis are recognized, but the most important is *atherosclerosis.* Although the etiology of atherosclerosis has not been established, the pathogenesis is well characterized. The vessels involved are primarily the large, elastic arteries which receive the blood more or less directly from the heart. These include the aorta, the carotid arteries and the arteries of the brain, the coronary arteries supplying the heart muscle, the renal arteries, the iliac arteries supplying the legs, and, to a lesser extent, the vessels supplying the abdominal viscera.

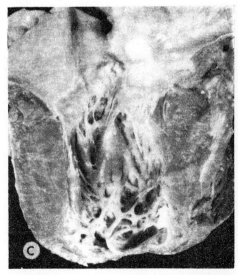

Figure 10-7 Old myocardial infarct affecting apex of the left ventricle at bottom of picture. Note the white scar tissue and the thinness of the ventricular wall as compared to the muscle just above, on the right and left sides of the picture. *(From R. P. Morehead, Human Pathology, McGraw-Hill, New York, 1965, p. 651. By permission of the publishers.)*

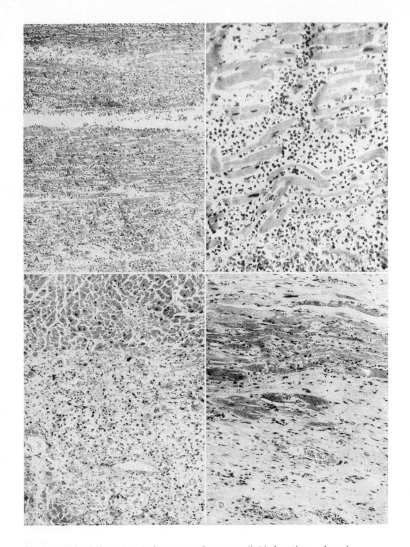

Figure 10-8   Microscopic features of myocardial infarction. A and
B: Infarct at 3 days.   In the low-power magnification, the muscle
fibers can be seen to be separated by an inflammatory exudate.
In the higher-power magnification, it is evident that the muscle
fibers are disrupted and necrotic and that the inflammatory exudate is composed largely of polymorphonuclear cells.   C: At 2
weeks the inflammatory reaction has subsided, but a large area of
muscle has been destroyed in the lower portion of the illustration.
D: At 6 weeks the infarcted muscle has been replaced by a fibrous
scar.   (From R. P. Morehead, Human Pathology, McGraw-Hill,
New York, 1965, p. 652.   By permission of the publishers.)

Pathogenesis

The first lesion is the deposition of fatty material, chiefly cholesterol, immediately beneath the intima (Fig. 10-9). It is not certain whether this deposit arises from the blood vessel itself or, more likely, from the lipids in the bloodstream. As the cholesterol accumulates, there is some fibrous reaction and disorganization of the adjacent vascular wall. The intima is displaced into the lumen of the blood vessel by the increasing cholesterol deposit. At this time, microscopic examination of the blood vessel shows the presence of cholesterol crystals. Eventually, calcium is deposited in the lesions, and often the amount of calcium deposited is sufficient to outline the affected artery so that it is visible on x-ray.

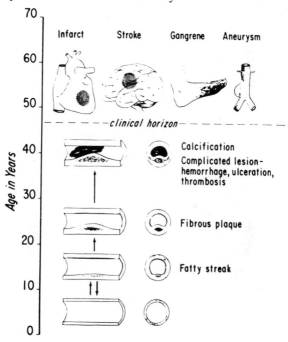

Figure 10-9 Diagramatic sequence of the development of atherosclerosis. Relatively early in life, fatty streaks appear underneath the intima. These become fibrous plaques containing cholesterol and eventually progress to calcification. Finally, hemorrhage, ulceration, and thrombosis resulting from the vascular lesions produce the clinical manifestations of infarction, stroke, gangrene, and aneurysm. [*From H. C. McGill, Jr., J. C. Grier, and J. P. Strong in M. Sandler and G. H. Bourne (eds.), Atherosclerosis and Its Origin, Academic Press, New York, 1963, p. 16. By permission of the publishers.*]

Atherosclerosis leads to a number of complications which produce the clinical manifestations of the disease. The increasing mass of the lesion may directly occlude the vessel. However, the most frequent manifestation is the formation of thrombi on the intima, which has been made irregular by the underlying process (Fig. 10-10). This in turn occludes the vessel, producing ischemia of the tissues which would normally have been supplied. Embolization is not uncommon as a further complication of these thrombi. The large accumulations of cholesterol may erode the intima and may themselves become artheromatous emboli. The word *atheroma* derives from the Greek and refers to the fact that the material in the lesions looks like gruel, or porridge. Finally, the disruption of the vessel wall may lead to a hemorrhage in the wall between the lesion itself and the media. The hematoma which forms may then also narrow the vessel lumen and impair blood flow.

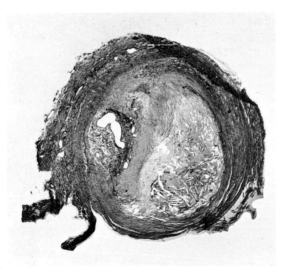

Figure 10-10 Severe atherosclerosis with thrombosis. On the right, the light area is where cholesterol has deposited between the intima and the media. There is much fibrosis and the clear, angular slits on the lower right are due to cholesterol crystals which are dissolved during preparation of the section. On the left, the small remaining passage was occluded by a thrombus which has further reduced its size. *(From B. D. Fallis, Textbook of Pathology, McGraw-Hill, New York, 1964, p. 401. By permission of the publishers.)*

Factors Predisposing to Atherosclerosis

Although the precise etiology of atherosclerosis is not known, a number of factors have been established which predispose to or accelerate the development of the process. Men are more susceptible than women, particularly before the age of 50 years. Age itself is a factor, since atherosclerosis requires time to develop. The blood concentrations of cholesterol, other fats, and uric acid are important; high values increase the risk. There is a wide normal distribution of these concentrations. Hereditary factors seem most important in setting the level, but in most instances the interplay of diet and heredity is not entirely understood. There are several well-defined specific hereditary disorders in which the blood level of one or another of these compounds is clearly elevated, and in each of these instances frequent premature complications due to atherosclerosis have been documented. Despite the fact that the blood levels can be brought down by diet, and as a result dietary regimens have been widely prescribed, there is no clear evidence that diet will affect the course of the process.

Personality variables have been thought to play an important role. Several groups of investigators have presented data suggesting that atherosclerotic complications are more common in persons with driving personalities than in those who are more relaxed. Other studies show no significant socioeconomic variation, and successful executives are reported to have relatively less premature atherosclerosis than the average. Occupations and personal habit patterns leading to reduced physical activity are associated with an increased risk. Hypertension clearly increases the risk. Since atherosclerotic lesions occur at sites of vascular stress, such as the takeoff sites of tributary vessels, the contribution of hypertension is understandable.

Diabetes mellitus increases the risk, probably due to the effects of the generally observed increase in blood cholesterol and fat and the less frequently observed increase in the blood pressure. The presence of diabetes and of hypertension tends to eliminate the differential in risk between men and women. Obesity has been considered a contributory factor, but recent data indicate that it is the commonly associated hypercholesterolemia, hypertension, lack of exercise, and related conditions rather than the obesity per se which are responsible.

Finally, there is the well-documented but still unexplained observation that cigarette smoking predisposes to premature atherosclerotic complications.

Complications of Atherosclerosis

The complications of atherosclerosis, primarily those leading to heart disease and stroke, account for approximately half of all deaths in the United States. Arteriosclerosis of the coronary arteries supplying the myocardium (heart muscle) leads to three different clinical manifestations. The *coronary occlusion* is the sudden obstruction of a coronary artery by a thrombus on an atherosclerotic plaque. This causes the classic heart attack, with sudden death or the more gradual development of a myocardial infarction. Recovery usually leaves a scarred muscle, which may then become subject to heart failure, which is the inability of the muscle to function as an adequate pump. *Coronary insufficiency* is caused by slower rates of arterial narrowing and may produce myocardial fibrosis and scarring without the acute manifestation of a myocardial infarction. *Angina pectoris* is another manifestation of coronary vascular insufficiency; cardiac pain is produced by increased work demand upon the muscle, and the pain is relieved by rest.

Strokes cause 15 percent of all deaths. Since they are not always fatal, they affect an even larger portion of the population. *Cerebral thrombosis* is the commonest lesion, but the combination of atherosclerosis and hypertension often leads to *cerebral hemorrhage.* Mortality is high, especially with hemorrhage. The residual brain damage in those who survive is variable, often hardly discernible, but is usually marked by *hemiplegia,* or paralysis on one side of the body.

Atherosclerosis of the lower aorta and iliac arteries supplying the legs leads to ischemia, with symptoms like those of angina pectoris (Fig. 10-11). The patient gets pain in the legs after walking a short distance, but the pain is relieved in a few minutes after resting. This phenomenon is called *intermittent claudication.* Thrombosis of the aorta or iliac vessels often leads to gangrene of one or both legs (Fig. 10-12). Dilatation or actual rupture of the lower aorta is not uncommon and is being recognized with increasing frequency now that surgical methods of treatment are possible. Finally, atheromatous lesions may occlude the orifices of the renal (kidney) arteries as they arise from the aorta. Narrowing of these vessels is one of the causes of hypertension; complete occlusion results in infarction and loss of kidney function. Although there are many other regions affected by atherosclerosis, these are the principal ones which demonstrate the importance of the process.

Prevention and Treatment

In the absence of known etiology, prevention is not really possible. The slow development of the lesions makes extremely difficult the evaluation

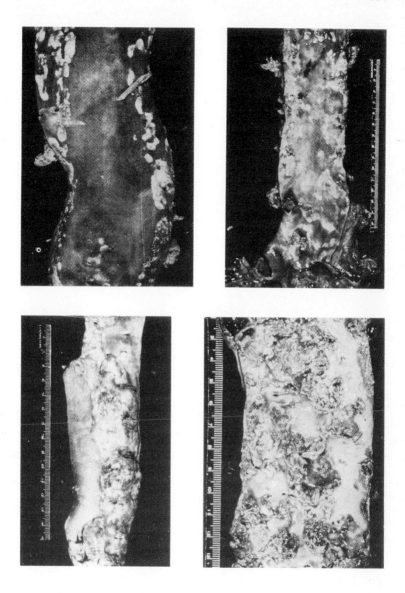

Figure 10-11   Progressively severe atherosclerosis of the abdominal aorta.   The widely scattered, shallow intimal plaques increase in size and number, becoming confluent and deeper. Eventually, the endothelial surface becomes ulcerated and a thrombus can be seen on the most advanced lesions in the illustration on the lower right.   *(From S. L. Robbins, Pathology, 3d ed., Saunders, Philadelphia, 1967, pp. 579–580.   By permission of the publishers.)*

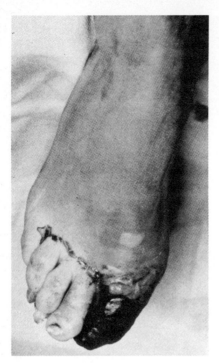

Figure 10-12   Ischemic gangrene of great toe. Ischemic complications in the feet and legs frequently follow severe arteriosclerotic lesions. [*From E. N. Hall in W. A. D. Anderson (ed.), Pathology, 6th ed., Mosby, St. Louis, 1971, p. 745. By permission of the publishers.*]

of the effect of any regimen.   It seem reasonable to avoid obesity, maintain reasonable physical activity, give up cigarette smoking, treat diabetes and hypertension, attempt to lower the blood cholesterol, lipids, and uric acid, and to cultivate a placid state of mind.   However, with the possible exceptions of the cessation of cigarette smoking and the treatment of hypertension, there is little evidence as yet that control of these factors will reduce the incidence of this disease.   Probably it is too early to evaluate the data.   Atherosclerosis usually occurs late in life, and prevention will probably have relatively little effect on overall longevity; it has been estimated that total eradication of atherosclerosis may increase average life expectancy only 4 or 5 years (See Chap. 12).   However, many people develop lesions prematurely, and there appears to be an increase in the frequency of early involvement, particularly of the coronary arteries. Identification and preventive treatment of this group might produce demonstrable results.   The criteria for identification are increasingly accurate, and large-scale preventive programs are being planned.   The difficulty of such study should not be underestimated.

Once atherosclerosis has become manifest, treatment is directed at the specific lesion.   The management of myocardial infarctions in coronary care units already demonstrates that it is possible to modify the unfavorable course in many patients. The development of x-ray techniques which make it possible to visualize blood vessels and to identify lesions, coupled with surgical procedures which either clear the atheromatous plaques and thrombi out of the vessel or which replace the occluded vessels with living or synthetic grafts, has revolutionized our approach and has improved the outlook for the patient.

BIBLIOGRAPHY

BLUMENTHAL, H. T. (ed.): *Cowdrey's Arteriosclerosis,* 2d ed., Springfield, Ill.: Charles C Thomas, Publisher, 1967.

SANDLER, M., and G. H. BOURNE (eds.): *Atherosclerosis and Its Origin,* New York: Academic Press, Inc., 1963.

SHERRY, S., K. M. BRINKHOUS, E. GENTON, and J. M. STENGLE (eds.): *Thrombosis,* Washington, D.C.: National Academy of Sciences, 1969.

SHOEMAKER, W. C.: *Shock: Chemistry, Physiology and Therapy,* Springfield, Ill.: Charles C Thomas, Publisher, 1967.

SPAIN, D. M.: "Atherosclerosis," *Scientific American,* August, 1966.

THAL, A. P.: *Shock: A Physiologic Basis for Treatment,* Chicago: Yearbook Medical Publishers, Inc., 1971.

WEIL, M. H.: *Diagnosis and Treatment of Shock,* Baltimore: The Williams & Wilkins Company, 1967.

Neoplasia

A *neoplasm,* literally "new tissue," is an inappropriate, excessive growth of cells. When malignant, the characteristics are local invasion, metastasis (distant spread), and ultimate somatic death. Although the word *tumor* was originally used in the general sense of a mass, its present use is now usually restricted to neoplasms. The suffix *oma* generally indicates a tumor, and there are still a few examples residual from previous usage, for example, *granuloma* referring to a chronic inflammatory process and, more specifically, *tuberculoma* referring to a tuberculous granuloma. The term *cancer* is a nonspecific term which includes all types of malignant neoplasms. The term is most apt since it derives from the Greek word for crab, and it is the clawlike extension of neoplastic cells into normal tissue that is one of its most characteristic features.

Cancer is extremely common. It will affect one in every four individuals. There are almost half a million new cases in the United States every year. One-third are successfully treated and the remainder die. Cancer is thus responsible for about one-sixth of all deaths, second in frequency to arteriosclerosis. Experts in *oncology,* the study of tumors, believe that if present knowledge were applied by both patients and physicians, the successful treatment of cancer could increase from one-third to one-half of the total.

THE CHARACTERISTICS OF NEOPLASIA

Benign Tumors

Benign tumors are extremely common and almost all individuals have several scattered in various parts of the body. These tumors may take on different forms depending upon the tissues from which they arise and their location within the body. One of the commonest is the simple fleshy wart or mole, which is called a *papilloma.* If the tumor consists of only a lump of thickened epithelium, it is described as *sessile,* or broad-based. Not infrequently the papilloma may develop in such a way that there is a narrow stalk, or pedicle, which then expands into a boarder tumor. These papillomas are said to be *pedunculated.* A pedunculated mass is also termed a *polyp* (Fig. 11-1). If the benign tumor arises not on the surface but in the depths of tissue, the shape is somewhat different.

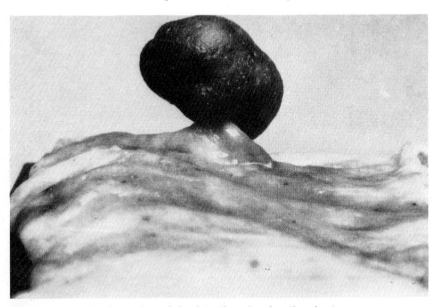

Figure 11-1   A benign polyp of the intestine showing the short pedicle by which it is attached to the mucosa. *(From L. V. Acker-man and J. A. DelRegatto, Cancer, 4th ed., Mosby, St. Louis, 1970, p. 651. By permission of the publishers.)*

As the tumor cells develop, their spread is limited by the pressures of surrounding tissues. If the pressures are equal in all directions, the tumor will take on a spherical form. If the tumor arises where the pressures are unequal, as within a space bounded by connective-tissue fascial sheaths, the tumor may be ovoid and compressed along the axis of major pressure. Perhaps the most common form of deep tumor is the *lipoma,* which is a benign tumor of fatty tissue. These frequently arise during middle age, grow very slowly, and are manifest as soft, movable, and spherical masses lying beneath but not attached to the skin. Benign tumors that are made up of glandular tissue are called *adenomas.*

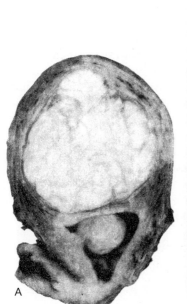
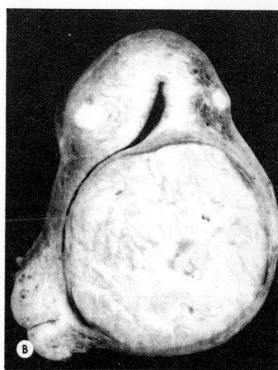

Figure 11-2   Leiomyomas of the body of the uterus. These benign tumors are commonly, although erronously, called fibroids. In *A* there is a large intramural ("within the walls") tumor and a smaller, pedunculated submucosal polypoid tumor in the lumen (cavity) of the uterus. In *B* two small and one large tumor can be seen. The sharply outlined borders of these tumors and the relatively homogenous gross internal structure are characteristic of benign tumors in general. *(From R. P. Morehead, Human Pathology, McGraw-Hill, New York, 1965, p. 877. By permission of the publishers.)*

Microscopic examination of a benign tumor reveals large numbers of normal cells, usually quite regularly arranged. The separation of the neoplastic and the normal tissue is usually quite sharp and easily defined (Fig. 11-2). Benign tumors growing within tissues cause necrosis of adjacent normal tissue, which then undergoes fibrosis. A capsule is thus produced, and if an attempt is made to remove the tumor, there is often a sharp line of cleavage between the normal and neoplastic tissue. In general, benign neoplasms do not tend to recur when they are carefully removed.

It should not be thought that, because they are not malignant in the usual sense, benign tumors are always innocent. First, the growth of a benign tumor may, by its local pressure, cause damage to a vital structure. A meningioma, which is a benign tumor of the meninges, can produce loss of function and eventual death as a result of its pressure on the brain within the rigid confines of the skull. This tumor can be removed and rarely recurs; often the relief of pressure allows restoration of integrity and function of the injured nerve cells. An extremely common tumor, the *uterine fibroid,* which is really a benign tumor of smooth muscle rather than of fibrous tissue, may interfere with pregnancy both by obstructing the passage of sperm into the fallopian tubes and by making the local uterine environment unfavorable for trophoblastic implantation. When they are large, fibroids may create problems in delivery, and in nonpregnant women they may cause local irritation leading to irregular uterine bleeding. A pedunculated tumor may twist on its stalk and become necrotic due to lack of blood. The most interesting complications produced by benign tumors are those caused by functioning endocrine adenomas. At least two different types of functioning adenomas of the pituitary, four of the adrenal, and one each of the thyroid, parathyroid, pancreatic islets of Langerhans, ovary, and testis have been described. These functioning adenomas often produce unusual syndromes and are difficult to diagnose, especially since the tumor may be quite small and inaccessible to direct examination. Yet removal of the appropriate tumor may result in a dramatic and sometimes lifesaving cure.

Malignant Tumors

Malignant neoplasms can generally be easily distinguished from benign tumors (see Table 11-1). The first important differentiating characteristic is the *invasiveness* of the malignancy (Fig. 11-3). Microscopic and often gross examination of the tumor shows fingerlike strands of neoplastic tissue extending into the normal tissue. This extension takes the path of least resistance; however, no tissue is immune from penetration. In

Table 11-1   Characteristics of Benign versus Malignant Tumors*

	Benign	Malignant
Cellular character	Relatively normal	Abnormal in varying degree
Tissue character	Relatively normal	Abnormal in varying degree or totally absent
Mitotic activity	Slight	Great
Rate of growth	Relatively slow and restricted	Rapid and unrestricted
Manner of growth	Expansive	Invasive and destructive
Limitation	Usually demarcated, often encapsulated	Not sharply demarcated or encapsulated
Recurrence after simple removal	Rare	Frequent
Metastases	Never	Usual
Vascularity	Relatively slight	Moderate to marked
Necrosis and ulceration	Unusual	Usual, often with hemorrhage
Constitutional effects	Uncommon	Usual

* Modified from Hopps

general, dense connective tissues such as fascia are not penetrated, and the walls of arteries are rarely involved. The nature of malignant invasiveness is obviously not merely quantitative but qualitative as well. A benign tumor may be just as large and its cells may be reproducing just as rapidly, but it expands and does not invade the normal tissues. Since the malignant tumor tissue remains continuous, it seems improbable that infiltration is due to tumor cell mobility of the type demonstrated by phagocytes. There is no evidence to support the concept of phagocytosis by tumor cells at the ends of the infiltrating cords. According to Berenblum, the most reasonable hypothesis is that the malignant tumor produces proteolytic enzymes which dissolve intercellular binding substances in its path. There is some support for this hypothesis from recent techniques that identify tissue enzymes by their response to stains used in microscopic examination. These stains suggest the presence of such enzymes at the borders of rapidly growing malignancies.

A second characteristic of malignant neoplasia is the ability to produce secondary tumors at a distance from the primary source. This phenomenon is termed *metastasis* and will be discussed in detail subsequently. The combination of invasiveness and metastasis results in *recurrence* subsequent to treatment, a third characteristic feature. This is undoubtedly a misnomer, since recurrence must be due not to the development of a new tumor but to initial failure to remove or destroy

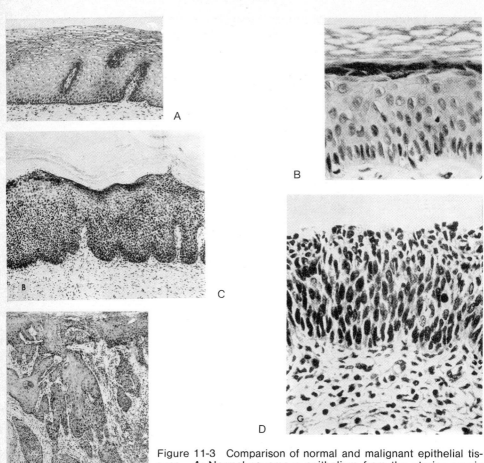

Figure 11-3   Comparison of normal and malignant epithelial tissues. *A:* Normal squamous epithelium from the uterine cervix
(X110). *(From R. P. Morehead, Human Pathology, McGraw-Hill,
New York, 1965, p. 189. By permission of the publishers.) B:*
Normal epidermis from forearm (X270). *(From R. P. Morehead,
Human Pathology, McGraw-Hill, New York, 1965, p. 188. By per-
mission of the publishers.) C:* Intraepithelial squamous cell car-
cinoma.   There is increased cellularity and disorganization of
epithelial cells which are still, however, restricted to the epidermis
(X110). *(From R. P. Morehead, Human Pathology, McGraw-Hill,
New York, 1965, p. 192. By permission of the publishers.) D:*
Higher-power magnification of intraepithelial carcinoma showing
increased cellularity and loss of organization (X270). *(From R. P.
Morehead, Human Pathology, McGraw-Hill, New York, 1965, p.
192. By permission of the publishers.) E:* Early squamous cell
carcinoma of tongue.   Note how cords of epithelial cells invade
the subepithelial tissues (X80). *(From R. W. Evans, Histological
Appearances of Tumors, 2nd ed., E. and S. Livingston, Ltd.,
Edinburgh and London, 1966, p. 948. By permission of the publishers.)*

all the malignant cells. Thus it is only the clinical evidence of the tumor which recurs.

Much has been said about the *rapidity of cellular* growth as a characteristic of neoplasia. Yet the rapidity of growth in neoplastic cells is no greater than that of cells undergoing repair and is probably considerably less than the rate of growth of cells during fetal development. In normal growth and in repair, however, there appear to be factors related to intercellular pressures and overall integrity of structure which decelerate cellular growth and maintain normal tissue structure and function. Apparently in neoplasia this restraint is either lost or interfered with and cellular proliferation continues. It is the inappropriate continuation of cellular proliferation, rather than the rapidity of growth, which is the important characteristic.

It is generally presumed that the neoplastic defect lies within the cells. *Cellular changes* would be expected and, in fact, are generally present. One of the most characteristic changes is a tendency toward structural reversion of the cell from its specialized to its less specialized state. This is known as *anaplasia* and may show varying degress of loss of specialization. In general, the more anaplastic the cells, the more malignant the tumor. As the tumor progresses, the component cells may become increasingly anaplastic; however, the reverse—that is, return to the more differentiated form—almost never occurs. Metastases tend to be somewhat more anaplastic than the parent tumor. In fact, sometimes extremely anaplastic metastases may be observed before the primary lesion has been identified, and it may be impossible to deduce the original site of the tumor from the metastasis. Another characteristic associated with anaplasia is an inconstancy of size and shape of the cell, called *pleomorphism*. The nucleus tends to be large and to stain more densely than normal, and the nucleolus, a small body within the nucleus, is also relatively enlarged and prominent. The nucleus may vary in size and shape, and there is generally an increased number of both normal and abnormal mitoses present. The overall size of the cell is increased, but most of this is due to the increased nuclear size rather than to an increase in cytoplasm. Recognition of the abnormalities in cells has now progressed to the point where it is possible, under favorable circumstances to recognize single neoplastic cells. This has become a useful adjunct to cancer diagnosis.

Tissue Changes

Despite the fact that the primary defect is in the cell and that neoplastic cells can now be readily identified, ultimate reliance is generally placed on tissue examination. The important characteristics of invasion and metastasis are, after all, tissue phenomena. The organization of neoplastic tissue is clearly different from normal. There is a loss of the usual cellular organization, and although the various components may be present, their arrangement is obviously dysfunctional. The normal stratification, or layering, of epithelium may be lost. There may be a loss of polarity of nuclei in columnar epithelium, with the nuclei randomly located within the cell rather than all regularly placed at the same end. There may be imperfect development and discontinuity of acini (glandular sacs) and ducts in glands, and secretory products may accumulate in cysts due to failure of drainage. There is evidence of disruption and destruction of adjacent normal tissue. The neoplasm itself may show areas of central necrosis due to the failure to develop an adequate blood supply. This is especially true in the liver. This process is responsible for central ulceration in surface tumors. Infiltration by inflammatory cells, especially lymphocytes, is not uncommon and does not necessarily indicate infection. The supporting structures for a cancer are not themselves neoplastic but develop in response to the tumor. There is a wide range. Tumors which are made up almost entirely of neoplastic cells are relatively soft and are occasionally called *encephaloid* (brainlike) because of the consistency of the tissue. Slow-growing tumors which produce large amounts of fibrous supporting tissue may be quite hard. They may be sufficiently dense at times to create a gritty sensation when cut with a knife. These tumors are known as *scirrhous* carcinomas from the Greek word *skirros,* meaning "hard."

The ultimate, most important characteristic of malignant tumors is the fact that they invariably cause death when untreated. Although there are occasional reports of confirmed cancers which have undergone spontaneous regression and cure, this probably does not occur more frequently than once in 100,000 times and is not a practical consideration. However, careful examination and documentation of such cases might provide interesting and important clues to the nature and treatment of other forms of cancer.

Physiological and Biochemical Effects of Malignant Tumors

Despite the fact that cancer is primarily a cellular defect and that there have been intensive studies of cellular physiology and biochemistry, surprisingly little useful information has been obtained. Most tumor cells have been found to metabolize sugar and carbohydrates only as far as lactic acid. This means that the cells are capable of performing the metabolic steps without oxygen, i.e., anaerobically, but are unable to perform properly the more energy-producing, oxygen-consuming, or aerob:c phase of carbohydrate metabolism. However, this variation is not u.nique and tends to be characteristic of rapidly growing tissues in general. The end result is an increased production of lactic acid and a decreased production of carbonic acid. Presumably the lactic acid is then metabolized by the normal tissues.

One of the striking characteristics of cancer is the continued growth of the tumor despite obvious wasting and malnutrition in the remainder of the body. This may be explained in part by the observation that cancer cells have a competitive advantage in taking up amino acids from the bloodstream. Thus the malignancy is said to act as a "nitrogen trap." There is also evidence to suggest that there may be a generalized vitamin B deficiency due to excessive use by the tumor. The overall picture of tumor metabolism is that the cellular activities are focused on those of growth with a reduction in their specialized activities. However, some function persists and some endocrine tumors, for example, put out measurable amounts of hormone. In fact, some malignant tumors may be characterized by excessive hormone production, just as are the benign adenomas. It is not clear whether this is due to increased activity on the part of the tumor cells or whether it is the result of a large mass of glandular tissue secreting at a normal or less than normal rate.

As yet no abnormal metabolic process has been identified for tumor cells. The only changes have been quantitative. The proteolytic enzymes found at the periphery of cancers have not been identified. One interesting manifestation of a variety of malignant tumors has been the elaboration of polypeptide hormones not usually associated with the original structure. It would be both interesting and important to know if these hormones are being produced in an abnormal site or if they are tumor products which mimic the hormone. If the former, it could merely mean that the genetic capacity to produce the hormone, usually repressed by cell specialization, has been derepressed. If the latter, it may represent a specific effect of tumor metabolism. Recent research demonstrates that some of the compounds with hormone effects are not identical with the true hormones and cannot be due to gene derepression.

The Clinical Characteristics of Malignant Tumors

At this point only general characteristics shall be described. Features which are the result of the location of specific primary or metastatic lesions will not be discussed. One of the most characteristic manifestations of a malignancy is weight loss, which often eventually leads to body wasting.

This may occur even when the size of the tumor is too small to account for significant alteration in the functions of any of the organs involved. At one time investigators thought that malignancies produced metabolic products which could account for this phenomenon. The failure to identify any abnormal metabolic product has made this hypothesis untenable at present. The nitrogen trapping may account for the weight loss, but it is difficult to believe that this can be the only explanation, since frequently the tumors are quite small in proportion to the total body size at the time that weight loss begins. The cause of death from many cancers is often obscure. There may be no evidence of sufficient interference with any of the vital processes to account for death. The fact that both weight loss and death occur indicates that there must be some fundamental relationship between the presence of the tumor and the function of the body which is as yet unknown.

Pain is a common accompaniment of cancer and depends upon the nature of the local involvement. Since there are no nerves in the cancer, pain is produced indirectly. The commonest cause is pressure and tension upon the nerves of adjacent normal tissue. The headache of brain tumors is due to the pressure upon the meninges; and in bone the pain is due to stretching of the periosteum, a membrane which covers the surface of the bone. Neoplastic ulcerations may cause pain because of direct irritation of exposed tissue. Obstruction of various passages results in pain characteristic of obstruction and not specific for neoplasia. Common sites of such obstruction are the intestinal tract and large bowel, urinary tract, and gallbladder. Pain is one of the most important and difficult problems in the management of patients with cancer. The minimization of pain is a major responsibility of those caring for cancer patients.

Fever, often present in cancer, is believed due to the release of necrotic material although, as in the case of weight loss, this causality has not been established. In this era in which prolonged and hidden infectious disease is rare, otherwise undiagnosed and prolonged fevers often turn out to be due to malignancies. The commonest tumors to cause fever are the tumors of the lymph nodes and blood cells and, less frequently, tumors of the kidney.

Disfigurement is a frequent complication of cancer. This may be due to the superficial location of the lesion with distortion of features, presence of a mass, ulceration, and occasionally infection. Disfigurement may be indirect as a result of ascites secondary to tumor implantations in the peritoneum, edema due to obstruction of lymphatic drainage, jaundice due to obstruction of the bile ducts, and severe body wasting.

Cancer produces a wide range of psychological problems. The average individual is all too well aware of the ultimate outcome of inadequately treated cancer, and he may be expected to show severe depression and withdrawal reactions. After all, the anxieties are certainly fully justified. In some patients psychiatric problems may arise before the recognition of the presence of cancer. It has been reported that some patients with carcinoma of the pancreas show personality changes and abnormal behavior even before the presence of a physical illness is recognized. Unfortunately, these observations have not yet been sufficiently documented to fully establish their validity.

CLASSIFICATION OF TUMORS

Tumors are classified by the organ from which they arise, the type of tissue involved, and whether they are benign or malignant. The type of tissue must, in almost all cases, be verified by microscopic examination. Classification by cell or tissue type has proved to be useful in predicting the clinical and pathological course of the tumor. Part of this identification includes the determination of the benign or malignant potential of the neoplasm. Thus, a gastric adenocarcinoma can be readily recognized as a malignant tumor of the glandular epithelium of the stomach which has a different course and outcome from a uterine leiomyoma, or fribroid. The classification presented in Table 11-2 is generally accepted.

The first category is that of epithelial tumors. Numerically these make up by far the majority of all cancers. Benign tumors of the skin have already been identified as papillomas. Those arising from the mucous membranes are called *polyps.* Since the mucous membrane is a glandular structure, these are also known as adenomatous polyps. Malignant tumors of the epithelium are known as *carcinomas.* The two major types of carcinomas are *squamous cell carcinoma,* made up from flat, layered cells such as are present in the skin, and *adenocarcinomas,* derived from the glandular epithelium of the intestinal tract and structures embryonically derived from it. Although most carcinomas originate from ectodermal and endodermal cells, not all do. For example, the lining cells of the uterus, which are derived from mesoderm, also produce tumors that are characteristically carcinomatous. Although the squamous cells are characteristic of the skin, a number of tissues can undergo change, so that there are squamous cell carcinomas as well as adenocarcinomas in a number of organs including, for example, the lung and the esophagus. The change of a cell from one type to another, in this case from mucous membrane to squamous epithelium, is known as *metaplasia.* Metaplasia is not a malignant change per se but is usually a response to irritation, and removal of the irritation often allows the cell changes to revert to

Table 11-2　A Simple Classification of Tumors

Tissue or origin	Benign	Malignant
Group I. Epithelial tumors		
Surface epithelium	Papilloma	Carcinoma
Glandular epithelium	Adenoma	Carcinoma (adenocarcinoma)
Group II. Connective tissue and muscle tumors		
Fibrous tissue	Fibroma	Fibrosarcoma
Cartilage	Chondroma	Chrondrosarcoma
Bone	Osteoma	Osteogenic sarcoma
Fat	Lipoma	Liposarcoma
Blood vessels	Hemangioma	Hemangiosarcoma
Lymph vessels	Lymphangioma	Lymphangiosarcoma
Smooth muscle	Leiomyoma	Leiomyosarcoma
Striated muscle	Rhabdomyoma	Rhabdomyosarcoma
Group III. Hemopoietic tissue tumors		
Lymphoid tissue		Follicular lymphoma
		Lymphosarcoma
		Lymphatic leukemia
		Reticulum cell sarcoma
		Monocytic leukemia
		Hodgkin's disease
Granulocytic tissue		Myelogenous leukemia
Erythrocytic tissue		Polycythemia vera
Plasma cells		Multiple myeloma
Group IV. Nervous tissue tumors		
Glial tissue		Glioma
Meninges	Meningioma	Meningeal sarcoma
Peripheral nerve cells	Ganglioneuroma	Neuroblastoma
Retina		Retinoblastoma
Adrenal medulla	Pheochromocytoma	
Neurilemmal sheaths	Neurilemmoma	Neurilemmal sarcoma
Group V. Tumors of more than one tissue		
Breast	Fibroadenoma	Cystosarcoma phylodes
Embryonic kidney		Wilms's tumor
Multipotent cells	Teratoma	Teratoma
Group VI. Tumors which do not fit easily in one of the other groups		
Melanoblasts	Pigmented nevus	Malignant melanoma
Placenta	Hydatidiform mole	Chorionepithelioma
Ovary	Cystadenoma	Cystadenocarcinoma
	Granulosa cell tumor	Granulosa cell tumor
	Fibroma	
	Brenner tumor	
		Carcinoma
		Arrhenoblastoma
Testis	Interstitial cell tumor	
		Seminoma
		Embryonic carcinoma
Thymus	Thymoma	Thymoma

SOURCE: Sir Howard Florey (ed.), *General Pathology*, 4th ed., W. B. Saunders Company, Philadelphia, 1970.

their normal type. However, metaplasia is often a premalignant change, and the resultant neoplasm is irreversible.

The second major category consists of tumors arising from connective tissue. Usually included within this group are also tumors of smooth and striated muscle, blood and lymph vessels, and mesothelium. Embryologically, these tumors are all derived from tissues that originated from the mesoderm. However, because there are exceptions to this generality, the germ layer of origin is not considered essential to the classification. Malignant tumors in this group are known as *sarcomas,* from the Greek word meaning "fleshy." Benign tumors are characterized by the name of the tissue involved followed by the suffix *oma,* and malignant tumors are similarly identified by the tissue name followed by the suffix *sarcoma.* Thus we have lipoma and liposarcoma, fibroma and fibrosarcoma, myoma and myosarcoma, and so forth.

The hematopoietic tumors are generally classified separately and make up a surprisingly heterogenous group. Some of these tumors, such as lymphosarcoma, Hodgkin's disease, and reticulum cell sarcoma, may appear to start in single fixed foci; however, frequently when these tumors are first recognized, many lymph nodes are already involved. It is then very difficult to determine whether the tumors arose in each of the lymph nodes by a separate process or whether they spread without evidence of infiltration of other tissues. The most widely known of the hematopoietic tumors, the leukemias, are characterized by large numbers of neoplastic cells in the bloodstream which are, of course, carried throughout the entire body. Thus it is impossible to identify a site of origin.

Tumors of nervous tissue make up the fourth major group. Nervous tissue is made up of two major components, the nerve cells, or neurons, and the supportive tissue, or glial cells. Mature nervous tissue does not multiply and therefore does not give rise to tumors. Immature or neuroblastic cells occasionally produce tumors of the eye (retinoblastoma) and of the adrenal gland (adrenal neuroblastoma). As would be expected, these are tumors of childhood. All other central nervous system tumors arise from the glial cells. They are unique in that, although certain forms show the invasiveness of other malignant neoplasms, they do not metastasize.

The last two categories are less rigidly defined and vary greatly in description from author to author. The first group consists of rare, unusual tumors arising from more than one tissue type. The second group includes a variety of tumors which cannot be classified with the preceding groups.

In the past, certain tumors have been characterized by the suffix *blastoma.* A blastic cell is considered to be an extremely undifferentiated cell which gives rise to a variety of more differentiated cells. Thus the suffix may be used in two ways: first, to indicate that the tumor arises from an embryonal type cell; and second, to indicate that anaplasia has resulted in cellular dedifferentiation to such an extent that the cell appears to have primitive and unspecialized characteristics. Present usage favors the restriction of this term to the former category.

GENERAL FACTORS AFFECTING THE INCIDENCE AND LOCATION OF TUMORS

Knowledge regarding biological relationships and the location and frequency of tumors is extensive and rapidly expanding. A large number of mechanisms which can produce cancer (carcinogenic mechanisms) are known, and these can be applied to the study of cancer in experimental animals. The clinical utility of this information is still limited to situations where strongly predisposing factors are known and can be avoided. As yet the specific mechanisms for clinical carcinogenesis are not known, and a more fundamental approach to prevention and treatment cannot be devised. It is probable that neoplasia represents not one but a number of diseases, which contributes to the complexity of the problem. Nevertheless, much is known which, if applied, could contribute greatly to a reduction in the incidence of cancer.

Age

Cancer is most frequent at the extremes of life. Most tumors of childhood are due to cancers arising from primitive cells and are undoubtedly related to embryogenesis. Between the ages of 5 and 15, cancer is now the second most common cause of death, following only accidents in frequency. However, since the death rate at this age is far lower than it will be at any subsequent age, the absolute number of tumors, although significant, is relatively small. The subsequent increase in the frequency of cancer progresses logarithmically in such a way that the numbers become substantial after the age of 45 and large after the age of 65. Of all cancers, 50 percent occur after the age of 65, although only 9 percent of the population is in this age range. When the number of cancers is related not to the total population but to the number of individuals in each age group, this relationship is quite striking. In 1850 only 2½ percent of the population was over the age of 65, and in 1900 only about 4 percent. It is obvious that the combination of the changing age structure of the population and the increased frequency of neoplasia with age accounts for most of the increased incidence of cancer.

Although the risk of cancer in general increases with age, the spec-

Table 11-3   Most Frequent Types of Cancer by Age (Except for Skin)*

Age	Sex	Site
0–10		Leukemia, cancer of the brain, kidney, eye, and bone
10–20		Leukemia, Hodgkin's disease, cancer of the brain and bone
20–30		Leukemia, Hodgkin's disease, cancer of the testes, uterus, ovary, brain, and breast
30–40	Males	Leukemia, cancer of the colon and rectum, genitals, and brain
	Females	Cancer of the uterus, colon and rectum, breast, and ovary
40–50	Males	Cancer of the lung, colon and rectum, and stomach
	Females	Cancer of the breast, uterus and ovary, colon and rectum
50–60	Males	Cancer of the colon and rectum, lung, and stomach
	Females	Cancer of the breast, uterus, and colon and rectum
60–70	Males	Cancer of the lung, stomach, colon and rectum, and prostate
	Females	Cancer of the breast, uterus, colon and rectum, and stomach
Over 70	Males	Cancer of the prostate, stomach, colon and rectum, lung, and bladder
	Females	Cancer of the breast, colon and rectum, stomach, and uterus

* Cancer of the skin is omitted from this table since there is seldom adequate reason for failure to diagnose it correctly and early.
SOURCE: A Cancer Source Book for Nurses, American Cancer Society, Inc., 1963.

trum of specific cancer types varies at different ages.   Table 11-3 indicates this changing age distribution.

Sex

The total incidence of cancer is slightly greater in men than in women. When the sex-related cancers of the testes and prostate and of the breasts, ovaries, and uterus are eliminated, the frequency of cancer in males is substantially higher.   The only exceptions are carcinoma of the thyroid, which is three times as frequent in women, and adrenal cortical tumors. Carcinomas of the lip, tongue, larynx, and esophagus are more frequent in men by a ratio of 10:1.   Carcinoma of the stomach is twice as common, bronchogenic (lung) carcinoma is five times as common, and carcinoma of the kidney is three times as common in men (Fig. 11-4).

Geographic Factors

One of the most fascinating aspects of the study of cancer is the fact that specific tumors have different frequencies in various parts of the world. In some instances the reason for this difference is known.   However, in many others it is unknown, and knowledge of the causes of these differences could be of critical importance in cancer control.   Some of the difference is accounted for by the difference in age structure of various

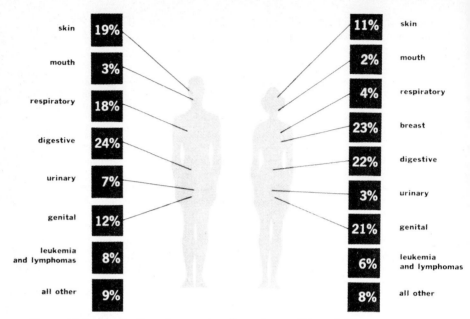

skin 19%
mouth 3%
respiratory 18%
digestive 24%
urinary 7%
genital 12%
leukemia and lymphomas 8%
all other 9%

11% skin
2% mouth
4% respiratory
23% breast
22% digestive
3% urinary
21% genital
6% leukemia and lymphomas
8% all other

Figure 11-4 Distribution of cancer by site and sex. [*From J. B. Aust in S. I. Schwartz (ed.), Principles of Surgery, McGraw-Hill, New York, 1969, p. 250. By permission of the publishers.*]

populations. The pattern in highly industrialized countries where old age is common results in a greater frequency than in less developed areas where old age is infrequent. Table 11-4 summarizes many of these differences.

Examples of regional differences where environmental factors are reasonably well known include the following: In Egypt there is a high incidence of carcinoma of the urinary bladder, which seems to be related to the almost universal infection with *Schistosoma hematobium*. Schistosomes are parasitic worms producing ova which, in the Egyptian variety, penetrate the bladder wall, where they encyst and cause local irritation. Cancer of the facial skin is common in light-skinned individuals who are occupationally exposed to large amounts of sunlight in tropical and desert areas. Negroes do not develop these types of skin cancers, but in tropical Africa skin cancers arise not on the face but on the legs, in the scars of ulcers whose etiology is not known. Cancer of the liver is common in Central Africa, Indonesia, China, and Japan. In these countries, hepatitis and cirrhosis are common and liver carcinoma is usually secondary to liver disease. However, the cause of the liver disease is often unknown, although it is suspected to be due to nutritional factors. There is recent evidence suggesting that a mold found on some grains and on peanuts

Table 11-4 Schematic Tabulation of the Relative Frequencies of Six Types of Cancer in Various Countries

	Breast	Cervix	Esophagus	Stomach	Liver	Oral cavity
Europe and United States	+++++	++	++	+++++	±	+
Japan	+	++++	+++	+++++	+++	++
China	+++	++	+++	+++	+++	++
Philippines	+++	++	+	++	+++	++++
Sumatra:						
a. Chinese	+	+	++	+++	+++	+
b. Malayan	++	+++	±	++	++++	+++
India	++	+++++	++	++	++	++++
South Africa (Bantu)	++	++++	±	++	+++++	+

SOURCE: I. Berenblum in Florey's *General Pathology*, p. 615.

produces aflatoxin, a chemical compound which may be the specific agent responsible in the African cases.

Many other variations cannot be explained on the basis of present information. Cancer mortality rates are similar in England, Holland, and Sweden. Yet the incidence of cancer of the stomach is only 40 percent as high in England as it is in the other two countries. The rate for carcinoma of the stomach is even higher in Czechoslovakia and Japan. Cancer of the breast causes 20 percent of all female deaths from cancer in England and Wales, 10 percent of such deaths in Italy, but only 3 percent in Japan. It is the consensus that these and other striking variations in cancer frequency are due to environmental factors. For example, the unique forms of cancer seen so frequently in African Negroes are rarely seen in the American Negro, whose distribution of tumors tends to approach that of the rest of the American community. Similarly, with the exception of carcinoma of the penis and the uterus, the distribution of cancer among Jews resembles that of their country of residence. It is believed that circumcision accounts for the decreased frequency of the genital carcinomas. The total incidence of carcinoma is about twice as great in New England as in the Southern states.

Socioeconomic Factors

Occupational cancer has given many clues to the nature of carcinogenesis. However, apart from specific occupation, there are certain variations in tumor incidence depending upon social class. In England it has been demonstrated that cancer of the exposed sites and of the upper alimentary canal from the mouth to the pylorus are about twice as frequent in the lowest classes as in the highest. The tumors of the skin are probably occupational in origin. On the other hand, the distribution of cancers of the upper alimentary tract were of the same order of frequency not only in the husbands, for whom an occupational factor might be suspected, but in their wives as well. Cancer of the breast showed a distinct class gradient, being greatest in the upper classes, but cancer of the uterus was more frequent in the lower classes. Failure to nurse the infant has been correlated with increased breast carcinoma and may be related to the increased frequency in the upper classes; failure to repair uterine cervical lacerations subsequent to delivery may predispose to uterine cervical carcinoma and would be more frequently observed in the lower classes.

Nutrition

The specific relationships of nutrition and carcinogenesis are not yet well defined. The probable sequence of diet, cirrhosis, and cancer of the liver has already been presented. Cancer of the liver, which can be produced in rats fed on azo dyes, can be prevented if the vitamin B intake is maintained at high levels at the same time. It has been suspected that smoked fish may be related to the high incidence of stomach cancer in Iceland. A known carcinogen (chemical capable of inducing cancer) has been identified in smoked fish. However, in Japan the fish are not smoked but are preserved in salt, and the incidence of stomach cancer is comparable. In northern Sweden there is a high incidence of cancer of the oropharynx. This is often preceded by the Plummer-Vinson syndrome in which there is anemia and esophagitis. The syndrome usually responds to iron and vitamin B therapy and is presumably of dietary origin. It is not certain whether this relationship is significant.

Occupation

Sir Percival Pott noted in 1775 that there was a high frequency of scrotal carcinoma in English chimney sweeps. At that time, as in the present, coal was the primary source of heat and therefore of the chimney soot. It was not until 1916 that Yamagiwa and Ichikawa were able to demonstrate that the chronic exposure of the epithelium of rabbit's ears to coal tar would produce a local epithelial tumor. Cook and Kennaway showed in 1932 that it was the benzathracene group of hydrocarbons which were responsible. Workers in the aniline dye industry have been known to have an unusually high frequency of papilloma and carcinoma of the bladder since the end of the nineteenth century. Rueper established in 1938 that 2-naphthylamine was the most important carcinogenic substance, although other aromatic amines are also suspected.

For three or four centuries it has been known that the miners in the south German and Bohemian mines of Schneeberg and Jáchymov had a high death rate from lung disease. Recent studies indicate that about three-fourths of the Schneeberg miners and nearly one-half of the Jáchymov miners die of carcinoma of the lung. The most generally accepted cause is the presence of a high content of radon in the ore and in the inspired mine dust. During the years after World War I, there was a unique increase in the incidence of bone sarcomas in adult women. All these women had been employed in painting the luminous numerals on watch faces and were in the habit of pointing their brushes by wetting them with their tongues. As a result they had ingested significant amounts of radium-containing paint which eventually settled in the bones and initiated the osteogenic sarcomas. From these few examples it can be seen that a large number of occupations may contain carcinogenic hazards. It may often take a number of years before these hazards are recognized. The epidemiological methods previously developed for infectious diseases are proving necessary and effective in this area as well.

Heredity

It has been possible to demonstrate in experimental animals that closely inbred strains can be developed which have either high or low frequencies of cancer. The data from studies of this type suggest that (1) there may be a genetic predisposition to a specific type of cancer and (2) that the quantitative distribution does not follow the proportions of a single gene relationship. Some caution must be taken in interpreting these data. In 1936 Bittner placed the litters of low-cancer-strain mice with nursing mothers of a high cancer strain and vice versa. Subsequently the breast carcinomas of the low cancer strain increased whereas those of the high cancer strain decreased. Further studies showed that the cancer was probably due to a virus transmitted through the milk from generation to generation. The genetic variations continued, although they were less marked when this procedure was used. The final conclusions were that in mouse breast cancer there were at least three factors operative: (1) the presence of genetic susceptibility, (2) the presence of a virus, and (3) female hormonal relationships, since the male mice were unaffected.

The relationship of genetic factors to human cancer is very unclear. Cancer will affect at least one of four individuals who live long enough, and therefore family histories showing the presence of cancer are not particularly significant. The presence of multiple cancers of the same type is much more suggestive but fortunately quite rare. For example, there is good evidence that Napoleon Bonaparte died at the age of 51 of scirrhous carcinoma of the stomach. His father died at the age of 39 with autopsy-proved stomach carcinoma, as did his youngest sister Caroline. His sister Elisa died at age 43, his sister Pauline at age 44, and his brother Lucien at age 65, all probably of carcinoma of the stomach. Recently, a rather unusual carcinoma of the thyroid has been reported which has been associated with an adrenalin-secreting tumor of the adrenal medulla (pheochromocytoma). In addition to this unusual combination, many of the cases have been reported in both mother and daughter. Despite the fact that many such instances can be cited, it seems probable that the hereditary basis for most carcinomas is relatively small as compared to the environmental influences.

However, there are a few rare situations for which genetic factors can be cited with reasonable certainty and neoplasia can be anticipated. Familial polyposis of the bowel is almost invariably associated with the development of bowel carcinoma. Several other syndromes seem to lead to bowel carcinoma. There are families in which retinoblastoma undoubtedly follows a genetic distribution. Xeroderma pigmentosum is an hereditary skin disease which is invariably followed by the development of skin cancer. Von Recklinghausen's disease, or neurofibromatosis, is associated with the development of sarcoma in about 5 to 10 percent of affected individuals. Down's syndrome may be due either to an additional chromosome 21 or to defects in chromosome 21. Many cases of chronic leukemia show a defect in a chromosome like 21, which is designated the Philadelphia chromosome. The excessive incidence of leukemia in children with Down's syndrome was thought to be related to these observations, but recent evidence that the Philadelphia chromosome is 22 has excluded this association.

Premalignant Lesions

Most benign tumors do not become malignant, although there are exceptions. Certain specific benign tumors frequently appear to be premalignant. Hereditary multiple polyposis of the intestinal tract has already been mentioned. Gastric polyps, serous cystadenomas of the ovary, papillomas of the urinary bladder and of the vocal cord, and neurofibromatoses often become malignant. Common epidermoid moles rarely become malignant; however, a certain type of blue nevus which is really made up of melanomatous tissue may become a melanosarcoma. All these lesions should probably be removed as a prophylactic measure when they are recognized. Many older individuals, especially those who have been exposed to excessive amounts of sunlight or to radiation, develop senile keratoses. These lesions, which are not themselves neoplasms, very frequently become carcinomatous and should be removed (Fig. 11-5A, B). Occasionally there is a thickening of the mucous membranes, especially of the mouth and of the vagina, known as leukoplakia. The incidence of carcinomatous change in leukoplakia is sufficiently high that it is usually recommended that these areas be removed.

Physical Trauma

The relationship of simple physical trauma to the development of cancer has been the subject of much speculation and investigation. Careful study has produced a consensus that the chance of a single trauma ever resulting in neoplasia is extremely remote. There is a somewhat better case for repeated trauma; there are many examples, such as the relationship of pipe smoking to cancer of the lip, and of carious, jagged teeth to

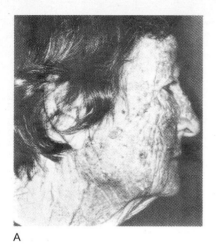

A

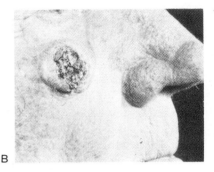

B

C

Figure 11-5 Carcinomas of the skin. *A:* Multiple squamous cell carcinomas arising in skin long exposed to sunlight. [*From H. Pinkus in T. B. Fitzpatrick (ed.), Dermatology in General Medicine, McGraw-Hill, New York, 1971, p. 412. By permission of the publishers.*] *B:* Nodular ulceration and invasive squamous cell carcinoma of the cheek. [*From H. Pinkus in T. B. Fitzpatrick (ed.), Dermatology in General Medicine, McGraw-Hill, New York, 1971, p. 414. By permission of the publishers.*] *C:* Typical and common squamous carcinoma of the lip. Early recognition almost invariably results in cure. [*From B. F. Rush, Jr., in S. I. Schwartz (ed.), Principles of Surgery, McGraw-Hill, New York, 1969, p. 439. By permission of the publishers.*]

cancer of the tongue (Fig. 11-5C). However, even in these instances, the case is not considered conclusive, and a combination of factors is believed to be involved in the carcinogenesis.

THE ETIOLOGY OF CANCER

It is apparent from the preceding discussion that a number of specific agents have been implicated in the production of neoplasms. We shall examine them more closely and attempt to evaluate them in relation to the current theories of carcinogenesis.

Chemical Carcinogens

The relationship of benzanthracine hydrocarbons to the production of scrotal carcinomas in chimney sweeps and experimental skin cancer in rabbits has already been mentioned. A carcinoma of the lip frequent in Scotch fishermen is probably due to the same cause; tarred lines are held in the lips as they are being repaired. Also mentioned have been the aniline dyes which produce bladder tumors. Azo dyes produce liver cancer when fed to vitamin-B–deficient rats. Urethane produces lung tumors in mice, but when painted on the skin it is apparently harmless. If the skin painted with urethane is later painted with croton oil, skin cancers are produced, although neither agent alone is effective. Recently 2-acetyl-aminofluorene was under investigation as an insecticide. Toxicity studies showed that it produced a variety of cancers in rats. At present several hundred casual, occupational, and experimental carcinogens are known. Fortunately most require repeated exposure or a unique combination of sequential exposures, which renders their accidental carcinogenesis relatively unlikely. When industrial carcinogens are recognized, procedures can be undertaken to prevent their action.

   The role of hormones in carcinogenesis has been noted because of the marked sex differences in the incidence of cancer and because about 25 percent of tumors are in hormone-producing or hormone-controlled organs, i.e., breast, uterus, and ovary in women and prostate in men. Experimental breast cancer in mice can be prevented by removal of the ovaries. In male mice breast cancer does not usually occur. However, if the mice are castrated and estrogens are then administered, breast cancer can be produced in males exposed to the Bittner virus. Administration of estrogens will produce a variety of tumors in mice other than breast cancer. Many women have been given estrogens for prolonged periods of time, but as yet there is no evidence that they have resulted in cancer. Cancer of the prostate is undoubtedly dependent upon the presence of testosterone.

Physical Carcinogens

The effect of actinic radiation, or sunlight, in producing skin cancer has already been commented upon. There are a number of cancers for which repeated exposure to heat has been implicated. One of these is the Chotta cancer of Southern India. According to local custom, the Chotta cigar is smoked with the burning end held inside the mouth. Frequent oral cancer is held to be due to the repeated local exposure to heat. Another possibly heat-induced cancer is the kangri cancer of Kashmir. The kangri is a small brazier that is held under the garments against the abdomen for warmth. Skin cancer often develops on the abdomen in the region where the kangri is carried. Although it is attractive to postulate that both these cancers are heat-induced, it is possible that chemicals from the cigar and coal-tar derivatives from the heater may be equally responsible, at least in combination. A similar combination of heat and trauma is thought to be responsible for the pipe smoker's carcinoma of the lip.

Ionizing radiations are well-established physical carcinogens. The most dramatic example was the increase in cancer, especially leukemia, which followed the atomic bomb explosions in Japan. This experience demonstrates that a single exposure, if sufficient, can precipitate neoplasia. The increased incidence of leukemia noted within the first few years after the bomb blast has subsequently subsided; whether there will be an increased late incidence is not yet determined. Chronic radiation exposure produces radiation dermatitis, hyperkeratosis, and finally skin cancer. In the early days of x-ray this hazard was not known, and many radiologists and x-ray technicians developed these tumors. Lung cancer has been produced by inhalation of radioactive dust in the miners of Schneeberg and Jáchymov and bone cancer in the bones of the girls working with radium paint. According to one report, radiologists have four times the incidence of leukemia as physicians not comparably exposed to x-radiation.

Viral Carcinogens

It was natural to expect that the infectious origin of neoplasms would be thoroughly investigated. Early studies were essentially unsuccessful. The epidemiology of cancer failed to follow an infectious pattern; no organisms were isolated, nor could cancer be produced by known agents, and there was no immunological response which would implicate a possible infectious agent. The first suggestive evidence was the observation by Rous in 1911 that an ultrafiltrate of fowl sarcoma would produce the same tumor when inoculated into another chicken.*   Later (in 1932) Shope demonstrated that a filtrate of the skin papilloma of the wild cottontail rabbit would produce a true cancer in a domestic rabbit, but that a filtrate of the cancer was not further transmissible.   In 1936 Bittner discovered that the previously supposed hereditary breast cancer of mice was, in fact, transmitted through the mother's milk.   Lucké demonstrated in 1938 that the adenocarcinoma of the kidney of the leopard frog was produced by a virus of great specificity; intravenous injection invariably produced the tumor in the kidney alone, although metastases to other tissues would occur when the primary was established.   Gross showed in 1951 that mouse leukemia was viral in origin, and Stewart demonstrated that the same virus could also produce carcinoma of the parotid gland and fibrosarcoma of connective tissue.   When this agent was grown in tissue culture, the culture extract produced a broad variety of tumors when injected into newborn mice.   Because of its multiple potentiality, this virus has been named the polyoma virus (*poly* for "many," *oma* for "tumor").

This and other evidence has made it difficult to deny that a virus or viruslike particle can induce neoplasia.   A number of deductions from the observations described provide a formulation for some of the mechanisms involved.   First, the virus can remain latent within the cell for a long time.   This situation is not without precedent, since the virus of herpes simplex is known to remain dormant for long periods of time until an acute lesion is triggered by a febrile infection.   Second, most acute viral infections are destructive of cells, but the cellular response to the carcinogenic virus seems to be one of increased proliferation.   Third, once neoplasia is induced, the continued presence of a virus or of a viral particle may no longer be necessary.

Although three major groups of carcinogens, chemical, physical, and viral, are well established, the mechanism of the neoplastic process and the relationship of the carcinogens to this process is not known.   It is attractive, as many are tempted, to ascribe all cancer to the activation of viral processes.   The neoplastic process consists of a change in an individual cell or group of cells which results in various anatomic changes associated with excessive reproduction and decreased physiological function.   One of the attractions of the virus theory is that viruses are known to resemble DNA and RNA chains and to be able to modify normal cellular metabolism.   Both DNA and RNA viruses have been implicated, and it follows that the metabolic changes could be either in the nucleus

---

*Disbelief was so great that it was not until 55 years later, in 1966, that Rous received the Nobel Prize.   Fortunately he lived long enough—the Nobel Prize is given only to living scientists!

or the cytoplasm. Yet so far no virus has been demonstrated in any human cancer. The well-established roles of chemical and physical carcinogens requires that their actions also be explained. Either they must be able independently to initiate the neoplastic process or they must activate a latent viral factor. It is clear that although many questions must be answered, a broad area for exploration is already available and should yield much of the essential information.

Immunity and Cancer

In the past several years evidence has accumulated that the immune mechanisms are related to the development of tumors. This has been most evident clinically as a result of the use of drugs which suppress immunity, such as those used for prevention of transplant rejection. The frequency of cancer has been definitely increased in this group and the incidence of virus-induced warts of several types has also increased. Several instances are recorded in which cancer was accidentally introduced with a kidney transplant and metastasized widely. When the immunosuppressive drugs were discontinued, the transplanted tumor regressed and disappeared. Antibodies have been found to a number of tumors. These antibodies may increase when the tumor is excised and decrease when the tumor recurs and spreads. These observations suggest that an uncontrolled tumor produces enough antigen to overwhelm the antibody response.

The recognition of the presence of altered immune mechanisms in cancer is of fundamental importance. Immunity may be a mechanism for controlling cell and tissue integrity as well as for combating infection. Therefore, alterations in immunity do not exclude the carcinogenic importance of any of the carcinogenic agents previously discussed. The carcinogen may merely exhaust the immune defense. It is attractive to speculate that the efficiency of immunity decreases with age and is correlated with the increasing frequency of neoplasia (see Chap. 12).

SPREAD OF TUMORS

Local invasion and metastasis are essential characteristics of malignancy. An understanding of these processes is important, not only theoretically but also practically, to provide insight into the clinical characteristics and course of cancer. The main routes of spread of cancer are (1) by direct extension, (2) via the lymphatics, (3) via the blood vessels, (4) through natural passages and cavities, and (5) by inoculation.

Direct Extension

Local invasion has been discussed at some length in association with the characteristics of malignant neoplasia (Figs. 11-6 to 11-8).

Lymphatic Spread

The lymphatics are relatively easily accessible vessels which drain lymph and macrophages from the extracellular, extravascular compartment. Infiltration of tumor cells into the lymphatics is extremely frequent, especially in the case of carcinomas (Fig. 11-9). Tumor cells then progress along the lymphatics to the regional lymph nodes. Willis believes that spread to the lymph nodes is by lymphatic emboli, since continuous cords of tumor cells are almost never seen. Tumor cells can then block

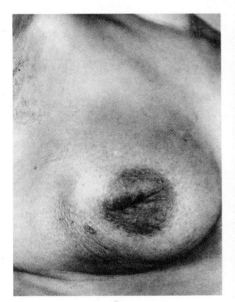 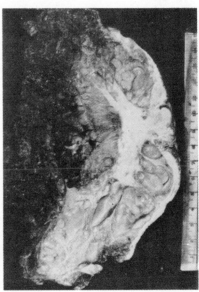

A   B

Figure 11-6   Carcinoma of the breast. *A:* Moderately advanced carcinoma with retraction of the nipple and dimpling of the tissue to the left of the areola. *(From L. V. Ackerman and J. A. DelRegatto, Cancer, 4th ed., Mosby, St. Louis, 1970, Figure 6-60. By permission of the publishers.)*   *B:* Cross-section of breast containing carcinoma. The invasion of the dense neoplastic tissue can be seen and the mechanism of dimpling and nipple retraction becomes evident. *(From Sir H. W. Florey, General Pathology, 4th ed., Saunders, Philadelphia, 1970, p. 689. By permission of the publishers.)*

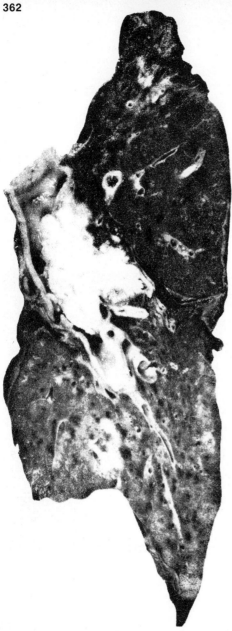

Figure 11-7 Carcinoma of the lung. This is the typical squamous cell carcinoma which is seen to arise in the bronchus rather than in the lung parenchyma. For this reason, it is known as a bronchogenic carcinoma. *(From R. P. Morehead, Human Pathology, McGraw-Hill, New York, 1965, p. 714. By permission of the publishers.)*

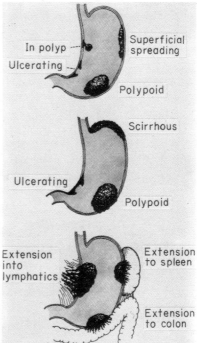

Figure 11-8 Stages in the development of carcinoma of the stomach. Upper figure: Early carcinomas involving only the epithelial layers of the stomach. Middle figure: Invasion of the submucosal tissues. The scirrhous carcinoma is infiltrating rather than polypoid and tends to be quite hard. Bottom figure: Extension of the tumor outside the stomach into adjacent organs. [*From N. H. Harkins, in J. G. Allen (ed.), Surgery, Principles and Practice, Lippincott, Philadelphia, 1957. By permission of the publishers.*]

the lymph node and cause retrograde flow of lymph, resulting in emboli going to alternate lymph nodes as well. In addition, tumor proliferation can proceed in the lymph nodes and further embolization can carry tumor cells into lymphatics draining centrally from the lymph node. Eventually, tumor cells enter the blood circulation. An especially important route of lymphatic drainage is via the thoracic duct, which delivers most of the lymph from the abdominal cavity and organs into the left subclavian vein just before its junction with the left jugular vein.

Hematogenous Spread

Hematogenous spread may be achieved by two routes: first, by progress through the lymphatics into the venous circulation; and second, by direct penetration into the veins. Willis believes that most venous penetration is via the lymphatics which enter the vein wall. Sarcomas rarely spread via the lymphatics but are almost entirely blood-borne. With the exception of sarcomas involving lymphoid tissue per se, lymph node enlargement is rarely seen. Once tumor cells enter the bloodstream, they may be disseminated to the organs supplied by that vessel. Tumors of the abdominal viscera which are drained by the portal vein generally

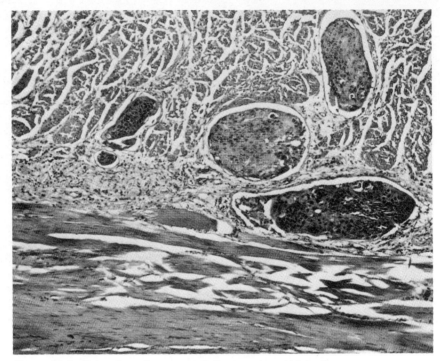

Figure 11-9 Extension of cancer of the esophagus into the lymphatic vessels of the muscular layers. Three large lymphatic vessels on the right and two smaller ones on the left can be seen plugged with tumor tissue. This tumor can now proceed to the lymph nodes either by direct extension or by embolization (X85). *(From L. V. Ackerman and J. A. DelRegatto, Cancer, 4th ed., Mosby, St. Louis, 1970, p. 87. By permission of the publishers.)*

metastasize first to the liver (Fig. 11-10). Other tumors are more likely to metastasize directly to the lungs. Since cancer rarely penetrates the arterial wall, special mechanisms must be provided to explain the systemic distribution of many metastases. Channels of up to 200 micrometers in diameter have been demonstrated in the lungs, therefore it is theoretically possible for small tumor emboli to traverse the lung. Occasionally there may be a paradoxical embolism in which the tumor cells enter the systemic circulation via a defect in the septum separating the right and left chambers of the heart. Retrograde flow in veins and lymphatics possibly explains other unusual localizations.

The most frequent sites of blood-borne metastases are the liver, lungs, and bones, which are involved in about 40, 30, and 15 percent respectively of fatal cases of malignant tumors of all kinds (Willis). Other common sites of metastasis are the adrenals (10 percent), kidneys (8 percent), brain

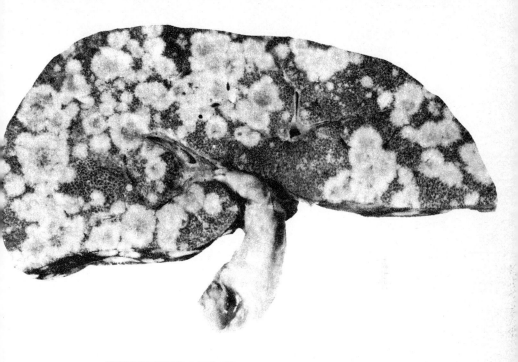

Figure 11-10 Multiple metastatic tumors to the liver. The lung and the liver, because of their large size and blood flow, are common sites for blood-borne metastases. *(From R. P. Morehead, Human Pathology, McGraw-Hill, New York, 1965, p. 55. By permission of the publishers.)*

(6 percent), and heart (5 percent). Carcinomas which commonly metastasize to bone include the prostrate, which frequently involves the sacroiliac area; the breast, which often metastasizes to the shoulder on the same side; the lung; the thyroid which frequently metastasizes to the skull; and the kidney. Carcinomas which frequently metastasize to the brain include the lung, the breast, the kidney, and less frequently the prostate and rectum. Metastases to the adrenals usually involve only the medulla, are most frequently from bronchogenic carcinoma, and rarely cause adrenal cortical insufficiency. Metastatic tumors to the kidneys are rarely clinically significant. Metastases to the spleen are rare.

Spread via Body Passages and through Body Cavities

On occasion it is possible that a tumor arising in the bronchus can become implanted elsewhere in the bronchus or that one arising in the renal pelvis can become implanted in the ureter or bladder. Although this type of spread is possible, it seems more probable that when such spread is seen it is the result of lymphatic extension. However, it is well established that cells from tumors of the abdominal cavity, especially the stomach, may become implanted elsewhere in the abdomen. Three sites deserve special comment: (1) Tumor cells may settle by gravity into the lower portion of the peritoneal cavity, which lies above and anterior to the rectum, 3 or 4 inches above the anus. Tumor cells may proliferate in this location and produce a hard tumor mass which is first detected on rectal examination. (2) Small tumor masses may implant throughout the peritoneal cavity and produce multiple small growths, a process which is referred to as *carcinomatosis*. (3) Cells may implant in the ovary and be associated with ascites. Not infrequently the ovarian metastasis is detected before the primary, which is usually in the stomach.

Inoculation

Finally, tumor cells may metastasize by implantation. This event is relatively rare, but many cases have been documented in which the surgeon's knife used to cut into the tumor has transplanted cells to another site during the same operation. For this reason special precautions are taken and the knife which has cut into tumor is not used again until it has been properly cleansed.

DIAGNOSIS OF TUMORS

The most important component of cancer cure is early diagnosis before spread beyond treatable limits. This requires that the patient be alert to possible signs of malignancy and that the physician effectively diagnose cancer if it is present. The American Cancer Society has embarked on an intensive educational program to alert the public to symptoms which may indicate cancer. It should be realized that these symptoms will occur far more frequently than will cancer itself. Vigilance, not panic, is the goal sought. The important symptoms are

1. Any sore that does not heal or that increases in size, particularly on the lips, tongue, ears, eyelids, or genital organs
2. A painless lump or thickening that persists, especially in the breast, tongue, lips, neck, armpit, or groin
3. Bleeding or abnormal discharge from any body opening, especially the mouth, rectum, vagina, or bladder
4. A change in bowel habits, particularly after the age of 40
5. Persistent hoarseness or sore throat
6. Persistent indigestion
7. Unintended loss of weight, continued unexplained fever, or a feeling of weakness

8. Progressive changes in the color or size of a wart, mole, or birthmark

9. ˙Persistent headache, sinusitis, or difficulty in vision

Clinical Examination

Whether or not the patient presents with symptoms which suggest to him the possibility of cancer, the physician should always be on the alert for this possibility. The fact that early cancers may be entirely asymptomatic is a persuasive argument for a routine annual examination, at least after middle age, when the incidence of cancer shows an abrupt increase. The physician must have time available for an adequate history and physical examination. In most instances, appropriate confirmatory studies will have to be performed. However, good judgment must be used to avoid excessive examination; overuse of x-rays is probably just as inappropriate as failure to perform the proper studies.

Radiology

Most of the common tumors will eventually be apparent on routine x-ray examination procedures. Unfortunately, a certain portion of tumors will not be detected, either because the lesion is too small or because it is inapparent for technical reasons. Should the clinical impression that an abnormality exists be sufficiently strong, the physician will continue with further studies, even in the presence of negative radiological findings.

Laboratory Tests

The past failure to find abnormal chemical and serological states in association with neoplasia has resulted in the paucity of specific laboratory diagnostic tests. One of the few useful procedures is the serum acid phosphatase which is specifically elevated in carcinoma of the prostate. Advanced cancer may demonstrate such nonspecific findings as leukocytosis, anemia, and increased sedimentation rate.

Exfoliative Cytology

One of the most useful screening procedures was the development of the procedure of exfoliative cytology. Papanicolau demonstrated that examination of cells from the uterine cervix gave information which correlated well with the presence of early carcinoma. Simple scraping or washing of the uterine cervix yields cells which can be placed on a slide, stained, and examined. Further, more definitive studies are carried out if the findings suggest cancer. The ease of the test, for both patient and technician, has resulted in its wide use. Success with the examination of uterine cells has led to similar examinations of bronchial washings, gastric aspirates, and urinary concentrates for tumors of the lungs, stomach, and urinary tract respectively. These have met with varying degrees of success but have been less useful than the test for uterine carcinoma.

Tissue Examination

Ultimately the diagnosis of cancer depends upon the microscopic examination of an appropriate piece of tissue. When taken from a living patient, such a piece of tissue is known as a *biopsy*. A biopsy may be taken by direct excision when the lesion is on an accessible surface, it may be removed by a special needle, or it may require an open operative procedure if the tissue is deemed inaccessible. In most instances it will be possible to make a positive diagnosis from a properly obtained specimen.

TREATMENT

Surgery

Excision of the tumor is the most common method of treatment. The effectiveness of surgery is limited when the lesion has extended beyond an area susceptible to removal, either for technical reasons or because of metastasis. The surgeon generally attempts a wide excision to get beyond the limits of the tumor. He also explores the regional lymph nodes to determine if they are involved. The possibility of cure is immediately greatly reduced when there is lymph node involvement. If this is the case, an attempt is made to remove as much of the affected lymph tissue as possible. Metastasis beyond the lymph nodes renders cure impossible. Local surgery may be performed, however, in order to ameliorate symptoms and to extend life. Occasionally metastases will regress to some extent if the primary tumor is removed.

Radiation

It is paradoxical that radiation not only produces tumors but is often effective in tumor treatment. Radiation therapy includes not only x-rays and related sources but also the use of radioactive isotopes. In general radiation sensitivity is inversely proportional to the degree of cellular differentiation. Thus, extremely anaplastic tumors are more sensitive than more highly differentiated ones. On the other hand, radiosensitivity is not equivalent to curability. Radiation has a direct effect on cells, causing death of the most rapidly multiplying ones and often impairing the reproduction of those not immediately destroyed. Radiation also causes damage to the blood vessels and impairs the blood supply to the radiated tissues. Finally, the radiation causes fibrosis and degeneration of the stroma and as a result further impairs the circulation and nutrition of the neoplastic tissue. Many tumors of the skin are effectively treated by irradiation, and some forms of carcinoma of the uterine cervix may be cured by local radiation or the application of radium or radon locally. In most other tumors, radiation is generally used in conjunction with surgery or as a palliative measure to cause regression of the tumor and temporary remission. Radioactive iodine has been used for the treatment of thyroid carcinoma, since iodine is preferentially absorbed by the thyroid gland. Radioactive phosphorus has been used extensively in the treatment of polycythemia vera and leukemia.

Because x-rays could be neither seen nor felt, their potency was not appreciated by the early radiologists. It took a considerable period of time before sufficient information was obtained to appreciate the complications which could ensue from the improper use of both diagnostic and therapeutic radiation. Previous reference has been made to radiation dermatitis. In the chronic form there are large dilated blood vessels visible on the surface. There is fibrosis beneath the skin with thinning, loss of dermal appendages, ulcerations, keratoses, and low-grade carcinoma. Patients receiving radium implantations into the uterine cervix may undergo an acute reaction about a year after treatment, with edema and the formation of an inflammatory mass in the adjacent tissues. This may subside after a time, but in a small percentage of cases necrosis ensues and a fistula may form between the rectum and the vagina. Pulmonary fibrosis may result from radiation to the chest. The radiation reaction of the kidney is also characterized by an acute response 6 to 12 months after radiation. This usually resolves, but it may leave permanent functional impairment. The development of extremely high-voltage equipment has made it possible to focus the radiation on the diseased tissue and to reduce the injury to adjacent structures.

Chemotherapy

The most recent development in cancer therapy is the development of chemicals which have effectively relieved symptoms and prolonged life, although none have resulted in a complete cure. However, the improvement in the course has been sufficiently impressive to warrant their use. For example, only 5 percent of children with acute leukemia will live for 1 year without treatment, whereas the combination of amethopterin, cortisone, and 6-mercaptopurine has resulted in 53 percent survival for 1 year.

The cancer chemotherapeutic drugs can be divided into four groups. The first of these are the alkalating agents of which the initial one was nitrogen mustard, a compound closely related to mustard gas. These agents react with DNA, producing mutation and cell death. They have been particularly effective in chronic leukemia, Hodgkin's disease, and lymphosarcoma. The second group of drugs are the antimetabolites, which act by interfering with a specific biochemical step in the metabolic pathway. Amethopterin interferes with the synthesis of folic acid, one of the vitamin B series. Amethopterin has been particularly effective in acute leukemia and choriocarcinoma. Other compounds in this series include 6-mercaptopurine and 5-fluorouracil. The third group includes the steroid hormones of the adrenal and sex glands. The adrenal cortical hormones (cortisone) have been useful in leukemias, Hodgkin's disease, lymphosarcoma, and multiple myeloma. Some patients with carcinoma of the breast have improved following removal of the ovaries and adminis-tration of androgens (male hormones.) Striking improvement has been obtained in carcinoma of the prostate by removal of the testes and adminis-tration of estrogens (female hormones). With this therapy many patients have lived a number of years and, in some instances, there has been demonstrable regression of metastases. A fourth group of drugs is a miscellaneous one including a number of unrelated drugs of variable utility.

Regional Perfusion

One of the difficulties in the use of cancer therapeutic drugs has been the limitation of dose due to general systemic toxic effects. Recently tech-niques have been developed which make it possible to infuse the drug directly into the tumor via the appropriate artery and to recover the excess drug from the draining vein. This technique is termed regional perfusion. Promising results have been obtained in this way for a number of tumors.

PROGNOSIS

The characteristic of cancer is that it inevitably causes death if untreated. It is difficult to speak of cure of cancer since recurrences have occured many years after apparently successful therapy. Fortunately such late recurrences are rare. However, it is generally the custom to evaluate treatment in terms of 5-year survival without evidence of disease. The prognosis for various cancers is different and depends upon the location and characteristics of the individual tumor. Almost all cancers of the skin should be successfully treated. There is approximately a 70 percent survival in cancer of the breast if there are no lymph node metastases; however, the 5-year survival drops to 40 percent if any lymph nodes are found to be involved. Cancer of the rectum, colon, and uterus, all quite common, have good prognoses when treated early. Increased vigilance for cancers of these sites should improve their outlook. On the other hand, treatment of cancers of the lung and stomach has been most unsatisfactory, although significant gains are being made. Until recently, palliative therapy was the best that had been achieved with the leukemias and lymphomas. The improved results in the treatment of acute leukemia, reports of possible irradiation cure of some cases of Hodgkin's disease, the use of melphalan in multiple myeloma, and similar developments are all encouraging. Fortunately, the chronic leukemias and lymphosarcomas arise late in life, and many of these patients live quite comfortably for a number of years.

The present outlook is that the success of treatment of the patients with cancer could possibly be increased from one-third to one-half if all the present methods of screening were put into active use and the best available treatment utilized. The incidence of cancer might be decreased if a more intensive attempt were made to eliminate premalignant lesions and to avoid exposure to known carcinogens. Carcinoma of the lung is presently responsible for 21 percent of all cancer deaths in men. This represents about $3\frac{1}{2}$ percent of all male deaths. Yet at the turn of the century, lung cancer was extremely rare. The evidence is overwhelming that cessation of cigarette smoking would drastically reduce the number of deaths from this particular cancer. The problem is to get the public to realize that cancer control requires active public participation. Finally, progress in oncology has been impressive during the past 5 years, particularly in the development of knowledge concerning basic tumor processes, the relationship of viruses to cancer, and the nature of the immune response to neoplasia. It is not unrealistic to expect major improvements in cancer control within the next generation.

BIBLIOGRAPHY

A Cancer Source Book for Nurses, American Cancer Society, Inc., 1963.

ACKERMAN, L. V. and J. A. DEL REGATTO: *Cancer,* 4th ed., St. Louis: The C. V. Mosby Company, 1970.

DULBECCO, R.: "The Induction of Cancer by Viruses," *Scientific American,* April, 1967.

FLOREY, SIR HOWARD: *General Pathology,* 4th ed., Philadelphia: W. B. Saunders Company, 1970.

HOPPS, H. C.: *Principles of Pathology,* 2d ed., New York: Appleton-Century-Crofts, 1964.

SHIMKIN, M. B.: *Science and Cancer,* U.S. Department of Health, Education and Welfare, Public Health Service Publication no. 1162, 1964.

WILLIS, R. A.: *Pathology of Tumors,* 4th ed., London: Butterworth & Co. (Publishers), Ltd., 1967.

Chapter 12

Aging

The problem of aging was not very important in primitive populations. Most individuals probably died of trauma and malnutrition. Those who were unable to provide for themselves, who performed no useful function within the group, or who were no longer sufficiently mobile did not survive. Under these circumstances the estimation of a natural longevity would have been difficult and undoubtedly invalid. Some individuals may have lived into old age, but anthropologists and archeologists have data suggesting that survival beyond the age of 40 was unusual. The development of agriculture and of fixed societies increased the security from both physical hazards and famine, and survival to an older age was possible. With greater contacts, infectious diseases probably became more common, thus nullifying some of this improvement.

   The average duration of life, or life expectation, in the early Iron and Bronze Ages was only 18 years and was only slightly longer during the Roman era (Table 12-1). This increased gradually to the Middle Ages, after which there was a plateau extending to the end of the eighteenth

Table 12-1   Average Length of Life

Time and place	Years
Early Iron and Bronze Age, Greece	18
2,000 years ago, Rome	22
Middle Ages, England	35
1687–1691, Breslau	33.5
Before 1789, Massachusetts and New Hampshire	35.5
1838–1854, England and Wales	40.9
1900–1902, United States	49.2
1945, United States	65.8
1957, United States	69.3

SOURCE: Metropolitan Life Insurance Company.

century, during which the average length of life was 35 years. The death rates during these periods were so high that in most European communities the population remained static from one century to the next. The population in the large cities would have been unsustained were it not for the constant influx of people from the countryside. Victor Heiser writes that as recently as 1900, eight out of ten infants born in the city of Manila died before the end of their first year of life. These conditions are undoubtedly true in all cities lacking modern means of sanitation and disease control. The results of public health measures and improvement in medical techniques is demonstrated by the tremendous change in average longevity in the past hundred years. In the place of malnutrition, infection, and trauma, the major causes of death are now degenerative diseases of the circulatory system, cancer, and a variety of metabolic disorders. Accidents are still important causes of death, although they are now most significant at the extremes of life.

Figure 12-1 shows the distribution of deaths in ancient Rome. The upper curve shows the percentage of those born who could expect to survive to a given age. The lower curve shows the percentage of those born who would die in each succeeding 5-year period. The extremely high infantile and juvenile death rate accounts for the rapid fall in the percentage of survivors. By age 20, more than 50 percent of those born had died, and by age 30 there were only 25 percent survivors. From this age on the chance of survival improved somewhat, and it appears that some individuals even managed to achieve significant longevity.

Figure 12-2 shows the death distribution in the United States for 1940. The important feature is that the number of deaths is moderate during the first few years of life, drops to a minimum between ages 10 and 15, and then gradually rises to a peak at age 75, after which it falls. Survivorship shows

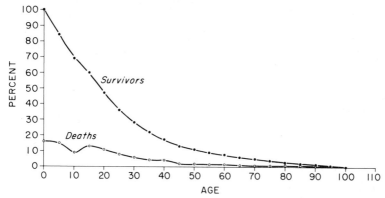

Figure 12-1   Survivors and distribution of death by age in ancient Rome. The lower curve shows the percent of total deaths which will occur in the subsequent 5-year period. The upper curve shows the percentage of survivors of an original group at 5-year intervals. Thus, the survival curve indicates the cumulative losses shown by period on the lower curve.

a modest neonatal and infantile drop, then levels off with a gradually increasing rate of loss after age 50. Fifty percent of the population can expect to reach age 70 and 25 percent to reach nearly 80 years.

Life-span is the maximum length of life, as opposed to *life expectation,* which is the average length of life. Extremely long life-spans have always been of great interest and a number have received wide publicity. One of the oldest was "Old Parr," who died in 1635 at the reputed age of 152 years. Incidentally, he was autopsied by William Harvey, who first conclusively demonstrated the circulation of the blood. Comfort and many others point out that all extreme examples of longevity are questionable by virtue

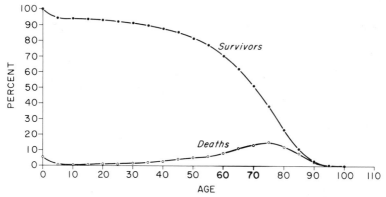

Figure 12-2   Survivors and death distribution of death by age in the United States, 1940.

of poor documentation. The three prerequisites are accurate knowledge of (1) the birthdate, (2) the death rate, and (3) the identity of the individual. Careful examination of most claims indicates that one or more of these prerequisites cannot be documented.

One of the first countries to introduce birth certificates was Great Britain, which did so as recently as 1837. It is traditional to send royal congratulations to Britons on their hundredth birthday, and the documents are checked at this time. Approximately one person in ten thousand survives to enter his second century. Since the initiation of this documentation, there has been no certified record of over 112 years. From all of the other records available there appear to be only four for whom reliable acceptance of an older age may be made. The oldest of these was one Pierre Joubert, 1701–1814, who was born and died in Quebec with a survival of 113 years and 100 days. Despite popular supposition to the contrary, there are only two mammals known to live longer than 50 years, the elephant and the rhinoceros. The life-span of the whale, also a mammal, is estimated at 40 to 60 years.

ANATOMIC CHANGES WITH AGING

The gross manifestations of aging are well known to all. Aging may proceed at different rates in different individuals. Yet in general, there is no confusion between youth, middle age, and senescence. Obvious characteristics include graying and loss of hair, wrinkling and irregularity of skin, wearing and loss of teeth, decreased muscle and increased fat. Although the fat increases, there is, in general, very little overall weight change until extremely old age. Height decreases gradually after age 30 and the loss averages about $\frac{1}{4}$ inch per decade, with an average decrease of an inch from age 30 to 70. Part of this loss is due to increased curvature of the spine and part to narrowing of the intervertebral spaces. Only in severe cases of osteoporosis (thinning of the bone), with collapse of the vertebrae, is there any actual shortening of the bones themselves.

Several types of cells in the body are incapable of replacement. These include the heart and skeletal muscle cells and the neurons. Studies in which counts of the relative number of cells in various portions of the brain were made at different ages indicate that there is a steady, progressive loss of cells which may amount to 20 to 25 percent as an average. Studies of muscle cells, both cardiac and skeletal, also indicate a decrease in number with age. Muscle cells can compensate by hypertrophy, but there is much evidence that the total muscle mass gradually decreases. Muscle cells and neurons accumulate pigment as they age, and this eventually may make up more than 5 percent of the cell mass. Because of their inability to reproduce, muscle cells and neurons are often referred to as *postmitotic* cells. Cells which actively replace themselves throughout life are known as *mitotic* cells. There is evidence that with aging, the rate of replacement by these cells decreases. The tissues of which they are a part also show increasing disorganization. This is manifested by a decrease in the regularity of cellular arrangement within tissue, a greater variability of nuclear size associated with a relative increase in cytoplasm, both contributing to a greater irregularity in structure of the individual cells, an accumulation of pigment within certain cells, and a greater number of gross chromosome abnormalities.

Gerontologists have paid considerable attention to the extracellular components of tissue. Most work has been done on the collagen fibers. These fibers are responsible for the creation of strength in tendons and fascial sheaths. Collagen increases in quantity and changes in quality with aging. As Comfort points out, it is the collagen content of the meat which enables us to tell whether we are eating veal or beef, lamb or mutton, a fryer or an old laying hen. The properties of collagen change with aging. The tension required to prevent thermal contraction of rat-tail collagen increases ninefold between birth and normal death. This may well be due to the lining up of the individual collagen strands into larger and larger uniform bundles. It seems probable that the increased collagen in arterial walls with aging is as much responsible for the loss of vascular elasticity as is arteriosclerosis.

Elastin is the second constituent of the intercellular space. Much less is known of it than of collagen. Presumably it is responsible for the elasticity of such structures as skin and the elastic blood vessels. There is evidence of change in the chemical composition of elastin with age. Microscopic examination of elastic fibers show thickening, fragmentation of the ends, and irregular arrangement associated with aging. Aged elastin appears to have a greater affinity for calcium, and this may be associated with the development of arteriosclerosis. Reticular fibers make up the smallest component of the extracellular supporting tissues. They are more intimately bound with the cells. These fibers have been reported to become increasingly coarse and numerous with aging.

There is a progressive loss of total body water after the age of 25 or 30 years. This decrease in total body water averages between 25 to 30 percent. Differential studies indicate that there is very little change in the extracellular component, and that the entire change is due to a decrease in the intracellular water. The quantitative data for this decrease are not precise, but are on the order of 30 to 35 percent. This decrement in intracellular water can be associated only with a proportionate decrease in active cell mass, a presumption that is supported by several other lines of evidence. Body potassium is largely contained within the cell, and the total body content of potassium can be determined by placing the individual in a whole-body radiation counter and counting the radioactive potassium 40 which is present as a normal component. Studies of total body potassium indicate a 20 to 25 percent decrease with age in proportion to weight. The decreased number of cells has been commented on previously.

Anatomic Changes in Organ Systems

Changes in the cardiovascular system include a decrease in cardiac size (except in association with heart failure), increased pigment in the heart muscle cells, increased collagen and decreased elastic tissue in the blood vessel walls with decreased vascular elasticity, and reduction in the extent of the vascular tree by reduction in number of functioning collateral vessels. The digestive system changes are characterized by the wearing and loss of teeth, although the latter may be due to peridontal disease and not to age-related change; decrease of the number of taste papillae; frequent presence of diaphragmatic hernias; and increased frequency of gastric atrophy and colonic diverticulosis. Respiratory changes include both loss of lung mass and increasing rigidity of the chest walls. It is generally appreciated that the lymphoid tissues in the respiratory system, especially the tonsils and adenoids, decrease in size with age and may even become inapparent. The urinary system changes are characterized by a 30 to 40 percent decrease in the number of functioning nephron units. The hematopoietic system is very little affected, although the blood cell mass is decreased in proportion to the decrease in the blood volume. The formation of ova in the ovary stops with the cessation of menses, but spermatogenesis continues in the male, although at a markedly reduced rate. It is not known the extent to which the demineralization and thinning of bones seen in osteoporosis represents a disease or is a result of the aging process. Changes in the nervous system have already been mentioned. There is usually a marked reduction in brain cells, yet the size and configuration of the brain is often normal even at advanced age.

In summary, there are a number of anatomical changes associated with aging which involve almost all the organ systems. Many of these changes are well known and readily apparent. The most consistent changes appear to be at the cellular level, and few tissues are spared. There is a decrease in the number of actively functioning cells, an increase in the irregularity of cell size and shape and of the arrangement of cells in tissues and progressive changes in the supporting intercellular substances. The extracellular fluid volume remains essentially constant, but the total body fat increases and approximately replaces the weight loss caused by the decrease in cellular mass.

PHYSIOLOGICAL CHANGES WITH AGING

Almost all the organ systems of the body show a progressive decrease in functional capacity after the attainment of maturity during the third decade. For example, the cardiac output at rest decreases at the rate of 0.6 percent per year from age 30 to age 80, a total decrement of 30 percent. It might be argued that this is merely a response to decreased body needs as a result of the decrease in the active cell mass. However, the maximum heart rate in response to physiological stress also decreases with age, indicating that even within the reduced need for cardiac output there is a reduced capacity to respond to stressful situations.

Figure 12-3, taken from Strehler, summarizes a number of physiological functions which have been measured. Each of these shows a linearly progressive decrease, although the rates of decrease vary from system to system. The reduction in the capacity of the cardiovascular system has already been mentioned. The figure also shows that the respiratory system

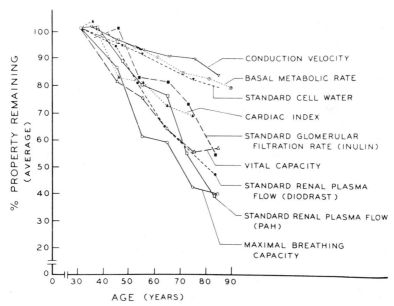

Figure 12-3   The decrement of various human functional capacities with age. *(From B. L. Strehler, Quarterly Review of Biology, 34:117, 1959. By permission of the publishers.)*

is similarly involved, with marked reductions in both the vital capacity (the maximum amount of air that can be gotten out of the lungs between forced inspiration and forced expiration) and, more importantly, in the maximal breathing capacity, which indicates the ability to obtain oxygen under the conditions of work stress. A decrease of the same order of magnitude is seen not only in the rate of blood flow through the kidneys but also in the rate of filtration by the glomeruli. Other studies, not charted, also indicate that the renal tubules are similarly impaired, and this reduction in both filtration and tubular function indicates a reduction in excretory reserve. The reduction of nerve conduction velocity, although of a much smaller order of magnitude than most of the other parameters presented, shows that the deterioration in function involves the nervous system as well. Several tests of muscular strength indicate that there is a progressive linear decrease of about 50 percent from age 30 to age 90. This is true in men and women and in both the dominant and subordinate hands.

Changes in the functional capacity of the endocrine system have received special attention. It has long been known that the basal metabolic rate, the rate of oxygen consumption at rest, decreases with age, and standard tables have been available to correct for this change. At the same time, the circulating thyroid hormone, as measured by the protein-bound iodine, shows no change with age. These observations can be reconciled by the observation that the oxygen consumption is proportional to the residual cell mass, which indicates that the rate of activity of individual cells is essentially unchanged with age. At the same time, thyroxine turnover studies indicate that the rate of thyroid hormone production is proportionately reduced. Thus, the constant blood level of thyroid hormone is due to a slower rate of turnover. There is no apparent change in the activity of the parathyroid hormone.

Recent evidence suggests that impairment of the ability to handle sugars with age depends on factors other than the amount of insulin present. The production of female sex hormones (estrogens) decreases with age until about 60 years and then levels off at a low rate of production. Estrogens are also produced in small amounts by men, and this rate of production does not seem to change. Production of male sex hormones (androgens) by men decreases gradually. Since some androgens are produced by the adrenals, they are present also in women, in whom the rate of decrease is relatively rapid until the sixth decade and then continues to decrease at a much slower rate. Cortisone, one of the hormones of the adrenal cortex, does not appear to be altered. However, the adrenal normally responds to stress by an increased production of cortisone, and this response is blunted.

Ordinarily there is a feedback system which operates much like a thermostat between the pituitary gland and the thyroid, adrenal, and sex glands. When the production of thyroid, adrenal, and sex hormones is adequate, the pituitary puts out little hormone to stimulate these glands. When their production is inadequate, the pituitary responds by increasing the production of the appropriate "tropic" hormone. After the menopause there is a marked increase in the gonadotropic hormone of women. This indicates that the pituitary is responding to the decrease in female sex hormones and that the decrease in their production is the result of a local change in the ovaries rather than of failure of pituitary stimulation.

One of the most sensitive areas of study has been that of intellectual capacity with age. Figure 12-4 shows the results of a number of IQ tests. These curves seem to follow the functional curves of many other systems. However, they are subject to a number of criticisms, since the individuals at age 70 were not comparable to those at earlier ages in terms of education and test experience. Intelligence as presently measured is a combination of several components, and a number of studies have been performed to separate these components. As might be expected, the

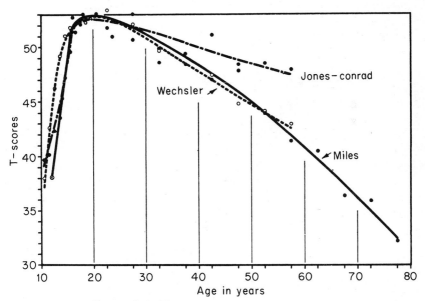

Figure 12-4   Mental test scores related to age. [*From Harold E. Jones and Oscar J. Kaplan, "Psychological Aspects of Mental Disorders in Later Life," in Oscar J. Kaplan (ed.), Mental Disorders in Later Life, 2d ed., Stanford University Press, Stanford, Calif., 1956, Figure 12, p. 104. By permission of the publishers.*]

capacity for learning and abstract reasoning appears to decrease with age, whereas those components associated with memory tend to increase. Where studies have been performed on the same individuals at varying intervals, the intellectual decrement has not been so apparent. However, as yet no group has been tested throughout a prolonged life-span. Lehman, in a very thorough and provocative study entitled "Age and Achievement," has shown that most creative achievements have been performed by individuals under the age of 35 or 40. He surveyed a vast literature of science, the arts, literature, and philosophy and found that the most significant scientific, artistic, literary, or philosophical contributions were made by individuals between the ages of 25 and 40, even when corrected for the number of individuals surviving at any age group. On the other hand, contributions in social and administrative areas were more frequently made by individuals in the older age groups.

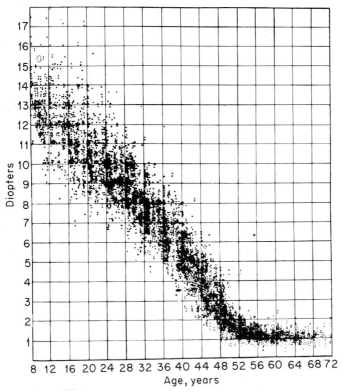

Figure 12-5 Age and the accommodative capacity of the eye. [*Duane, quoted by J. A. Friedenwald in Cowdry (ed.), Problems of Aging, 3d ed., Williams & Wilkins, Baltimore, 1952, p. 251. By permission of the publishers.*]

Very few physiological functions cease abruptly. The most characteristic of these, and one which appears to be unique to humans, is the cessation of ovulation and menstruation at the menopause. The relationship to decreasing levels of estrogen production and increasing levels of gonadotropic hormone production has been mentioned. Another such change is in the ability of the lens to accommodate to near vision. When the ciliary muscle is at rest, the lens is set to focus at distant vision. Accommodation to near vision requires contraction of ciliary muscles and a change in the shape of the lens, so that it becomes thicker and therefore more powerful. As the lens ages, its structure becomes more rigid, so that with muscular contraction the capacity to change shape decreases. Figure 12-5 shows the accommodation capacity of the human eye with age. The range of ability to accommodate at any given age is remarkably constant and could almost be used as an objective measure of age until age 50.

Despite the fact that numerous anatomical changes are seen in the cells with aging and that most theories of aging are based on cellular explanations, there is very little evidence of altered cellular function. Older mitotic cells replace themselves less rapidly. Specific metabolic functional changes have been difficult to discern. A few metabolic processes may be reduced 10 to 15 percent. It is interesting that nerve conduction time, which must be a cellular function in the neuron, is reduced only 15 percent between ages 30 and 80. Shock points out that this must be contrasted to decrements of 40 to 60 percent in total organ performances. These discrepancies must be reconciled in any general theory of the aging process.

SOME GENERAL CHARACTERISTICS OF AGING

Modern mortality statistics show that there is a rather large number of neonatal deaths and that the frequency of death decreases rather rapidly to a nadir at about age 10 or 11 (see Fig. 12-2). From this point, the number of deaths at each age increases gradually to a maximum in the seventies, and then it decreases again. Benjamin plotted the numbers of deaths at each age from English life tables for 1841 and 1950 to 1952 for males (Fig. 12-6A and B). He noted that the termination of each of these curves on the right resembled one limb of a normal distribution curve. By reconstructing a complete curve (dotted lines in the figures), he postulated that there could possibly be a "normal" life-span with a normal distribution as indicated by the curves. By this reasoning, all deaths not under the curve should be nonsenescent deaths. The data derived from this concept are of interest.

Between the years 1841 and 1950, life expectancy for men in England

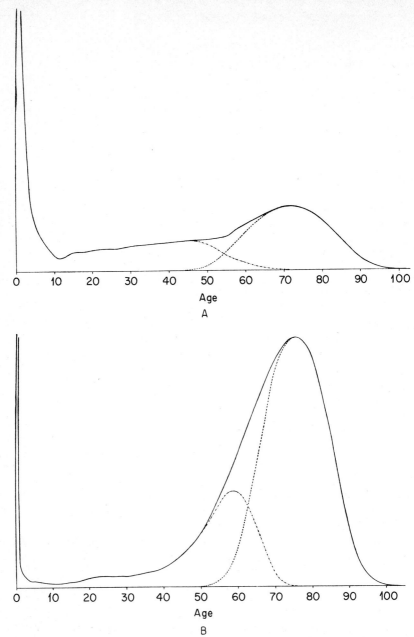

Figure 12-6 *A:* Distribution of deaths by age at time of death
(males), England, 1840. Solid line, total deaths at age; dotted line,
senescent deaths; dashed line, nonsenescent deaths. *B:* Distribution of deaths by age (males), England, 1950. *(From B. Benjamin in Ciba Colloquia on Ageing, J. A. Churchill, London, 1959,
p. 2. By permission of the publishers.)*

Table 12-2   Senescent Deaths, Males

Period of deaths	Peak age, years	Proportion of total deaths, percent
1841	72.0	39.9
1950–1952	75.7	69.4

SOURCE: B. Benjamin, in Ciba Colloquia on Ageing, J. A. Churchill, London, 1959.

increased from 41 to almost 70 years. However, during this period, the peak age of death increased only from 72.0 to 75.7 years. The increase of the life expectancy was entirely due to the decrease in the number of nonsenescent deaths. During this period the percentage of deaths within the senescent curve increased from 39.9 to 69.4 percent (Table 12-2). The slight increase in the peak age can be accounted for by the more abrupt slope which the survivorship curve would demonstrate if survivorship is plotted as in Fig. 12-2. If this concept is correct, a theoretical "ideal" distribution might be proposed as in Fig. 12-7. Under these circumstances there are no nonsenescent deaths, and all deaths would fall within the range of the curve. While this concept must be modified by further data to be presented, the death distribution obtained from the life tables suggests that there is a general factor operating to restrict longevity, a factor which is, to a certain extent, independent of the actual cause of death.

In 1825 Gompertz, a British actuary, proposed a formulation which is now known as Gompertz's function. Based on data then available to him, he noted that after the neonatal and juvenile deaths had decreased

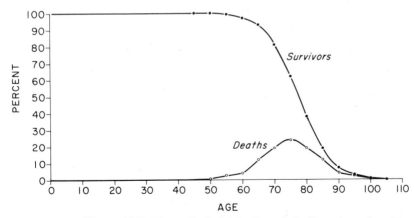

Figure 12-7   Theoretical distribution of death and survivorship, assuming that all deaths are due to old age alone.

to a minimum at age 10 or 11 years, the risk of dying subsequently doubled every 8½ years. Thus, if the risk were 1 in 1,000 at age 10, it would be 2 in 1,000 at age 18½, 4 in 1,000 at age 27, 8 in 1,000 at age 35½, and so forth. Plotting the logarithm of human mortality against age, one gets a straight line (Fig. 12-8). Some correction must be made for the excess of accidental deaths in young adults, particularly males. Subsequent studies have shown that all mammals and most other animals show death rates which conform to this principle. The variables are the origin, which depends upon the initial death rate, and the slope, which depends upon the doubling time. It is important to understand the significance of this concept. If death were due to random accidents and diseases alone, the risk of dying at any given year would be the same. The situation would then be like radiological decay, for which a half-life can be calculated. Only half the population would be eliminated during each half-life, and some individuals would live to an extremely old age. However, since

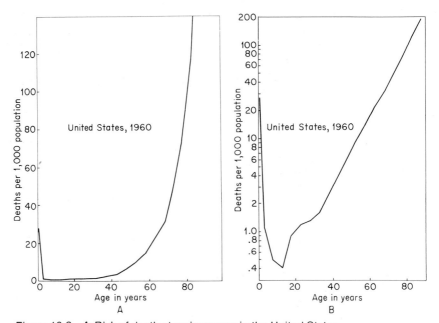

Figure 12-8   *A:* Risk of death at various ages in the United States, 1960. *B:* The Gompertz curve of the risk of death by age in the United States, 1960, on semilogarithmic coordinates. Note that from age 35 onward, the risk of death increases linearly with age. The excessive death rate between approximately ages 15 and 35 is due to accidental deaths. *(From J. P. Fox, C. E. Hall, and L. R. Elveback, Epidemiology, Man and Disease, Macmillan, New York, 1970, pp. 156–157. By permission of the publishers.)*

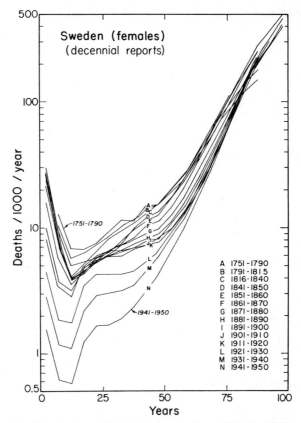

Figure 12-9   Death rates of Swedish women from 1751 to 1950.
[From H. B. Jones in J. Birren (ed.), Handbook of Aging in the Individual, University of Chicago Press, Chicago, 1960, p. 341. By permission of the publishers.)

the risk of dying actually increases, there is eventually an age at which the risk of dying is 100 percent and beyond which there can be no survivors.

Figure 12-9 is based on vital statistics data for Swedish women since 1751. Note that in the top curve the lowest point is that of about 7 deaths per 1,000 at age 12, whereas the most recent curve is at 0.6 deaths per 1,000 per year. This represents the reduction in juvenile and neonatal deaths in the past two centuries. Therefore it is apparent that environmental factors can alter the overall pattern of death risk. The curves show relatively little tendency to cross, and minor fluctuations may be due to inadequacies of data or to such environmental changes as famines, epidemics, or wars. Finally, note that the most recent curves ascend slightly more steeply than do the original. There is evidence suggesting that in modern countries the doubling rate is now 7 years rather than 8½. This is in agreement with the observations that while the death rate in early life has been markedly decreased, there has been very little modification in the life-span, as demonstrated in particular by Fig. 12-6A and B.

In order to clarify this concept, examine Table 12-3. When there is a doubling rate of 8½ years, as the initial death rate at age 10 decreases from 10 to 5 to 1 to 0.5 per 1,000, the age at which the population would be extinguished (i.e., the risk of dying is greater than 1,000 per 1,000 individuals per year) increases. However, if the doubling rate is 8½ years when the death rate is 1 per 1,000 per year at age 10 and the doubling rate falls to 7 years as the death rate is reduced to 0.5 per year at age 10, the death rate at younger ages is less, but it eventually catches up. Thus, the extinguishing age is approximately the same. This process has been gradual, so that the curves do not actually cross, but this phenomenon may be a clue to the reason for the failure of extreme longevity to increase in proportion to increasing life expectancy.

It has been pointed out that the configuration of the Gompertz curve is characteristic only for a given environment. The improvement in childhood mortality by the control of infectious diseases and malnutrition has created a large part of the total effect observed. On the other hand, data from prisoner of war camps during World War II indicate that a whole population may be moved to a less favorable curve when the environment is altered. Notice that the fundamental configuration of the curve is independent of the specific cause of death. Most deaths today are due to cardiovascular diseases, strokes, cancer, and accidents. Figure 12-10 shows that each of these conforms to the Gom-

Table 12-3 Expectation of Death (per 1,000 per Year) at Different Ages from Gompertz Curve at Various Rates and Doubling Times

Age (years)	Doubling rate 8.5 years				Doubling rate 7 years	
10	10	5	1	0.5	1	0.5
18.5	20	10	2	1	2.3	1.1
27	40	20	4	2	5	2.5
35.5	80	40	8	4	12	6
44	160	80	16	8	28	14
52.5	320	160	32	16	65	28
61	640	320	64	32	145	73
69.5	1,280	640	128	64	360	180
78		1,280	256	128	800	400
86.5			512	256	1,920	960
95			1,028	512		2,100

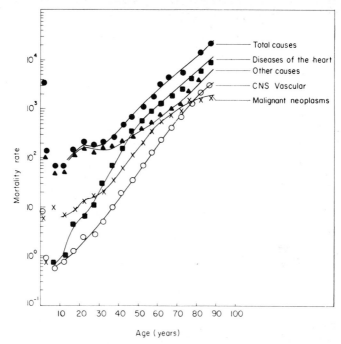

Figure 12-10   Gompertz plot of cause-specific mortality rates.
*(From B. L. Strehler and A. S. Mildvan, Science, 132:14, 1960.
By permission of the publishers.)*

pertz curve.   This would, of course, be expected, since these four conditions cause about 75 percent of all deaths, and any major discrepancy
would alter the curve for all deaths.   Equally striking, however, is Fig.
12-11, which shows that the risk of dying of pneumonia at any age follows the Gompertz curve, and similarly that the distribution of deaths
from accidents is comparable to the distribution of deaths at all ages
(Fig. 12-12).   The reason that the absolute number of deaths decreases
after age 75 is that the remaining number of individuals has decreased.
However, the risk to the survivors of dying of a given condition increases
in accord with the expectations.

THEORIES OF AGING

Strehler has pointed out that age changes must meet four basic criteria.
These are universality, progressiveness, intrinsicality, and deleteriousness.
Since all organisms age, it is necessary that the features of aging be present
in all.   Thus specific changes such as cancer, while they may be associated with aging, are not characteristics of aging per se.   Our experi-

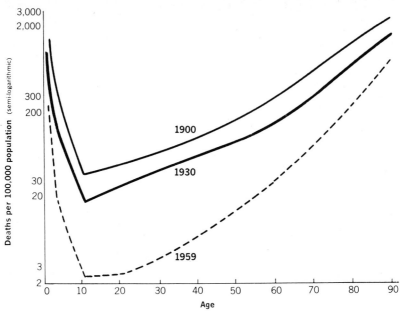

Figure 12-11   Age and mortality rates from pneumonia. *(From H. A. Reimann, Geriatrics, 18:433, 1963. By permission of the publishers.)*

ence, supported by the evidence of the Gompertz phenomenon, indicates that aging is a progressive phenomenon due to the accumulation of many small effects rather than to infrequent large episodes. Intrinsicality may be questionable. The possibility that some extrinsic factor, such as cosmic radiation, causes the universal, progressive, and deleterious changes of age cannot be completely excluded, although it seems improbable. Finally, the deleterious effects of aging are manifest not only in the observable changes but in the increased risk of illness and death as well.

Another series of criteria which must be met for a theory of aging have also been proposed by Strehler. First, the theory must account for the Gompertz phenomenon of a logarithmically increasing death rate. Second, it must be able to accept the observation that physiological functions decrease linearly rather than logarithmically with age. Finally, it must be compatible with the observation that as the initial values of the death rate are decreased in young individuals, the doubling time also decreases.

Theories of aging have been legion and only those with special relevance shall be discussed. A common defect in most theories has

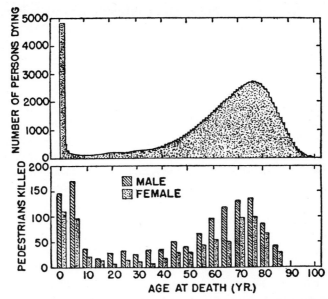

Figure 12-12 Comparison of distribution by age of all deaths and deaths of pedestrians. Note the general conformity of the two curves except for the excessive accidental deaths between 5 and 15 years. *(From A. Comfort, The Process of Aging, The New American Library, New York, 1964, p. 29. By permission of the publishers.)*

been an attempt to identify an observable aging change with the cause of aging. The best known of these was the theory that since gonadal activity decreases, aging is the result of deficient sex hormones. Testes extracts and implantations were attempted with little success. The recent availability of testosterone indicates that its use will temporarily increase muscle strength and sexual vigor. But this is not the equivalent of arresting or reversing the general effects of aging. That aging is not the result of sexual decline is easily demonstrated, since castrated animals live as long as intact ones. Sexual deterioration is one of the results of aging, not a cause.

The relationship of genetics to longevity is of great theoretical importance. It has been amply demonstrated that the offspring of long-lived parents have advantages in terms of longevity, although recent data suggest that since most individuals are living into old age, this factor may not be as important as was formerly thought. However, the inheritance of longevity raises interesting questions. Medawar pointed out that longevity per se has no survival value and selection for longevity would not be possible as long as the parents survive long enough to reproduce and to protect their offspring until they in turn were capable of independent survival. Animal senescence in nature is so rare as to be hardly natural. Following up on Medawar's thesis, Comfort suggests that the biological programming may go only so far as maturity and reproduction and then stop, leaving the organism to carry on as best it can without help. Comfort compares this to the rocket which is shot off to take pictures of Mars but which, on passing Mars, has no program and will continue on aimlessly until shattered by meteorites or some other cosmic accident. If the entire mechanism is intrinsic, as Strehler suggests, then there are minor defects built into the system which can be altered only by environmental factors and which tend to accumulate until the organism can no longer cope with an environmental stress.

Serious attention is being given at the present time to only a few of the many possible theories. The *somatic mutation theory* is based on the demonstration that with age there is an increase in the number of mitotic cells with definitely demonstrable chromosomal abnormalities. Presumably this may be the reflection of an even greater number of invisible abnormalities involving single genes or groups of genes. This theory is particularly popular because it can be demonstrated that irradiation increases the number of abnormal chromosomes and that measurable amounts of radiation will produce predictable life shortening in some experimental animals. Since all individuals are exposed to some natural radiation, this could account for the observed effects. However, not all the radiation effects are comparable to the natural changes with aging. It seems most probably that in the experimental situation, at least, radiation acts as an environmental influence unfavorably affecting the characteristics of Gompertz's function. Genetic change as a cause of aging is not eliminated by the possibility that is is not produced by irradiation.

A theory closely related to the somatic mutation theory proposes that with time there is an increasing frequency of translational errors in the step between RNA and protein synthesis. These errors could accumulate in both mitotic and postmitotic cells, but while errors of transcription due to defective genes would probably occur most frequently in mitotic cells, errors in translation would be expected to be more frequent in postmitotic cells.

Some interesting and important data have recently been presented by Hayflick. He demonstrated that embryonic human fibroblasts could be maintained on cell culture for only 50 generations, and that the older the source of the fibroblasts, the fewer the possible generations. He also demonstrated that previous studies which had suggested that cells could be carried in culture indefinitely had been misinterpreted. These apparently immortal cells had transformed into cells analogous to cancer cells and therefore were not normal. The implication of this information is that each cell line, independent of all other factors, has a limited capacity for survival, and that defects must be passed from generation to generation of mitotic cells until further replacement is no longer possible.

The *immunological theory* proposes that, with age, abnormal proteins are produced and precipitate an immune response or that some of the immunologically competent cells, the lymphocytes, become altered so that they fail to recognize normal proteins as "self" and react to them. This condition has been compared to the chronic rejection reaction in transplantation where the antigenic gene is relatively weak. This theory then can be coupled with the somatic mutation theory and overcomes some of the objections to it.

The so-called *"clinker theory,"* in distinction to the first two, relates only to the fixed postmitotic cells. These cells, principally the neurons, heart muscle, and voluntary muscle cells, are known to accumulate pigment with age. Since these cells are irreplaceable, the included granules may interfere with their function.

An early theory of aging, the *overspecialization theory,* calls attention to the fact that there is differentiation and specialization of cells in all complex organisms and that, while most unicellular animals can reproduce by simple division, multicellular animals must start over again with sexual union and the redifferentiation of the whole system of cells. The integration of function of groups of extremely differentiated cells may gradually develop small inapparent errors which cumulatively reduce the ability to adapt to stress.

Finally, there are *theories of cross-linkage* between long molecules, of which the most extensively studied have been those of collagen. Long molecules possess many points where chemical reactions can occur and result in their aggregation. The result would be the interference in normal molecular functions, as is noted in the loss of tissue elasticity with the increase in collagen deposition with age. Similar aggregations within cells might either bind components or physically block normal reactions.

None of these theories successfully answers all the experimental objections, yet at the same time each has considerable data in its support. It is possible that they may not be mutually exclusive. It also seems probable that aging is not a designed characteristic but rather results from the fact that life prolonged beyond successful reproduction is not an evolutionary consideration.

SYNTHESIS AND SPECULATION

A number of generalizations might be made at this point:

1. Aging is a specific general process which produces observable changes in structure and function.

2. Aging results in an increasing vulnerability to environmental stress and disease and is associated with a logarithmically increasing risk of death.

3. The evidence suggests that the life-span is about 110 years and maximum average life expectancy is no greater than 80 to 85 years.

4. The underlying mechanism of the aging process is not known. Genetic constitution is probably important, but its role is undetermined. The improvements in life expectancy may be due to modification of the aging process, or they may be due to an overall reduction in the number of life-threatening situations.

5. It is possible that eventually the aging process will be modified and that life-span and life expectancy will be lengthened.

Figure 12-13 shows a comparison of survivorship curves in ancient Rome, the United States in 1940, and in an "ideal" situation. The absence of neonatal and accidental deaths is improbable and possibly undesirable. In addition, the Gompertz formulation indicates that the death frequencies will rise very gradually from age 10 rather than all being distributed in a normal distribution curve. Therefore the ideal limit is unquestionably beyond what can be achieved. On the other hand, the current survivorship data show that there has already been considerable progress toward the ideal since 1940. The difference between these two curves represents the probable maximum that can be achieved without altering the process of

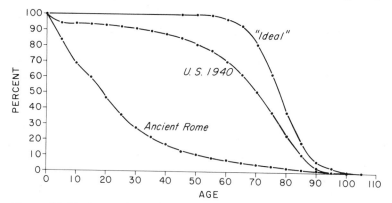

Figure 12-13 Comparison of survivorship: ancient Rome, The United States (1940), and ideal.

aging itself. If this is the case, and much evidence indicates that it is, then we have reached the point where the study of the aging process is more pertinent than are extensive studies of specific disease processes in age.

Concern regarding the increased number of older persons in the population is expressed because of the possibility that modern society will have increasing numbers of decrepit individuals who will survive for indefinite periods of time. It is probable that this concern is unfounded. More people are reaching old age because they have been well until old age. There is evidence that diseases associated with old age, such as heart disease and cancer, are actually appearing at comparable frequencies in individuals who are older than their counterparts in earlier generations. In other words, as the Gompertz function is shifted more favorably, the functions for these major diseases are shifting proportionately. A biologically aged individual is vulnerable because he is aged, and he will continue to be vulnerable for the same reason. Although more people will reach old age, the evidence suggests that senescence itself will not be prolonged.

This preoccupation with the possibility that the incapacitated aged will be disproportionately preserved points out a problem which is not often considered. If life is to be prolonged, at what age range is this most likely to occur? If given a choice, most individuals would choose to have this prolongation during the period of active maturity. Undue prolongation at either end of life would probably not be in the general interest. Fortunately, the evidence indicates that life prolongation will probably be during the desired period. For the past century, the onset of puberty, as indicated by the initiation of menses, has been decreasing in age at the rate of approximately 4 months per decade, that is, it has decreased approximately $3\frac{1}{2}$ years in a century. It has already been demonstrated that with improvement in the Gompertz function, death decreases during youth and middle age but rises steeply with the approach of old age. If these interpretations are valid, future generations can hope for longer and healthier mature and productive years.

A final consideration. The population explosion which is causing great social and political concern is the result of a decreasing death rate, not an increasing birthrate. Birth control was no problem as long as most children died before the reproductive age. Even if the birthrate were to remain constant over a long period of time, a sudden increase in life expectancy from 70 to 140 years would double the population by the time the death rate had again stabilized. Since life expectancy increased from 40 to 70 years in the past century, this alone has accounted for much of the population gain in advanced countries. An ever greater proportionate increase in life expectancy, particularly the decrease in juvenile mortality, accounts for the gain in underdeveloped countries benefiting from immunizations, malaria control, vitamins, and penicillin. However, now that most people will survive through the reproductive age, a rational program of population control has become imperative. In addition, scientific and social developments not only allow most individuals to approach the normal human life span, but promise that a way to slow the aging process itself will be found. It may not be too soon to consider the implications of such a development.

BIBLIOGRAPHY

ANDREW, W.: *The Anatomy of Aging in Man and Animals,* New York: Grune and Stratton, 1971.

COMFORT, A.: *The Process of Aging,* New York: New American Library, 1964, London: Weidenfeld and Nicolson, 1965.

FREEMAN, J. T. (ed.): *Clinical Features of the Older Patient,* Springfield, Ill.: Charles C Thomas, Publisher, 1965.

HAYFLICK, L.: "Human Cells and Aging," *Scientific American,* March, 1968.

POWERS, J. H. (ed.): *Surgery of the Aged and Debilitated Patient,* Philadelphia: W. B. Saunders Company, 1968.

ROSSMAN, I. (ed.): Clinical Geriatrics, Philadelphia: J. B. Lippincott Company, 1971.

SHOCK, N. W. (ed.): *Aging: Some Social and Biological Aspects,* publication no. 35, Washington, D.C.: The American Association for the Advancement of Science, 1960.

STREHLER, B. L.: *Times, Cells and Aging,* New York: Academic Press, Inc., 1962.

VERZAR, F.: "The Aging of Collagen," *Scientific American,* April, 1963.

WALFORD, R. L.: *The Immunologic Theory of Aging,* Copenhagen: Munksgaard, 1969.

Index